Nursing the Adult with a
Specific Physiological Disturbance

Nursing the Adult with a Specific Physiological Disturbance

Patricia Hunt
Bernice Sendell

SECOND EDITION

MACMILLAN

First published 1983
Reprinted (with corrections) 1984 (twice), 1986
Second edition 1987

Published by
MACMILLAN EDUCATION LTD
Houndmills, Basingstoke, Hampshire RG21 2XS
and London
Companies and representatives
throughout the world

Printed in Great Britain by
Scotprint Ltd,
Musselburgh, Scotland

ISBN 0-333-44079-X

**To all the Staff and Learners of the
Bristol and Weston School of Nursing**

Contents

** Including care plan and evaluation/progress notes.
 * Including care plan.

** Including care plan and evaluation/progress notes.
 * Including care plan.

** Including care plan and evaluation/progress notes.
 * Including care plan.

Foreword to the series

This series of textbooks offers a fresh approach to the study of nursing. The aim is to give those beginning a career in nursing, and those already qualified, opportunities for reflection to broaden their approach to nursing education and to identify their own nursing values. The text includes material currently required by those preparing for qualification as a nurse and offers a basis for developing knowledge by individual studies. It should also assist qualified nurses returning to nursing, and those wishing to gain further insight into the nursing curriculum.

The authors of each book in the series are from widely differing nursing backgrounds, and, as experienced teachers of nursing or midwifery, they are well aware of the difficulties faced by nursing students searching for meaning from a mass of factual information. The nurse has to practise in the real world, and in reality nursing students need to learn to practise with confidence and understanding. The authors have therefore collaborated to illustrate this new perspective by making full use of individual nursing care plans to present the knowledge required by the nursing student in the most appropriate and relevant way. These textbooks can therefore be used in a wide variety of nursing programmes.

The practice of nursing — as a profession and as a career — and the education of the nurse to fulfil her role are both affected by national and international trends. The Nurses, Midwives and Health Visitors Act 1979 in the United Kingdom, the Treaty of Rome and the European Community nursing directives 1977, as well as the deliberations and publications of the International Council of Nurses and the World Health Organization, all make an impact upon the preparation and the practice of the nurse throughout the world.

Nursing values may not have changed over the past one hundred years, but society and the patterns of both life and care have changed, and are constantly changing. It is particularly important, therefore, to restate the essentials of nursing in the light of current practice and future trends.

Throughout this series the focus is on nursing and on the individual — the person requiring care and the person giving care — and emphasises the need for continuity between home and hospital care. 'Neighbourhood Nursing — a focus for care', the Report of the Community Nursing Review under the chairmanship of Julia Cumberlege (HMSO, 1986), has drawn attention to this need. The developing role of the nurse in primary care and in health education is reflected throughout this series. The authors place their emphasis on the whole person, and nursing care studies and care plans are used to promote understanding of the clinical, social, psychological and spiritual aspects of care for the individual.

Each book introduces the various aspects of the curriculum for general nursing: the special needs (1) of those requiring acute care; (2) of the elderly; (3) of children; (4) of the mentally ill; and (5) of the mentally handicapped. The latter is a new text in the 'Essentials of Nursing' series — edited by a well-known and respected nurse for the mentally handicapped and with contributors experienced in differing aspects of caring for people with mental handicap. The text on maternity and neonatal care, written by a midwifery teacher, provides the material for nursing students and would be helpful to those undertaking preparation for further health visiting education.

The authors wish to acknowledge their gratitude for the assistance they have received from members of the Editorial Board, and from all those who have contributed to their work — patients and their relatives, students, qualified nurses and colleagues — too numerous to mention by name. To all those nurse teachers who have read some of the texts, offering constructive criticism and comment from their special knowledge, we offer our grateful thanks. Lastly, we thank Elizabeth Horne for her contribution to the physiology material in the text, and Mary Waltham for her help with this second edition.

1987   Sheila Collins

Preface

We have great pleasure in introducing the 2nd edition of this nursing text, which we hope will continue to be useful and stimulating for all nurses and nursing students concerned with the giving of patient care both in the hospital and in the community.

An attempt has been made to develop the nursing model related to a patient's specific needs rather than to the care of a patient with a medical condition, and we have been guided in our choice of chapters by V. Henderson's *Pathological States that Modify Basic Needs*: for example, Chapter 1 — Nursing patients with disturbances of fluid and electrolyte balance.

Within the Introduction to this edition we have highlighted the concept of adulthood and how it can be perceived.

Within each chapter we illustrate some of the factors which always affect basic needs, as identified by V. Henderson, including age, social and cultural states, temperament, and physical and intellectual capacity. These always need to be considered when modifying nursing care to meet the patient's needs caused by his pathological condition.

No attempt has been made to cover every pathological state or physiological disturbance, but we hope that our choices have given you a basis for further development of the nursing model of care.

A series of patient histories are included with self-testing questions and some guidelines for suitable answers, which we hope will stimulate further discussion and encourage self-directed learning.

A development of this edition has been the insertion of four Evaluation of Care and Suggested Record of Progress Sheets in Chapters 1 and 2.

1987

Patricia Hunt
Bernice Sendell

Acknowledgements

The authors would like to extend their thanks to the following people: Miss M. W. Watson, Director of Nurse Education, Bristol and Weston School of Nursing, who started us off as teachers and is determined to see us through; Mrs Margaret Bawn for her expertise in deciphering our writing and bringing order out of chaos; Miss Anne Betts for reading our efforts and giving us heart to continue; Miss Elizabeth Horne of Macmillan Publishers for her unbounded enthusiasm for our ideas and guidance through, for us, uncharted waters, and also for her major contribution to the text as the author of the normal physiology at the commencement of each chapter (this provides a comprehensive base from which the nurse can learn the normal physiology and use to compare with the abnormal physiology described later); Mrs Shirley Stevens and Mrs Ann Lawrence for librarian support; Ms Mary Waltham for her guidance to this second edition; all the patients we have tried to nurse; and all the nurses we have tried to teach.

A note on the series style

Throughout this book, in keeping with the other titles in this series, the term *nursing student* has been used to mean *both* student or pupil nurses *and* trained nurses who are undertaking post-basic training or who are keeping up to date with the recent literature. For clarity and consistency throughout the series the nurse is described as *she;* this is done without prejudice to men who are nurses or nursing students. Similarly, the patient is sometimes referred to as *he,* when the gender is not specifically mentioned.

Care plans, which are used throughout the books in this series, are indicated by a colour corner flash to distinguish them from the rest of the text.

Introduction

As this book is concerned mainly with nursing the adult, we would like you to pause and take part in several activities to remind you of the various perceptions of adulthood.

What marks the transition from childhood to adult status?

Can you list any events which are recognised as marking this transition?

Social/status
Biological/physical
Psychological/emotional
Cultural
Intellectual
Others

Now ask a friend or relative who is much older, or younger, than you to do the same exercise and compare your answers.

Is there any difference in your responses? Why do you think this is? Can you now say that there is a clearly defined transition from childhood to adult status, or would you agree that the process can depend to some extent on an individual's make-up, status, cultural background or circumstances.

At what age do you consider people enter:

Adolescence? . . . .
Adulthood? . . . .
Middle-age? . . . .
Old age? . . . .

Do you know anyone of roughly the same ages as you have chosen? If so, could you now ask them to answer the same questions? Do your answers match? If there are discrepancies, why do you think this is?

At what age would you expect the following to have occurred in the 'average person':

	Average age	Your personal profile
1. Left home?		
2. Got married/chose a partner?		
3. Had first child?		
4. Reached maximum physical fitness?		
5. Ceased being sexually active?		
6. Went on holiday with peers?		
7. Became happy with self?		
8. Active in politics?		
9. Concerned with religion?		
10. Involved in community affairs?		
11. Started to prepare for retirement?		
12. Successful in relating to — the elderly? — the young?		
13. Adventurous in leisure activities?		
14. Capable of caring for others?		

Now use the second column and answer the same questions as they apply to you personally or how you would expect them to apply to you.

Age norms and age expectations operate as prods and brakes upon behaviour, in some instances hastening an event, in others, delaying it. Men and women are not only aware of the social clocks that operate in various areas of their lives, but they are also aware of their own timing and readily describe themselves as 'early', 'late', or 'on time' with regard to family and occupational events.

(Neugarten, 1977, page 45)

Attempting to define adulthood isn't easy. Is there a legal definition or requirement to help us?

Below is a list of activities/responsibilities which have a minimum legal age. Can you correctly match the activity to the list of minimum ages? (See page xviii for some suggested answers.)

Key no.	Activity		Age/ years	Enter the key number of your matching activity here
1.	Leaving school	A	10	
2.	Stopping of entitlement to free medicines	B	16	
3.	Able to marry	C	16	
4.	Drive a car	D	16	
5.	Criminal responsibility	E	16	
6.	Age of sexual consent	F	17	
7.	Buy an air rifle	G	17	
8.	Buy a drink in a public house	H	18	
9.	Drive a heavy goods vehicle	I	18	
10.	Be President of United States of America	J	18	
11.	Vote for Member of Parliament	K	21	
12.	Take out a hire purchase agreement	L	35	

We have tried to reach a definition of adulthood but have seen that it cannot be totally dependent on age and/or culture but is largely concerned with maturity — that is, how an individual uses his/her adult rights and responsibilities within a particular environment.

Having considered some of the aspects of 'being an adult', we now include examples of Patients' Profiles to assist in assessing a patient's needs. The examples were taken from three patient histories which appear later in the text.

A Patient Profile to assist in assessing patients and the development of a problem-solving approach to care

Name _Mr George Watson_   No. _012345_

Address _100 Tack Road, Grenville_

1 Circle any conditions that are present in your patient in each of the five columns. Remember that more than one is possible in most of the columns

2 Starting with the age column, take your selected condition and consider each of the 14 functions requiring assistance and tick in the box(es) those appropriate to your patient's needs, e.g. an elderly patient may require assistance with 2, 3 and 5

3 Repeat the same procedure with subsequent columns

Conditions Always Present that Affect Basic Needs				Physiological Disturbances
Age	*Temperament*	*Social/Cultural*	*Physical/Intellectual Capacity*	1. Fluid and electrolyte imbalance (circled)
Newborn	Emotional state or passing mode:	(Member of a family unit with friends and status) (circled)	(Normal weight) (circled)	2. Oxygen want
Child	(a) normal	A person relatively alone	Over-weight	3. Shock
Adolescent	(b) euphoric, hyperactive	Maladjusted	Under-weight	4. Consciousness
Adult	(c) (anxious,) fearful, agitated, hysterical	Destitute	Normal mentality	5. Local injury/ disease
(Middle aged) (circled)		(Smoker) (circled)	Gifted mentality	6. Metabolism
Elderly	(d) depressed/ hypoactive	Drinker	Normal sense of: hearing sight equilibrium touch	7. Seeing, hearing, smell and touch
Aged			Loss of sense of: hearing sight equilibrium touch	8. Communicable conditions
			Normal motor power Loss of motor power	9. Immobilisation: disease/treatment

Functions requiring assistance	Age	Temperament	Social/Cultural	Physical/Intellectual Capacity	Physiological Disturbance
1. Breathing			✓		
2. Eating or drinking					✓
3. Elimination					✓
4. Sleep or rest					✓
5. Movement		✓			✓
6. Maintenance of body temperature					✓
7. Keeping body clean					✓
8. Dressing suitably					✓
9. Avoiding dangers and injury					✓
10. Communication		✓			✓
11. Worship		✓			✓
12. Work					✓
13. Participation in recreation		✓			✓
14. Learning to satisfy curiosity					✓

A Patient Profile to assist in assessing patients and the development of a problem-solving approach to care

Name _____ *Miss Mary Clark* _____ No. _____

Address _____

1 Circle any conditions that are present in your patient in each of the five columns. Remember that more than one is possible in most of the columns

2 Starting with the age column, take your selected condition and consider each of the 14 functions requiring assistance and tick in the box(es) those appropriate to your patient's needs, e.g. an elderly patient may require assistance with 2, 3 and 5

3 Repeat the same procedure with subsequent columns

Conditions Always Present that Affect Basic Needs				Physiological Disturbances
Age	*Temperament*	*Social/Cultural*	*Physical/Intellectual Capacity*	
Newborn	Emotional state	Member of a family	*Capacity*	1. Fluid and electrolyte imbalance
Child	or passing mode:	unit with friends	(Normal weight)	2. Oxygen want
Adolescent	(a) normal (circled)	and status	Over-weight	3. Shock
Adult	(b) euphoric,	(A person relatively alone) (circled)	Under-weight	4. Consciousness
(Middle aged) (circled)	hyperactive	Maladjusted	Normal mentality	5. Local injury/ disease (circled)
Elderly	(c) anxious, fearful,	Destitute	Gifted mentality	6. Metabolism
Aged	agitated,	Smoker	Normal sense of:	7. Seeing, hearing, smell and touch
	hysterical	Drinker	hearing	8. Communicable conditions
	(d) depressed/		sight	9. Immobilisation: disease/treatment
	hypoactive		equilibrium	
			touch	
			Loss of sense of:	
			hearing	
			sight	
			equilibrium	
			touch	
			Normal motor power	
			Loss of motor power	

Functions requiring assistance	Age	Temperament	Social/Cultural	Physical/Intellectual Capacity	Physiological Disturbance
1. Breathing					
2. Eating or drinking					✓
3. Elimination					✓
4. Sleep or rest			✓		✓
5. Movement					✓
6. Maintenance of body temperature					
7. Keeping body clean					
8. Dressing suitably					✓
9. Avoiding dangers and injury					
10. Communication					✓
11. Worship					
12. Work					✓
13. Participation in recreation					✓
14. Learning to satisfy curiosity					

A Patient Profile to assist in assessing patients and the development of a problem-solving approach to care

Name _Simon Matthews_   No. _____

Address _____

1 Circle any conditions that are present in your patient in each of the five columns. Remember that more than one is possible in most of the columns

2 Starting with the age column, take your selected condition and consider each of the 14 functions requiring assistance and tick in the box(es) those appropriate to your patient's needs, e.g. an elderly patient may require assistance with 2, 3 and 5

3 Repeat the same procedure with subsequent columns

Conditions Always Present that Affect Basic Needs				Physiological Disturbances
Age	*Temperament*	*Social/Cultural*	*Physical/Intellectual Capacity*	1. Fluid and electrolyte imbalance
Newborn	Emotional state	(Member of a family)	Normal weight	2. Oxygen want
Child	or passing mode:	unit with friends	(Over-weight)	3. Shock
(Adolescent)	(a) normal	and status	Under-weight	4. Consciousness
Adult	(b) euphoric,	A person relatively	Normal mentality *	5. Local injury/ disease
Middle aged	hyperactive	alone	Gifted mentality	6. Metabolism
Elderly	(c) anxious, fearful,	Maladjusted	Normal sense of:	7. Seeing, hearing, smell and touch
Aged	agitated,	Destitute	hearing	8. Communicable conditions
	hysterical	Smoker	sight	(9. Immobilisation: disease/treatment)
	(d) depressed/	Drinker	equilibrium	
	hypoactive		touch	
			Loss of sense of:	
			hearing	
			sight	
			(equilibrium)	
			touch	
			Normal motor power	
			(Loss of motor power)	

* Mentally handicapped

Functions requiring assistance	Age	Temperament	Social/Cultural	Physical/Intellectual Capacity	Physiological Disturbance
1. Breathing					
2. Eating or drinking		✓	✓	✓	
3. Elimination		✓	✓		✓
4. Sleep or rest				✓	✓
5. Movement		✓	✓		✓
6. Maintenance of body temperature				✓	✓
7. Keeping body clean				✓	
8. Dressing suitably				✓	✓
9. Avoiding dangers and injury				✓	✓
10. Communication				✓	
11. Worship				✓	
12. Work					✓
13. Participation in recreation				✓	
14. Learning to satisfy curiosity				✓	✓

The items ticked in the Patient Profiles should assist you to formulate a care plan which includes the functions which require assistance for your patient from both the physiological disturbances and the conditions which are always present.

An essential part of planning and implementing care is the inclusion of a clearly defined record of the patient's progress and response to care with an ongoing evaluation of what we do to and for patients. Short- and long-term goals for implementing care should be discussed and agreed with the patient and/or relatives, suitable monitoring methods should be chosen, and a realistic review period should be set.

Evaluation

What *is* evaluation?
    Determination of the value of.
So what makes you decide this value (of nursing care)?
How do you value care?
Who values it?
How do you put a value on something?
What is value?
    Value is worth . . . . . .
    That which renders anything useful or estimable.
    The degree of this quality.
    Relative worth.
    To esteem or rate at a price.
    To prize.

'Evaluation is dependent upon the comparison of information collected *before* nursing action has been taken with information collected after nursing action has been taken. It is the comparison that makes it different from assessment.'
Kratz (1979)

What are we evaluating?

Things we do to and for patients and the patient's progress and response to care could fall into three categories: nursing activities related to patient comfort, safety and well-being; nursing activities pertaining to observations and measurements; and nursing actions relating to diagnosis and treatment.

What can help you evaluate care and record the patient's progress and response to care?

To assist you, we have given you some questions to ask yourself when writing progress reports under each of these headings.

Nursing actions relating to patient comfort, safety and well-being

You need to ask the patient and family (if possible) whether the present nursing actions are needed to maintain the patient's level of information and safety.

Nursing actions pertaining to observations and measurements

For what purposes are these measurements required?
Who wants the results of the measurements?
What happens to the results?
Are different measurements required?
If yes, what is required and how often?

Nursing actions relating to diagnosis and treatment

Do the treatments require altering — i.e., in type and frequency?
Do the medicines require stopping, starting, changing?
Are the nursing activities still necessary?
Have the course/s of treatment, medicines been completed?

We now include a suggested aid to writing patient progress notes. Give some thought to how you could use this in your own work setting, and then compare your results with how we have tried to use the form with Mr Watson and Mrs Jones in Chapter 1 and Mr Jones and Mr Brittain in Chapter 2.

EVALUATION OF CARE AND SUGGESTED RECORD OF PROGRESS

Patient's Name ....

Date .... Time ....

QUESTIONS TO HELP YOU WITH EVALUATING CARE AND PROGRESS

Nursing actions relating to patient comfort, safety and well-being

- What is the patient's response to his/her condition?
- Are the present nursing actions still required?
- Is the patient, and his/her family, informed?

Nursing actions pertaining to observations and measurements

- What is the patient's response to the observations and measurements being made?
- Are the present measurements/observations still required?
- Have results been seen or relayed to the appropriate practitioner/carer?
- Has the patient been informed of the changes?

Nursing actions relating to diagnosis and treatment

- What is the patient's response to diagnosis and treatment?
- Are the patient's treatments still required?
- Have the course/s of treatment been completed or discontinued?
- Has the patient been informed?

* * * * * * *

- Who has visited the patient?
- What information has been given to relatives/visitors?

* * * * * * *

- Has the care plan been updated?
- Are the objectives/goals of care still relevant?

Signature of
Reporting Nurse ....

Designation ....

Signature of
Supervising Nurse ....

Designation ....

Within this book you will find suggestions and methods for recording assessment, planning and evaluation of nursing care which we hope you will think about and from which we hope you will use those points which you feel would be helpful to you and beneficial to your patients now and in the future.

ANSWERS to activities/minimal age of responsibility exercise (page xiii).

10 years	key number 5	criminal responsibility
16 years	key number 1	leaving school
	key number 2	stopping of entitlement to free medicines
	key number 3	able to marry
	key number 6	age of sexual consent
17 years	key number 4	drive a car
	key number 7	buy an air rifle
18 years	key number 8	buy a drink in a public house
	key number 11	vote for a member of parliament
	key number 12	take out a hire purchase agreement
21 years	key number 9	drive a heavy goods vehicle
35 years	key number 10	be President of United States of America

Chapter 1

Nursing patients with disturbances of fluid and electrolyte balance

Normal maintenance of fluid and electrolyte balance

(a) The digestive system

Fuel (food) is taken into the body and processed so that it can be used for the maintenance of function, repair and growth. Waste material is eliminated. The digestive system consists of the alimentary canal—a 9 m tube running from mouth to anus—and adjoining accessory organs (teeth, salivary glands, liver, biliary system and pancreas).

As food progresses through the alimentary canal (Figure 1.1), different constituents are broken down chemically by the action of different *enzymes* produced by the various digestive *glands*. Enzymes are proteins produced and secreted by special cells within the glands. Different parts of the digested food, and also water, minerals and vitamins, are absorbed into the blood by the absorptive wall of the alimentary canal.

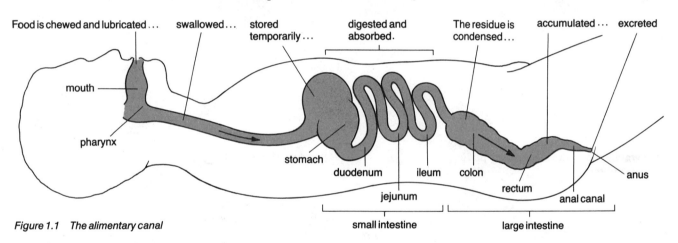

Figure 1.1   The alimentary canal

1   The mouth

Teeth

The dentition of an animal is adapted to its diet. Man is omnivorous (eats all types of food) and possesses, on each side, upper and lower, the teeth shown in Figure 1.2. In the adult there are eight teeth in each quarter, making a total of

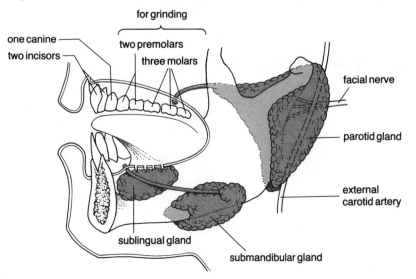

Figure 1.2   The mouth. Only the right upper row of teeth is described

thirty-two. These are called the permanent teeth. Between the sixth year and adolescence, the twenty deciduous or milk teeth of the child are shed and replaced by the permanent teeth. The third permanent molar (wisdom tooth) of each quarter normally comes through after the age of 17. Further replacement can only be artificial; therefore permanent teeth should be well cared for.

Salivary glands

Saliva is produced by the *parotid, submandibular* and *sublingual* glands, and in small quantities by glands in the mucous membrane of the mouth and tongue. It contains a protein called *mucin,* which lubricates the processes of eating and speaking, and salivary amylase, an enzyme which begins the breakdown of starch. Salt, sweet, acid and sour substances dissolve in saliva to stimulate the taste buds of the tongue. A decrease in body fluid causes a decrease in the flow of saliva (normally over a litre a day) and a feeling of thirst.

2 The oesophagus

Once food has been masticated (chewed) by the teeth, and formed into a soft ball *(bolus)* by the tongue, it is passed along the *oesophagus* to the *stomach*. This process is shown in Figure 1.3. Swallowing, although aided by gravity, is not dependent on it, as the bolus is moved along the oesophagus by the process of *peristalsis*.

1 Swallowing — the voluntary phase

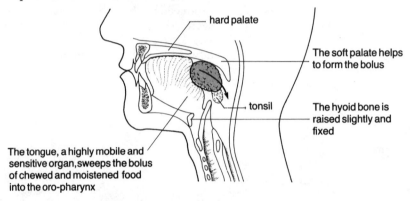

hard palate

The soft palate helps to form the bolus

tonsil

The hyoid bone is raised slightly and fixed

The tongue, a highly mobile and sensitive organ, sweeps the bolus of chewed and moistened food into the oro-pharynx

2 Swallowing — the involuntary phase — beginning

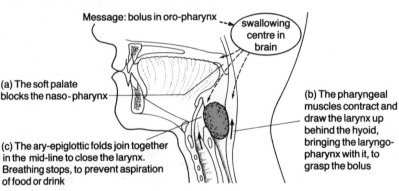

Message: bolus in oro-pharynx

swallowing centre in brain

(a) The soft palate blocks the naso-pharynx

(b) The pharyngeal muscles contract and draw the larynx up behind the hyoid, bringing the laryngo-pharynx with it, to grasp the bolus

(c) The ary-epiglottic folds join together in the mid-line to close the larynx. Breathing stops, to prevent aspiration of food or drink

3 Swallowing — the involuntary phase — continuation

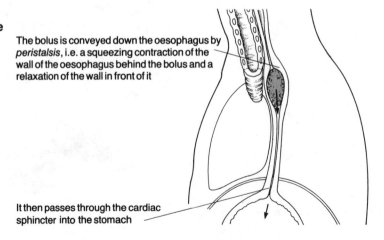

The bolus is conveyed down the oesophagus by *peristalsis*, i.e. a squeezing contraction of the wall of the oesophagus behind the bolus and a relaxation of the wall in front of it

It then passes through the cardiac sphincter into the stomach

Figure 1.3 Swallowing

3 The stomach

The stomach is a muscular bag of variable shape, size and position and has a maximum capacity of about 2.5 litres. Here, food is churned up by the contraction of the muscular wall, and mixed with the acidic *gastric juice* which is secreted by the gastric glands in the mucous lining of the stomach. The various secretions which make up the gastric juice are shown in Figure 1.4.

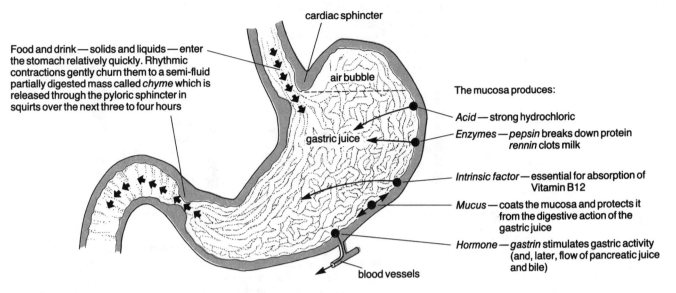

Food and drink—solids and liquids—enter the stomach relatively quickly. Rhythmic contractions gently churn them to a semi-fluid partially digested mass called *chyme* which is released through the pyloric sphincter in squirts over the next three to four hours

cardiac sphincter

air bubble

gastric juice

blood vessels

The mucosa produces:

Acid—strong hydrochloric

Enzymes—*pepsin* breaks down protein
rennin clots milk

Intrinsic factor—essential for absorption of Vitamin B12

Mucus—coats the mucosa and protects it from the digestive action of the gastric juice

Hormone—*gastrin* stimulates gastric activity (and, later, flow of pancreatic juice and bile)

Figure 1.4   The stomach

The acidic environment of the stomach, provided by the secretion of hydrochloric acid, is essential for the functioning of the enzyme *pepsin*, which breaks down protein. The acid also acts as a disinfectant, by killing most of the bacteria taken in with food.

The control of stomach activity, including the secretion of the various components of the gastric juice, is effected by both nervous and hormonal mechanisms, as shown in Figure 1.5.

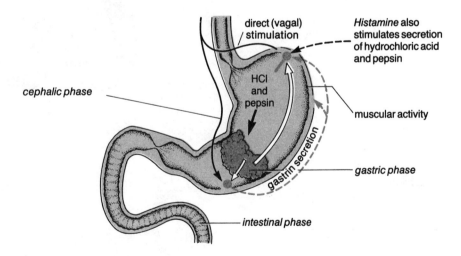

direct (vagal) stimulation

Histamine also stimulates secretion of hydrochloric acid and pepsin

HCl and pepsin

cephalic phase

muscular activity

gastrin secretion

gastric phase

intestinal phase

Figure 1.5   Control of gastric secretion

The sight, smell and thought of food can initiate gastric secretion, which is stimulated by the vagus nerve five or ten minutes later. Secretion stimulated in this way lasts for about one and a half hours and reaches a peak after half an hour; this is called the *cephalic* phase of gastric secretion. Once food arrives in the stomach the slight distension of the stomach walls further stimulates the flow of gastric secretions, an effect which lasts about four hours with a peak after two hours. This is the *gastric* phase. As the partially digested contents of the stomach *(chyme)* reach the small intestine, a hormone which *inhibits* the flow of gastric secretion is produced. This is the *intestinal* phase.

4 The small intestine

The digestive process continues and is completed in the small intestine, which is a convoluted tube about 5 m long. The intestinal juice containing the enzymes responsible for this final breakdown of food substances is alkaline.

The other important function of the small intestine is that of absorption of the small molecular glucose, amino acids, fatty acids and glycerol which have resulted from the breakdown of nutrients. Projecting from the lining of the small intestine are millions of little finger-like processes called *villi*. Inside each villus are blood capillaries and a lymphatic capillary (called a *lacteal*). Glucose and amino acids pass into the blood, and the fatty acids and glycerol are transferred into the lymph within the lacteal.

Figure 1.6 shows the four different ways in which the cells of the mucosa (the lining of the small intestine) effect the absorption of small molecules.

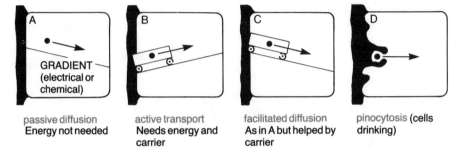

Figure 1.6 Absorption of small molecules by cells

In B and C, the wagon represents a *carrier*—an unknown substance that can take water-soluble molecules through the lipid membrane of the cell. If the carrier is used for another job, absorption is reduced.

Many substances are absorbed throughout the small intestine, e.g., folate, but some are absorbed more at one site than another, as shown in Figure 1.7.

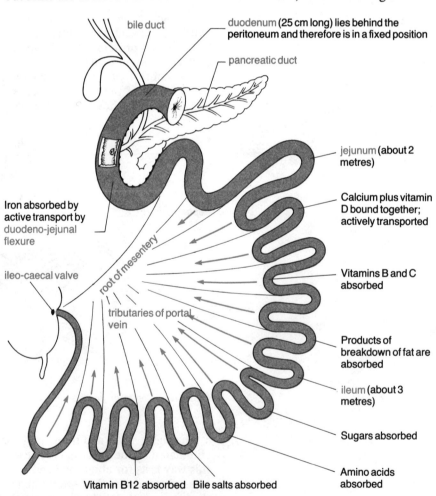

Figure 1.7 Absorption by the small intestine

The fluid contents pass rapidly through the small intestine—so rapidly that peristalsis, persisting briefly after death, empties the jejunum, and gave rise to its name (*jejunus*, Latin for 'empty', 'hungry').

The details of the whole process of digestion are summarised in Figure 1.8.

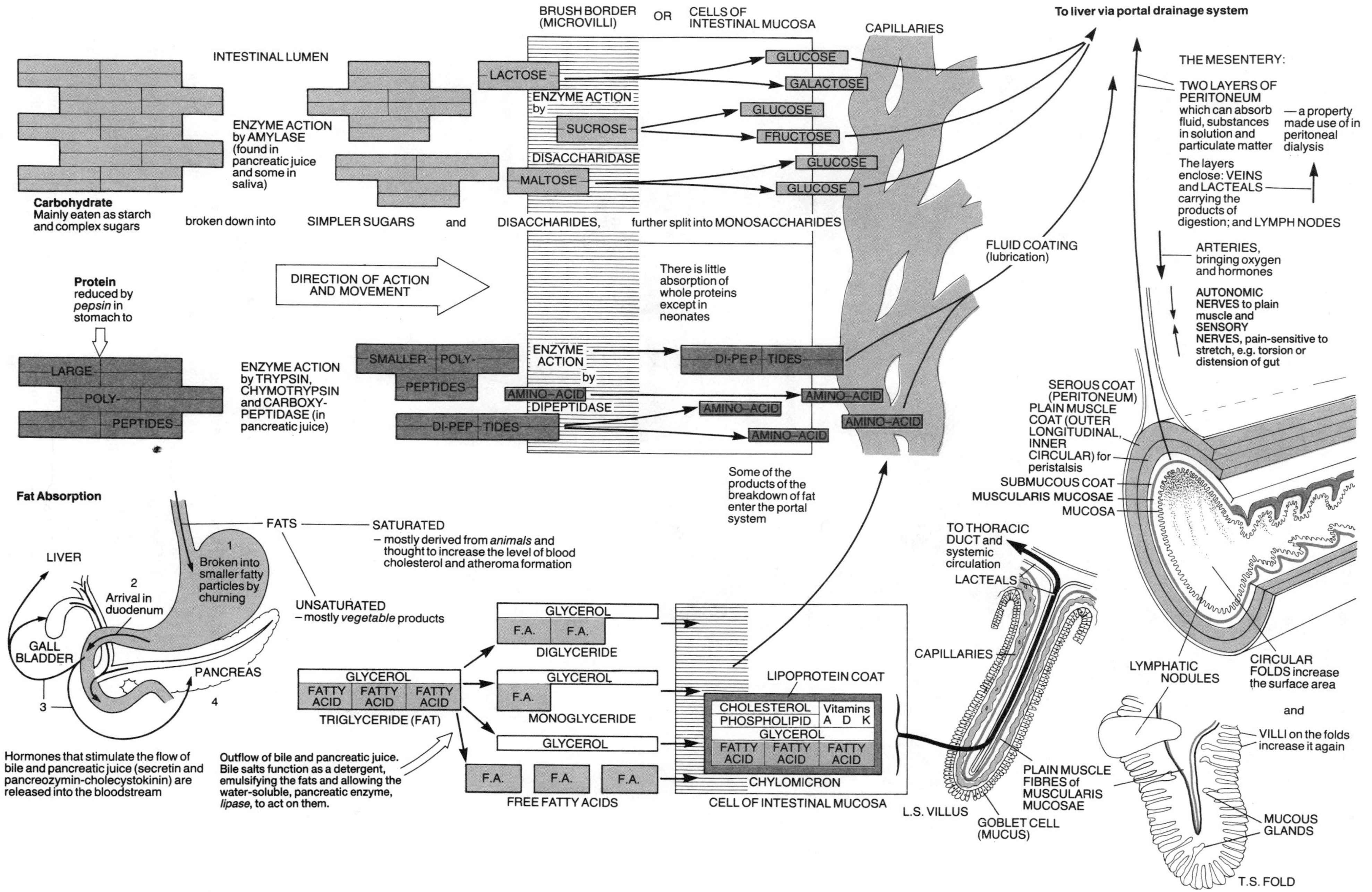

Figure 1.8 Process of digestion

5 The large intestine

The chief functions of the large intestine (Figure 1.9) are the absorption of water and some salts, and the periodic voiding of its contents (defaecation).

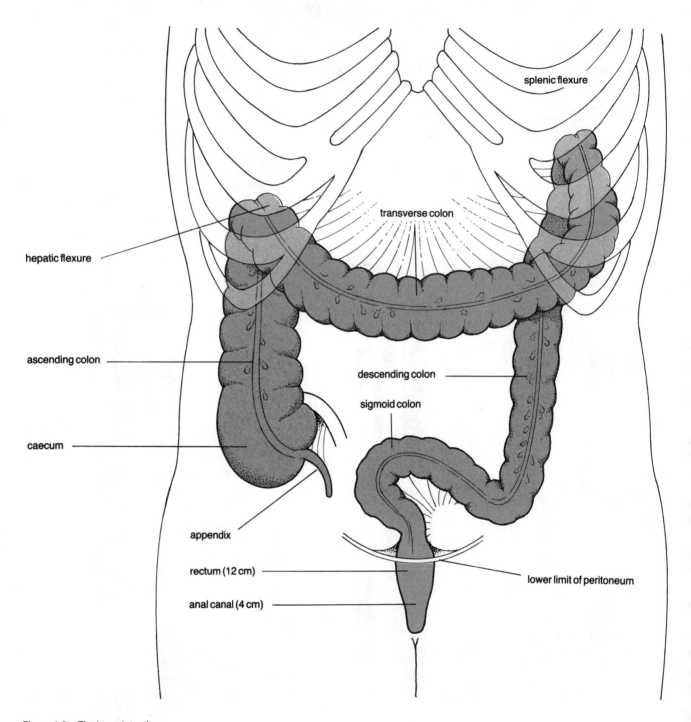

Figure 1.9   The large intestine

The colon (Figure 1.10) consists of the following parts:

1. The *caecum,* attached to which is the appendix.
2. The *ascending colon,* which is about 15 cm long and bound to the posterior abdominal wall.
3. The *transverse colon,* about 50 cm long, which has a mesentery (the mesocolon) and can therefore vary in position.
4. The *descending colon,* about 25 cm long, which has a constant position because, like the ascending colon, it is bound to the posterior abdominal wall.
5. The *sigmoid colon,* which is variable in length and position because it has a mesentery. At the end of the sigmoid colon, and below the lower limit of the peritoneum, are the *rectum* and the *anal canal.*

The colon is not essential for life. Total colectomy was briefly fashionable early this century to prevent constipation. The operation soon fell out of favour because severe diarrhoea resulted. Nowadays colectomy is sometimes performed for generalised colonic disease, usually ulcerative colitis, and the patient's health often improves considerably.

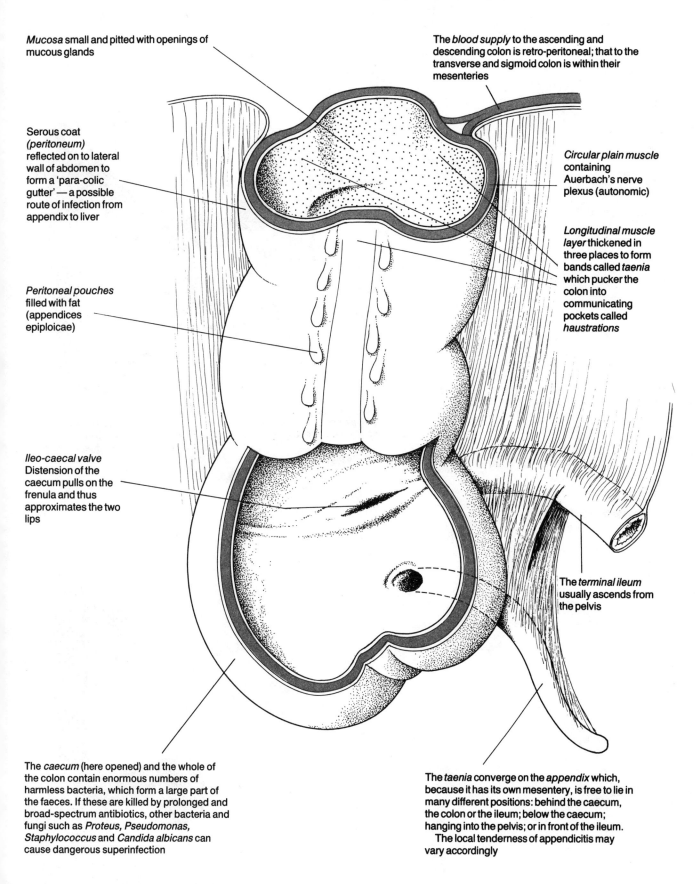

Mucosa small and pitted with openings of mucous glands

The *blood supply* to the ascending and descending colon is retro-peritoneal; that to the transverse and sigmoid colon is within their mesenteries

Serous coat (peritoneum) reflected on to lateral wall of abdomen to form a 'para-colic gutter' — a possible route of infection from appendix to liver

Circular plain muscle containing Auerbach's nerve plexus (autonomic)

Longitudinal muscle layer thickened in three places to form bands called *taenia* which pucker the colon into communicating pockets called *haustrations*

Peritoneal pouches filled with fat (appendices epiploicae)

Ileo-caecal valve Distension of the caecum pulls on the frenula and thus approximates the two lips

The *terminal ileum* usually ascends from the pelvis

The *caecum* (here opened) and the whole of the colon contain enormous numbers of harmless bacteria, which form a large part of the faeces. If these are killed by prolonged and broad-spectrum antibiotics, other bacteria and fungi such as *Proteus, Pseudomonas, Staphylococcus* and *Candida albicans* can cause dangerous superinfection

The *taenia* converge on the *appendix* which, because it has its own mesentery, is free to lie in many different positions: behind the caecum, the colon or the ileum; below the caecum; hanging into the pelvis; or in front of the ileum.
The local tenderness of appendicitis may vary accordingly

Figure 1.10 The structure of the large intestine

7

Defaecation

The process of defaecation is outlined in Figure 1.11. Healthy people vary considerably in how often they open their bowels—from three times a day to twice a week. A change in usual habit may indicate a disease process and should be investigated.

Many people believe, wrongly, that they will become ill if they do not defaecate daily. In reality, so-called 'auto-intoxication' occurs only in patients with severe liver failure. Much more harm is done by the unwise use of aperients than by the 'constipation' they are designed to relieve.

1   First phase

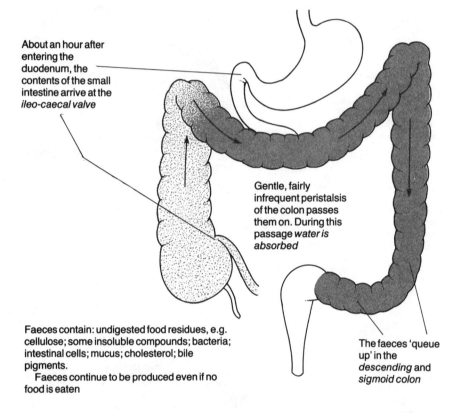

About an hour after entering the duodenum, the contents of the small intestine arrive at the *ileo-caecal valve*

Gentle, fairly infrequent peristalsis of the colon passes them on. During this passage *water is absorbed*

Faeces contain: undigested food residues, e.g. cellulose; some insoluble compounds; bacteria; intestinal cells; mucus; cholesterol; bile pigments.
   Faeces continue to be produced even if no food is eaten

The faeces 'queue up' in the *descending* and *sigmoid colon*

2   The gastro-colic reflex

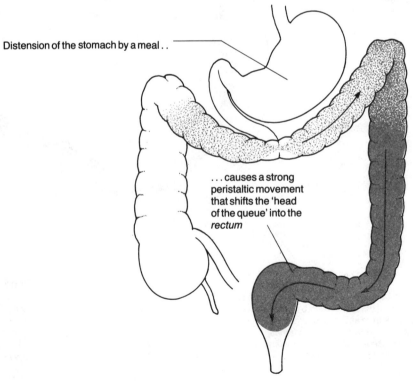

Distension of the stomach by a meal . .

. . . causes a strong peristaltic movement that shifts the 'head of the queue' into the *rectum*

Figure 1.11   Defaecation

3a In infants

Afferent impulses from the distended rectum, via a simple spinal reflex of the *parasympathetic N.S.*, trigger the emptying of about half the large intestine

As the child grows older, voluntary control from higher centres is superimposed as the nervous system matures. Toilet training is not possible until the nervous system is sufficiently developed, but convenient use may be made of the gastro-colic reflex by holding the baby over a 'potty' after feeds.

During the first two or three years of life, tone develops in the *external* anal sphincter, and defaecation comes under voluntary control.

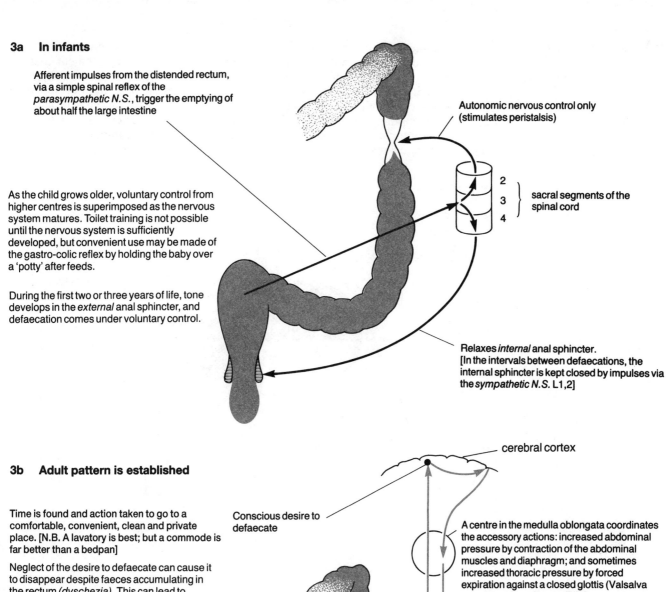

Autonomic nervous control only (stimulates peristalsis)

2
3 } sacral segments of the
4   spinal cord

Relaxes *internal* anal sphincter. [In the intervals between defaecations, the internal sphincter is kept closed by impulses via the *sympathetic N.S.* L1,2]

3b Adult pattern is established

Time is found and action taken to go to a comfortable, convenient, clean and private place. [N.B. A lavatory is best; but a commode is far better than a bedpan]

Neglect of the desire to defaecate can cause it to disappear despite faeces accumulating in the rectum *(dyschezia)*. This can lead to constipation, impaction (with scybala) and spurious diarrhoea (see later), especially in paralysed patients and the elderly

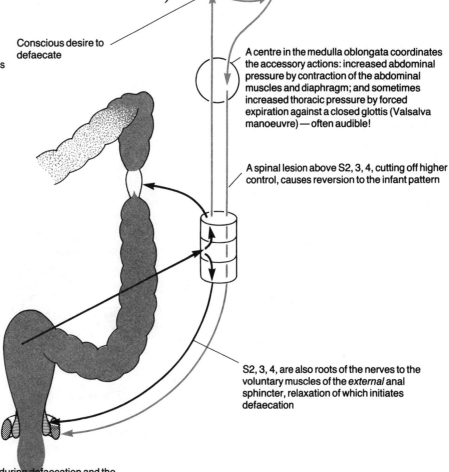

cerebral cortex

Conscious desire to defaecate

A centre in the medulla oblongata coordinates the accessory actions: increased abdominal pressure by contraction of the abdominal muscles and diaphragm; and sometimes increased thoracic pressure by forced expiration against a closed glottis (Valsalva manoeuvre) — often audible!

A spinal lesion above S2, 3, 4, cutting off higher control, causes reversion to the infant pattern

S2, 3, 4, are also roots of the nerves to the voluntary muscles of the *external* anal sphincter, relaxation of which initiates defaecation

The anus pouts during defaecation and the levator ani helps to restore it to its indrawn position

Figure 1.11 (continued)

(b) The urinary system

Some animals are so closely adapted to their particular environment that they are dependent on it. They fail to live successfully if the environment changes (for example, dinosaurs became extinct) or if they move to a different environment. Man, in common with many other animals, has developed an 'internal environment' which makes him less dependent on the external one, i.e., optimal physical and chemical conditions for body cells are maintained despite changes in the outside world. One of the most important organs of chemical regulation for man and other vertebrates is the *kidney* (Figure 1.12).

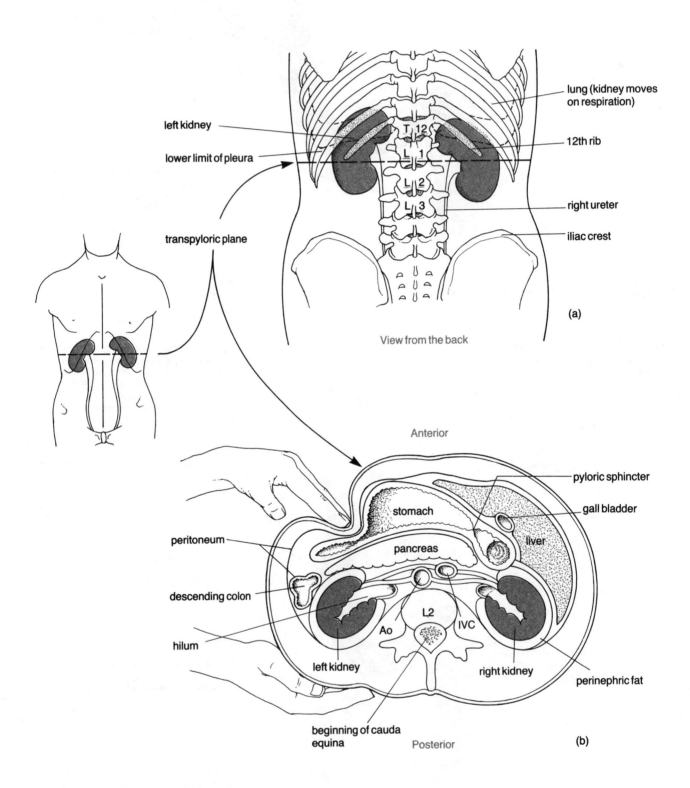

Figure 1.12   Position of the kidneys. (a) Longitudinal view and (b) transverse cross-section

The two kidneys are positioned against the posterior abdominal wall, alongside the aorta and the inferior vena cava, to which they are joined by blood vessels (Figure 1.13). The lower pole of the kidney is palpable in a thin person. On the left it can be differentiated from the spleen, as the kidney has no notch and the hand can be pressed in above it.

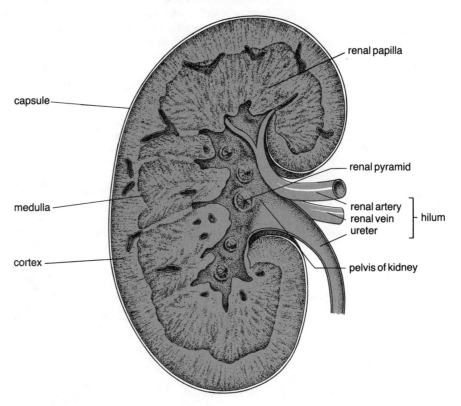

Figure 1.13   Section through the right kidney

The most important function of the kidney is to maintain constant composition and volume of the body fluids, primarily the blood, from which the other fluids are formed. This control is effected by the production of urine.

The kidneys also produce two hormones, *erythropoietin*, which stimulates the production of red blood cells, and *renin*, which helps to stimulate vasoconstriction.

(c) Maintenance of constant composition and volume of body fluids

Production of urine by the healthy kidney has the following effects:

1. Maintenance of the correct water content of the blood.
2. Maintenance of the correct electrolyte content of the blood. An electrolyte is a charged ion resulting from the dissolving of a simple salt, and the kidney is primarily involved with the regulation of sodium (Na^+), potassium (K^+) and chloride (Cl^-) ions.
3. Maintenance of the correct acid–base balance of the blood. This is measured as the pH.
4. Disposal by excretion of the waste products of metabolism (primarily urea) and drugs and other toxic substances.

The functional unit of the kidney is the *nephron* and there are approximately one million nephrons in each kidney. These undertake the two important functions, filtration and selective reabsorption, which result in the formation of urine.

1   Filtration

This occurs in the glomerulus of each nephron. Blood pressure in the glomerular capillaries is higher (70 mmHg) than in tissue capillaries elsewhere in the body because the diameter of the afferent (approaching) arteriole is greater than that of the efferent (departing) arteriole, and so water and small molecules are forced out of the blood vessels and into the Bowman's capsule.

In a healthy kidney, the large molecules, including plasma proteins and the blood cells, are retained within the bloodstream, but in disease some of these proteins and red blood cells may be forced out of the bloodstream and may appear in the urine. Figure 1.14 shows the route of the filtered molecules (including water) from the bloodstream into the Bowman's capsule of the nephron. All molecules forced out of the blood pass between breaks in the cytoplasm of the endothelial cells of the blood vessel, through the basement membrane of the capillary and between the foot-like processes of the podocyte cells of the nephron.

It has been estimated that 170 litres of fluid per day are filtered through the glomerular membranes of the two kidneys.

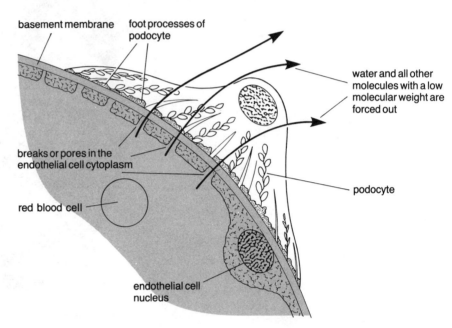

Figure 1.14   The filtration process

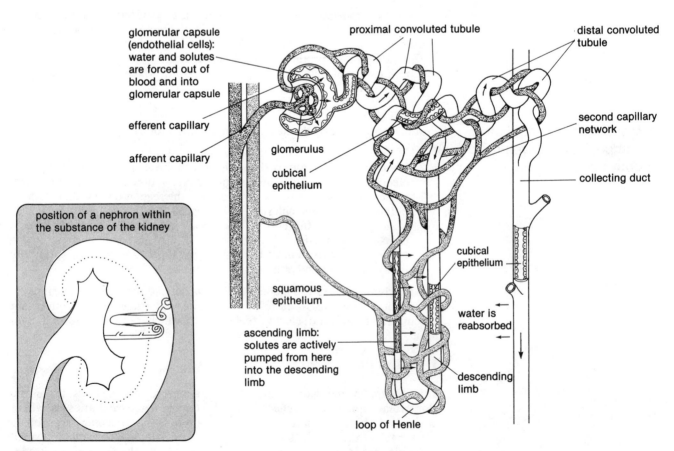

Figure 1.15   A single nephron

2 Selective reabsorption

The filtrate from the Bowman's capsule passes through the tubule of the nephron (Figure 1.15), and throughout its progress various molecules—including water—are reabsorbed from the filtrate back into the bloodstream. The tubule of the nephron is arranged so that it has a long loop (the loop of Henle) which dips down into the medulla of the kidney towards the point of a renal pyramid. At each end of the loop of Henle, the tubule is convoluted, thus providing an enlarged surface area, to increase the contact between capillaries and the tubule and thus facilitate the necessary reabsorption of solutes. About two-thirds of the water and sodium ions (Na^+) are reabsorbed in the *proximal* convoluted tubule. The absorption of Na^+ is an active process, requiring energy, and water follows by osmosis.

Reabsorption of some solutes and water continues from the loop of Henle and from the distal convoluted tubule, and the remaining fluid passes into a collecting tubule.

Solutes (mainly NaCl) in the filtrate are actively pumped from the ascending limb of the loop of Henle into the descending limb (and some into the blood) (Figure 1.15). This results in the overall tissue concentration of NaCl increasing towards the apex of the renal pyramids, so that further water is reabsorbed (by osmosis) from the fluid passing through the collecting tubules which run through the medulla.

This selective reabsorption ensures that, in a healthy kidney, all substances of nutritional importance (including glucose and amino acids) are reabsorbed, together with the correct quantities of water and the various ions—particularly

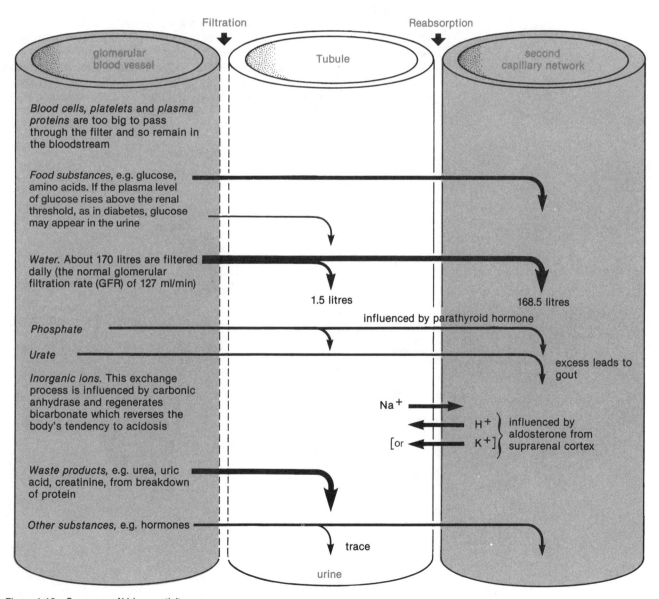

Figure 1.16 Summary of kidney activity

Na^+, K^+, Cl^- and Ca^{2+} —to maintain the body's correct salt balance. Waste substances, including urea and creatinine, are not absorbed, and so stay in the urine, which is the remaining fluid.

The reabsorption of water is controlled by a hormone called *antidiuretic hormone* (ADH), which affects the permeability of the distal convoluted tubules and the collecting tubules. ADH is produced by the posterior lobe of the pituitary gland, in the brain, in response to the concentration of the blood, which is monitored by osmoreceptor cells in the hypothalamus. If the concentration of salts in the blood is higher than is optimal (i.e., less water is present than usual), ADH production is increased.

This, in turn, increases the permeability of the walls of the collecting and distal convoluted tubules, and so water reabsorption is increased, thus rebalancing blood concentration. As the blood concentration returns to normal, ADH production drops. If ADH is deficient, insufficient water is reabsorbed, large quantities of dilute urine are passed, and the body becomes dehydrated. This condition is known as *diabetes insipidus*. Figure 1.16 provides a summary of the kidney activity described above.

3   The ureters

The ureters (Figure 1.17) are muscular tubes, about 25 cm long, which actively convey urine from the kidneys to the bladder. Small volumes of urine are squeezed along the ureters by peristaltic waves which originate in a pacemaker at the renal end of the ureter, and urine arrives in the bladder at an average rate of four or five jets per minute.

The urine formed in the renal tubules passes along the collecting tubules which open onto the *renal papillae*, and urine passes into the calyx and then the pelvis of the kidney. The outer coat of the ureter is fibrous and is continuous with the renal capsule, which surrounds the kidney, and with the outer coat of the bladder. The lining of the ureter is called the *mucous coat* and this is continuous with the covering of the renal papillae. When the ureter is not stretched, the mucous coat lies in five or six longitudinal folds. Between the fibrous coat and the mucous coat of the ureters lies a thick muscular layer.

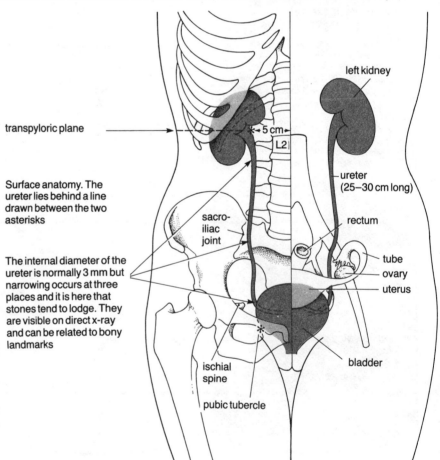

Figure 1.17   Position of the organs of the urinary system of the female

The ureters pass obliquely through the thick muscular wall of the bladder, forming a valve-like opening which prevents urine flowing back into the ureters when pressure in the bladder is raised during micturition.

4 The bladder and urethra

The bladder (Figure 1.18) is a muscular bag which stores urine, and the urethra is the passage which conveys the urine from the bladder to the outside of the body. The muscle of the bladder (called the *detrusor* muscle) consists largely of interlacing bundles of smooth or *involuntary* muscle fibres. At the base of the bladder, these smooth muscle fibres pass round the urethral opening to form the *internal sphincter*, which is stimulated by sympathetic and parasympathetic nerves from both lumbar and sacral parts of the spinal cord.

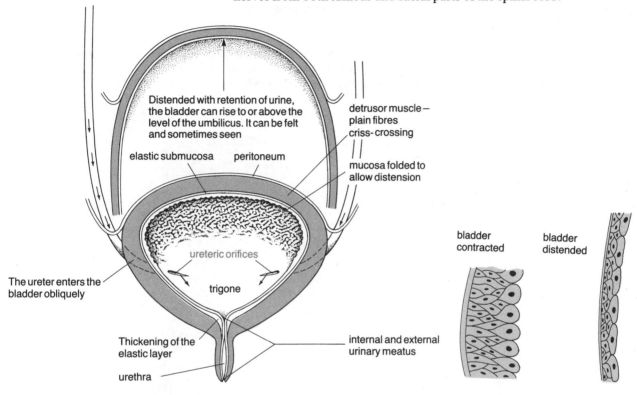

Figure 1.18   The bladder

Figure 1.19   Transitional epithelium

The inner lining of the bladder is called the *mucosa*, and consists of several folds of *transitional epithelium* (see Figure 1.19) which allow expansion as the bladder fills.

The triangle of the mucosa between the two openings of the ureters and the urethra is called the *trigone* and is smooth and free from folds, and does not expand with the bladder.

The *external sphincter*, at the external end of the urethra, consists of two *striated* or *voluntary* muscles, and so this sphincter is under voluntary control. When the bladder is empty, the sphincters are tonically contracted so that the urine from the ureters gradually expands the bladder. At first, this filling does not cause the intravesical pressure (pressure within the bladder) to rise significantly, because of the elastic properties of the bladder wall. As filling continues, however, the tension in the wall increases in proportion to the contained volume. Figure 1.20 shows the development of sensations as the bladder fills. The bladder is usually allowed to fill until it contains nearly 300 ml.

5 Control of micturition

In the healthy adult, micturition is under voluntary control. As the bladder fills, the pressure within it rises. Contraction waves appear in the muscular coat, stimulating pressure receptors and sending afferent impulses to the brain, where 'desire to micturate' is recorded. The procedure then depends on whether or not micturition is convenient.

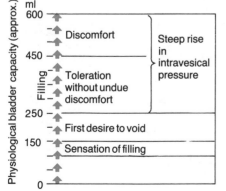

Figure 1.20   Filling of the bladder

If not convenient

Impulses from the cerebral cortex cause inhibition of the detrusor muscle, enlarging the bladder to accommodate the increasing volume of urine. The pressure in the bladder falls and the desire to micturate passes off for a time. The bladder can be 'trained' to hold large volumes of urine. Eventually the pressure rise becomes painful and the bladder is emptied.

If convenient

Impulses from the cortex pass down the spinal cord to the sacral segments and along the relevant parasympathetic nerves, stimulating the detrusor muscle to contract and thus opening the internal sphincter. Voluntary relaxation of the perineal muscles and external sphincter occurs. Intra-abdominal pressure rises as a result of the contraction of diaphragm and abdominal muscles, and the bladder empties.

The fact that women urinate less frequently than men is not due to greater bladder capacity but to a greater ability to suppress the emptying urges.

Figure 1.21 summarises normal nervous control of micturition. Voluntary control of micturition develops as the nervous system of the child develops, and

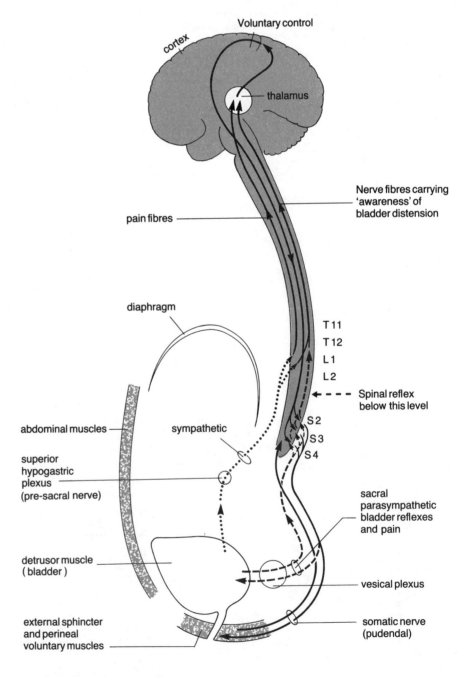

Figure 1.21   Control of micturition

a progressively increasing intravesical pressure (and therefore an increasing volume of urine in the bladder) can be tolerated, as shown in Figure 1.22.

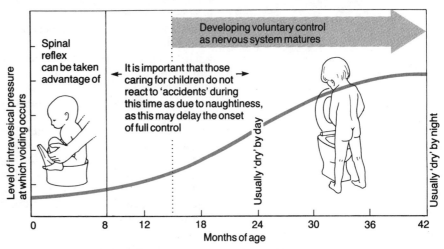

Figure 1.22 Development of the voluntary control of micturition

The patients with disturbances of fluid and electrolyte balance

(a) Fluid and electrolyte disturbances in patients with conditions of the digestive system

1 Patient study and care plan for an adult with acute intestinal obstruction

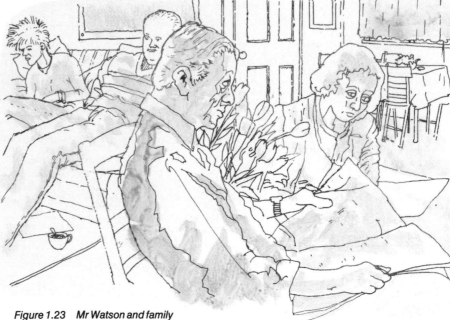

Figure 1.23 Mr Watson and family

History of social, psychological and physical events leading to the present condition

The patient chosen for this section to illustrate fluid and electrolyte disturbance has an acute intestinal obstruction due to a strangulated inguinal hernia.

Mr Watson, aged 50 years, lives with his wife and two teenage children (Figure 1.23) in a small terraced house with a large rear garden. He is employed as a postman and his leisure activities include gardening and holidays with his family. He smokes 40 cigarettes a day and drinks moderately.

During the last two winters Mr Watson has had episodes of acute bronchitis. He was first diagnosed two years ago as having an inguinal hernia. His name was added to the waiting list for surgery at this time. One week ago he started to complain of:

- Colic — spasmodic abdominal pain.
- Less frequent bowel actions.
- Loss of appetite.
- Feeling of abdominal distension.

Twelve hours ago he started to complain of:
- Nausea.
- Vomiting.
- Severe abdominal pain.
- Increasing abdominal distension.
- Inability to open bowels.
- Dry tongue and mouth and unpleasant taste in mouth.

During this time Mrs Watson observed that her husband was becoming anxious and frightened and appeared pale and sweating. She noticed that the vomit had altered from a clear to a greenish-brown, foul-smelling fluid. He seemed to be unable to keep anything down even though he complained of increasing thirst. Mrs Watson contacted their general practitioner in the morning. He visited Mr Watson at home and arranged for an ambulance to take him to hospital. Mrs Watson followed her husband to hospital with the help of a neighbour after ensuring the children had left for school.

At the accident and emergency department, Mr Watson's condition was assessed, diagnosis confirmed and treatment initiated on the basis of the following:
- History.
- Physical examination.
- Straight abdominal x-ray.
- Blood samples for cross matching.
- Electrolytes and urea estimation.

Immediate treatment involved:
1. Starting an intravenous infusion.
2. Passing a nasogastric tube.
3. Giving an intramuscular analgesic following confirmation of diagnosis.

Explanation of abnormal physiology and pathology

It is advised that you revise the normal structure and function of the gastro-intestinal tract (pages 2–9), and see Table 1.1.

Table 1.1

Related normal physiology	Abnormal physiology
(a) Appetite good; ingestion possible	Loss of appetite and reduced fluid intake due to interruption of normal function by mechanical obstruction
(b) *Stomach* (i) Secretion of gastric juice and hydrochloric acid (ii) Absorption of water and glucose (iii) Peristalsis	(i) Secretions continue (ii) Reduced absorption leading to accumulation of fluid (iii) Reversed causing vomiting
(c) *Small Intestine* (i) Peristalsis (ii) Secretion of intestinal juices (iii) Absorption of nutrients	(i) Increased, causing colic, and later absent (ii) Continues (iii) Reduced (refer to later explanation of pathology)
(d) *Large Intestine* (i) Peristalsis (ii) Absorption of water	(i) Dormant (ii) None available
(e) *Rectum* Defaecation	Stops

MECHANICAL OBSTRUCTION

It is advised that you refer to the normal structure and function of anterior abdominal wall, inguinal canal and blood circulation of the small intestine.

A hernia is a protrusion of viscus (e.g., an organ) or part of a viscus through a weakness of its surrounding structures (Figure 1.24).

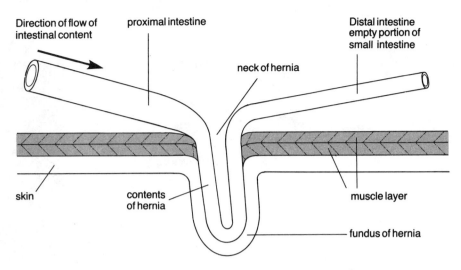

Figure 1.24   A hernia

Explanation

In order for a hernia to be defined as strangulated, the following sequence of events takes place:

1. Loop of small intestine protrudes through weakness in the muscle of the abdominal wall.
2. The neck of the hernia causes constriction of the lumen of the small intestine, causing mechanical obstruction.
3. Local oedema of the wall of the intestine causes further constriction at the neck, which impairs venous return.
4. This causes even more oedema, which eventually causes obliteration of the arterial blood supply.
5. This diminished arterial supply causes necrosis of the herniated portion of the small intestine.
6. The lack of blood supply and the mechanical obstruction at the hernia site cause gross distension of the proximal intestine and risk of perforation.

FLUID AND ELECTROLYTE DISTURBANCE

Explanation

As fluid accumulates in the proximal portion of the intestine, the patient starts to vomit contents of the stomach (containing possibly a past meal) (Figure 1.25 a, b). As vomiting persists vomitus becomes a clear fluid containing mucus; later it becomes bile stained and then faeculent, as intestinal contents continue to regurgitate through the pyloric sphincter due to reverse peristalsis from the site of obstruction.

As secretions into the intestine continue the blood volume decreases, leading to a drop in blood pressure, raised pulse, and reduced kidney perfusion causing oliguria. Tissue cells in turn become fluid-depleted, causing dry skin and mucous membranes, and sunken eyes.

With water, sodium levels are reduced, causing potassium to move out of the cells. The effects on the body are general fatigue, muscular weakness and gastro-intestinal distension.

Perpetual emptying of contents of the stomach leads to loss of hydrochloric acid and resulting disturbance of acid–base balance.

Further reading

Bell, G. B., Emslie-Smith, D. and Paterson, C. R., *Textbook of Physiology and Biochemistry*, 10th edition, Churchill Livingstone, London, 1980.
Green, J. H., *Basic Clinical Physiology*, 3rd edition, Oxford University Press, London, 1979.
Pathology textbook: refer to your teacher for guidance.

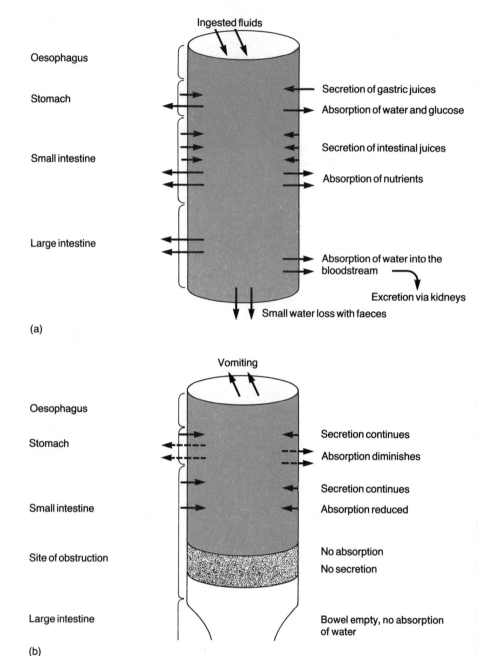

Figure 1.25 Fluid and electrolyte disturbance. (a) Normal circulation of fluid through the bowel and (b) abnormal circulation of fluid through the bowel

Care Plan

PREPARATION FOR PATIENT WITH STRANGULATED INGUINAL HERNIA

Preparation of staff
The nurse in charge needs to ensure that all staff are aware that an emergency admission of a patient with a strangulated hernia is imminent. She also needs to allocate a nurse to receive Mr Watson into the ward and to carry out the necessary care, ensuring that adequate supervision is available.

Preparation of environment
The nurse allocated to the care of Mr Watson arranges to attend to the following:
- Prepare bed for easy observation.
- Collect the necessary stationery.
- Collect the necessary linen for preparation for transfer to the operating theatre.
- Prepare equipment, including intravenous infusion stand, equipment for aspirating the stomach, dentures container.

Nursing history and assessment

After settling Mr Watson into bed, the nurse assesses his condition and records and reports her findings in the admission report as follows:

Mr Watson appears pale, sweating and anxious, with tongue and mouth dry. He is complaining of abdominal pain and nausea, and states that he has recently vomited green-coloured fluid. He has not had his bowels open for the past 3 days and shows signs of abdominal distension. He has had nothing to eat or drink since 7 am. He last passed urine at 2 am and noticed it was darker in colour than normal. The following observations were measured and recorded:

- Temperature 37.8°C.
- Pulse 100 beats per minute.
- Respirations 16 per minute.
- Blood pressure 100/70 mmHg.

The nurse gains further information from Mr and Mrs Watson by completing the nursing history and assessment sheet (Table 1.2).

Table 1.2   Nursing history and assessment sheet for Mr George Watson

---

NURSING HISTORY AND ASSESSMENT SHEET

Record No. _012345_

PATIENT LABEL

Mr/Mrs/Miss _George Watson_

Address _100 Tack Road, Greenville_

Male/Female   Age _50 years_

Date of Birth _5.9.36_

Date of admission/first visit

_10.11.86_

Time _____

Type: ☐ Routine ☑ Emergency

Transfer from: _____

Religion _C/E_

Practising/baptised _Non-practising_

Minister _____

Telephone number _____

Next of kin (name) _Mrs Alice Watson_

Relationship to patient _Wife_

Address _Same address_

Telephone numbers _____

Contact at night/in emergency   YES/NO

Occupation (or father) _Postman_

Marital status _Married_

Children (or place in family) _2 (teenage)_

Other dependants _____

Pets _____

School (children only) _____

Hobbies _Gardening_

Clubs _____

Favourite pastime _Family holidays_

Does patient smoke?   YES/NO _(40 cigarettes per day)_

Speech difficulty/language barrier

Dysphasia   Dysarthria

Accommodation

Lives alone   YES/NO

Part III/EMI/Old People's Homes/Rented

Other _Small terraced house_

Consultant _Mr North_

House officer _Dr Henderson_

Presenting condition _Intestinal obstruction_

History of present complaint and reason for admission

One week ago started colic, abdominal distension, loss of appetite, less frequent bowel actions. 12 hours ago started vomiting, severe abdominal pain, increasing abdominal distension, constipation

Past medical history

Acute bronchitis last 2 winters. Inguinal hernia for 2 years

Allergies _None_

Current medication

None

What patient says is the reason for admission and attitude to admission

Severe abdominal pain and vomiting

Patient's expectations _Surgical operation_

Any problems at home while/because patient is in hospital?

None

Relevant home conditions (e.g. stairs)

_____

Visiting problems

_____

Table 1.2 (cont.)

Care at home

Community nurse _____

No. _____

Name of GP _____ *Dr Davidson* _____

Address _____ *The Health Centre, Greenville* _____

Other services involved

Home help _____	Day hospital _____
Laundry _____	Day centre/club _____
Inco supplies _____	Health visitor _____
Aids _____	Social worker _____
Meals on wheels _____	Voluntary worker _____

Daily living

Diet

Special _____

Food or drink dislikes _____ *Milk* _____

Appetite: ☑GOOD ☐POOR

Remarks _____

Sleep

How many hours normally? _____ *7* _____

Sedation _____

What else helps? _____ *2 pillows* _____

Elimination

Bowels: Continent/Incontinent

How often opened? _____ *Daily usually* _____

Any medication? _____

Urinary: Continent/Incontinent

If incontinent; Day/Night/If not taken, how frequently? _____

Nocturia/Dysuria/Frequency/Urgency

Remarks _____

Female patients — Menstruation

Post-menopausal	Taking the pill
Regular	Irregular
Amenorrhoea	Dysmenorrhoea

Next period due: _____

Uses: STs Tampons

Hearing

Hearing aid: YES/NO

Remarks _____

Vision

Glasses/Contact lens: YES/NO

Remarks _____ *For reading* _____

Oral

Dentures or crowns: YES/NO

Any problems with mouth or teeth?

_____ *Upper and lower* _____

Mobility

Help needed with:

Walking/Standing/In/Out of bed/Bathing/Dressing

In/Out of chair/

Feeding/Other: _____

Remarks _____ *Normally active* _____

Prosthesis/appliance

Type of appliance _____

Help needed _____

General appearance

Normal	Dehydrated	Acutely ill
Obese	Thin	Emaciated

Remarks _____

Skin

Satisfactory	Broken areas	Dehydrated
Rash	Oedematous	Jaundiced
Pallor	Other *Dry mouth and*	
	(including bruising) *tongue*	

Remarks *Sweating* _____

Level of consciousness

Orientated	Semi-conscious
Confused	Unconscious

Remarks _____

Mental assessment (if appropriate)

Mood

Elated	Irritable	Agitated
Cheerful	Anxious	Aggressive
Miserable	Withdrawn	Suspicious
Apathetic		

Thought content

Hallucinations/Delusions/Paranoid Ideas

_____

Orientation

Time/Place/Person *Yes*

Very confused   Slightly confused

Any particular time of day? _____

Confabulation _____

Remarks _____

Surveillance   Physical/Emotional

Information obtained from _____ *Patient and wife* _____

Relationship to patient _____

By _____ *L. Johnson* _____

Position/level of training _____

Date _____ *10·11·86* _____

Time _____

Mr Watson's pre-operative care plan is shown in Table 1.3.

It has been decided that Mr Watson is to be transferred to the operating theatre in 3 hours' time.

The anaesthetist has been to examine Mr Watson and to order pre-medication.

Table 1.3   Pre-operative care plan for Mr Watson

Problem	Objective	Plan of care	Rationale
1. Emergency admission of an anxious patient accompanied by wife	Reduce anxiety of relative and patient	(a) Explanation and reassurance to be given to both	(a) Reduces problem
		(b) Give opportunity for wife to see medical staff and senior nursing staff	(b) Develops relationships and communications. Increases confidence in staff
		(c) Exchange information (including telephone numbers)	(c) Ensures later communication
2. Emergency admission of a clinically shocked patient	Alleviate shock	(a) Elevate foot of bed	(a) Increases blood flow to brain and vital centres
		(b) Prepare for and assist the setting up of intravenous infusion	(b) Replaces fluid lost and corrects electrolyte imbalance
		(c) Insert nasogastric tube, aspirate stomach contents. Observe and record aspirate	(c) Empties stomach, reduces vomiting and distension and allows accurate measurement of gastric fluid lost
		(d) Administer analgesia as prescribed and record its effect	(d) Reduces pain and neurogenic shock
3. Severe abdominal pain	Reduce pain	(a) Ensure comfortable position in bed	(a) Relieves abdominal muscle spasm
		(b) Give opportunity for husband to express fears	(b) Reduces anxiety
		(c) Administer analgesia and monitor and report effects	(c) Diminishes conscious awareness of pain
4. Dehydration and electrolyte imbalance	Replace lost fluid and correct electrolyte imbalance	(a) Record rate of intravenous infusion	(a) Prevents under- or over-hydration
		(b) (i) Record urinary output using fluid balance chart	(b) (i) and (ii) Monitors effects of treatment on blood volume and circulation
		(ii) Record temperature, pulse, respiration, blood pressure	
		(iii) Report significant changes of the above	(iii) Permits reassessment of the patient's condition
5. Vomiting faeculent fluid	Remove accumulating fluid in the stomach and prevent further vomiting	(a) Aspirate nasogastric tube frequently at regular intervals (½–1-hourly)	(a) Prevents accumulation of gastric fluid in stomach and prevents distension and discomfort
		(b) Observe, measure and record the amount, type, colour of aspirate using fluid balance chart	(b) Measures fluid loss and enables accurate replacement
6. Discomfort of naso-gastric tube	To relieve the discomfort	(a) Re-attach tube daily	(a) Prevents traction and abrasion to nostril
		(b) Nasal toilet as appropriate	(b) Prevents crusting and/or infection
7. Dry mouth	Relieve discomfort and detect early signs of the complications of a dry mouth	Inspect mouth and offer antiseptic mouthwashes	Relieves discomfort and reduces tendency to abrasions and infection
8. Dry and inelastic skin	Protect the skin from trauma	(a) Observe pressure sites 2-hourly and change patient's position	(a) and (b) Skin is more prone to damage by pressure and friction
		(b) Avoid friction when lifting and moving patient	

Table 1.3 (cont.)

Problem	Objective	Plan of care	Rationale
9. Sweating as temperature rises	Reduce patient's discomfort and prevent maceration of skin folds	Cool bed clothes, frequent hands and face wash	Reduces discomfort and the likely sites for the growth of micro-organisms
10. Susceptibility to infection following surgery	To reduce susceptibility	(a) Administer prescribed antibiotics (intramuscularly or intravenously) (b) Wash and shave operation site according to local procedures. NB Check that umbilicus is clean	(a) Reduces likelihood of infection resulting from contamination of peritoneal cavity during surgery (b) Reduces the number of skin surface micro-organisms
11. Patient smokes 40 cigarettes a day	To prevent post-operative chest infection	Teach deep breathing and coughing exercises with help of physiotherapist	Enables adequate ventilation and diffusion in post-operative period
12. Patient for emergency surgery	Prepare for operation	(a) Empty bladder, test urine for abnormalities, record result and amount (b) Dress patient in operation gown (c) Place stretcher canvas in bed (d) Attach identification label to patient's wrist (e) Remove valuables and place in safe keeping (f) Remove prosthesis (teeth) and place in labelled container (g) Check consent for operation has been given by patient (h) Have notes and x-rays available (i) Give pre-medication, usually an analgesic and parasympathetic system inhibitor (j) Check that fluid balance and observation charts are up to date	(a) Prevents involuntary emptying of bladder, checking for abnormalities of the urine (b) Reduces infection risk (c) Eases movement of patient (d) Assists checking correct patient (e) Prevents loss or damage (f) Prevents swallowing/choking and prevents loss (g) Legal requirement before operation (h) Required for medical staff (i) Reduces pain, anxiety and secretions (j) Provides information for operating theatre staff

RETURN OF MR WATSON TO THE WARD FOLLOWING RESECTION AND ANASTOMOSIS OF SMALL INTESTINE

The recovery ward nurse hands over details of surgical procedure and immediate recovery period care to the ward staff (see Table 1.4).

Mr Watson has an intravenous infusion of dextro-saline with antibiotics and potassium added in progress. The nasogastric tube is still in place and he has received 20 mg papaveretum intramuscularly. He has a lower abdominal wound with silk sutures to skin and vacuum suction drainage tube. His skin is pale, cool and dry and he is conscious and awake. Observations are:

- Temperature 37°C.
- Pulse 90 beats per minute.
- Respiration 16 per minute.
- Blood pressure 120/75 mmHg.

Mrs Watson has telephoned and intends to visit later this evening after arranging an evening meal for the children.

Table 1.4   Post-operative care plan for Mr Watson

Problem	Objective	Plan of care	Rationale
NB Potential Problems			
1. Shock, dehydration vomiting, dry mouth	Same as before operation	Plan of care continues as before	Unchanged
2. Surgical incision with drainage tube	Detect early signs of infection	(a) Observe temperature and pulse 4-hourly and record	(a) Temperature and pulse rise indicates infection present
		(b) Observe for changes in character of pain	(b) Local infection causes inflammation, swelling and pain
		(c) Report systemic effects, e.g., lethargy, reluctance to move	(c) Infection reduces defence mechanism of the body
	Ensure wound drainage	(a) Observe wound drainage, record amount and character	(a) Monitors fluid loss
		(b) Check and re-vacuum drainage apparatus daily or as necessary	(b) Ensures drainage tube is patent and that suction is adequate
	Ensure wound healing	(a) Redress wound aseptically as appropriate and report and record findings	(a) Monitors blood loss and reduces infection risk
		(b) Remove drainage tube when drainage is minimal and on doctors' instructions	(b) Ensures primary wound healing
		(c) Remove sutures when skin healed and/or on doctors' instruction	(c) Removes foreign body and risk of infection
3. Surgical intervention on the small intestine	Detect recovery of normal functions	(a) Check for return of bowel sounds daily and record	(a) Checks that peristalsis has returned
		(b) Continue measuring and recording amount of aspirate	(b) Checks rate of absorption of small intestine
		(c) Continue monitoring vital signs, including urinary output	(c) Enables correct timing for removal of nasogastric tube and intravenous infusion
	To reintroduce oral feeding	(a) Give 15 ml of water hourly, progressing to fluids as desired	(a) and (b) Promotes gradual recovery of functions of small intestine
		(b) Remove nasogastric tube and intravenous infusion when adequate daily oral intake of fluids is reached	
		(c) Introduce light diet leading to normal diet by discharge from hospital	(c) Ensures adequate nutrients for wound healing and maintenance of health
	To check the return of normal lower bowel function	Record flatus and incidence and character of bowel actions	This is a final check that normal function has returned
4. Previously smoked 40 cigarettes daily	Prevent chest infection	(a) Reinforce teaching, breathing exercises and coughing	(a) Promotes good ventilation, encourages expectoration
		(b) Encourage early mobility	(b) Increases muscular activity and venous return
		(c) Encourage reduction in smoking	
	Detection of chest infection	(a) Observe for alterations in respiration rate, depth and difficulty	(a) Indicates response to infection
		(b) Observe for skin cyanosis (blue-grey skin colour)	(b) Indicates reduced diffusion of gases

Table 1.4 (cont.)

Problem	Objective	Plan of care	Rationale
		(c) Observe increase in amount of sputum and/or colour or character of sputum	(c) Indicates response to infection
		(d) Observe for rise in temperature and pulse, sweating and mental confusion	(d) Indicates systemic effects of infection
5. Reluctance to move following operation	(a) To encourage mobility (b) To reduce risk of venous stasis, pressure sores, chest infection and urinary stasis	(a) Help patient to sit out of bed on first day after operation (b) Take short walk second day and increase to full mobility by discharge	(a) and (b) (i) Muscle pump aids venous return and prevents deep vein thrombosis (ii) Mobility increases chest expansion and ventilation, and diffusion (iii) Mobility reduces prolonged pressure on sacrum and other pressure sites (iv) Mobility promotes good bladder emptying (v) Mobility promotes a sense of well-being and independence

EVALUATION OF CARE AND SUGGESTED RECORD OF PROGRESS

Patient's Name Mr Watson

Date 11.11.86

Time 1400 hours

QUESTIONS TO HELP YOU WITH EVALUATING CARE AND PROGRESS

Nursing actions relating to patient comfort, safety and well-being

- What is the patient's response to his/her condition?
- Are the present nursing actions still required?
- Is the patient, and his/her family, informed?

Mr Watson is still lethargic and reluctant to move, has abdominal discomfort and has been anxious about the presence of wound drainage tube and intravenous infusion. Still requires nursing assistance with individual needs. He has seen the doctor this morning and he has been told what was done at operation.

Nursing actions pertaining to observations and measurements

- What is the patient's response to the observations and measurements being made?
- Are the present measurements/observations still required?
- Have results been seen or relayed to the appropriate practitioner/carer?
- Has the patient been informed of the changes?

Wants to sleep and is disturbed by frequent monitoring of his condition. Wound has leaked, requiring re-dressing and increase in frequency of observation to 1-hourly. The amount of gastric aspirate has reduced over the past 3 hours and the doctor has not yet been informed. Mr Watson has been told that no changes can occur until he has been seen again by the doctor this afternoon.

Nursing actions relating to diagnosis and treatment

- What is the patient's response to diagnosis and treatment?
- Are the patient's treatments still required?
- Have the course/s of treatment been completed or discontinued?
- Has the patient been informed?

Mr Watson is relieved to have the operation over and to know that there should be no long-term effects. There is a need for the intravenous infusion and oral fluids regime to be revised with the doctor this afternoon. The prescribed analgesia was last given at 12 noon and appears to be effective; further doses need to be prescribed for overnight cover.

* * * * * * *

- Who has visited the patient?
- What information has been given to relatives/visitors?

Mrs Watson — his wife
Present when doctor spoke to Mr Watson regarding operation performed.

* * * * * * *

- Has the care plan been updated?
- Are the objectives/goals of care still relevant?

Yes — frequency of wound observation increased.
Objectives unchanged.

Signature of Reporting Nurse *R. Green*

Designation *Student Nurse.*

Signature of Supervising Nurse *P. Philips*

Designation *Staff Nurse*

Before Mr Watson is discharged from hospital, the nurse needs to check that he is able to carry out all the basic functions that previously needed assistance (refer to V. Henderson, *Fourteen Basic Components of Nursing Care*). Mr Watson should also be advised to avoid lifting and heavy digging in the garden for the next 2 months and to attend the outpatient clinic for a follow-up examination in 1 month's time. If he experiences problems regarding return to work or any financial difficulty, he should be referred to the medical social work department.

2 Patient histories illustrating further problems related to fluid and electrolyte disturbance in patients with conditions of the digestive system

An adult with carcinoma of the stomach

Mrs Brown is a 60-year-old widow living in a bungalow on her own. She has a married son, who lives 100 miles away. Her interests show an involvement in Townswomen's Guild and Women's Fellowship with her Church.

Her past medical history consists of an abdominal hysterectomy when 45 years of age for fibroids and menorrhagia and treatment for depression following the death of her husband last year. Since last year Mrs Brown has shown disinterest in food which she attributed to her reluctance to cook for herself. In the past 6 months she has felt some upper abdominal pain and a feeling of fullness even after a small meal.

Mrs Brown also noticed her clothes becoming loose and ill-fitting, and when checking her weight she discovered she had lost 7 kg. During this period she felt increasing lethargy and a reluctance to participate in local activities. One morning she experienced a severe bout of upper abdominal pain, which was partly relieved by vomiting, and necessitated a call to her doctor. He decided that her symptoms required urgent investigation and arranged for her to see a consultant at the local hospital.

During the week Mrs Brown was seen by the consultant, who diagnosed a possible carcinoma of the stomach and recommended that she should be admitted to hospital for exploration and possible partial gastrectomy the following week.

During the next few days Mrs Brown arranged with her neighbour to look after her bungalow and garden but did not feel she wanted to tell her son about her admission to hospital.

On admission Mrs Brown appears worried and withdrawn. There are signs of recent weight loss and she looks pale and tired. After completion of the admission documents she is introduced to some of the other patients. Mrs Brown complains of poor appetite and infrequent bowel actions. Her temperature is 37.8°C, pulse 90 beats per minute, blood pressure 130/90 mmHg. Even with encouragement from the nursing staff Mrs Brown remains reluctant to inform her son of her admission.

Barium meal and endoscopy confirm the presence of a tumour partially blocking the pylorus, and this results in the decision to perform a partial gastrectomy in 3 days' time.

1. Devise a care plan for the preparation of Mrs Brown for her operation.

Question 1

Care plan should include reduction of anxiety by explanation and reassurance. Preparation of stomach by low residue diet, possible stomach washout(s), emptying of the bowel.

Care before, during and after the following investigations:

(a) Chest x-ray.
(b) Collection of blood sample for cross-matching, haemoglobin, electrolytes.
(c) Electrocardiogram.
(d) Urine ward test.
(e) General preparation for surgery.

2. Discuss how you would manage Mrs Brown's reluctance to inform her son.

Question 2

Gaining trust of Mrs Brown and enabling her to discuss her fears and possible reasons for her reluctance.

Discuss with Mrs Brown why it would be an advantage for contact to be made with her son.

Discover if there is another relative or friend she would prefer to inform.

Allow Mrs Brown to make her decision.

Accept Mrs Brown's decision.

3. Describe the changes in the normal structure and function of the stomach resulting from a malignant tumour.

Question 3

Refer to your teacher for guidance.

4. Describe the possible routes of spread and malignancy from this site to elsewhere in the body.

Question 4

Refer to your teacher for guidance.

5. Devise a care plan for post-operative management following a partial gastrectomy.

Question 5

Care plan should include the following observations and management.

(a) Post-operative observations of:
   ● vital signs
   ● wound
   ● mental state
   ● pain
(b) Management of:
   ● nasogastric tube
   ● intravenous infusion
   ● return to normal nutrition and mobility.

6. Discuss the reasons for and against whether Mrs Brown should be made fully aware of her diagnosis and prognosis.

Question 6

In your discussion you need to consider the medical, legal, psychological, religious and moral implications of either decision.

7. Discuss the facilities that could be made available for Mrs Brown to return to her own home.

Question 7

These need to include financial, social, psychological and physical provisions.

A young person with ulcerative colitis

Susan is a 17-year-old schoolgirl who lives with her parents and 10-year-old brother. She attends the local Technical College and plans to take her General Certificate of Education 'A' level examinations next term. In her free time she has a part-time Saturday job at the local newsagent and usually goes to a nearby weekly disco.

Her past medical history consists of one previous admission to hospital at the age of 13 years when investigation was required for her history of diarrhoea and recent weight loss. At this time she was diagnosed and treated for ulcerative colitis. For the following six months Susan required medication of Salazopyrin and Lomotil, during which time her general condition returned to normal and she has since remained fit and well.

On Monday Susan didn't feel well enough to go to school because of lower abdominal discomfort and diarrhoea. These symptoms persisted for the next few days with anorexia and increasing lethargy. By the end of the week Susan's bowel actions were becoming more liquid and containing increasing mucus and some blood. On Friday morning Susan's mother noticed that Susan was weaker, flushed and unwell and called the GP. He examined Susan and arranged for her immediate admission to hospital.

On admission to a medical ward, Susan appears tense and worried. She is flushed, feels weak and lethargic and shows signs of dehydration and anaemia. Susan is admitted to a bed with easy access to a toilet and a bell in order to call a nurse when required. The nurse admitting Susan assesses her present condition and obtains the following information:

- Bowel actions are liquid and contain mucus and blood.
- The frequency of bowel action has increased to 15 times a day.
- Lower abdominal pain is relieved by defaecation.
- Excoriated skin is present around the anus.
- Appetite is poor but a feeling of thirst persists.
- Lethargic condition.
- Skin and tongue dry.
- Urinary output diminished.
- Urine dark in colour.
- Temperature 39°C.
- Pulse 100 beats per minute.
- Respirations 22 per minute.
- Blood pressure 90/65 mmHg.
- Weight: 45 kg.

The nurse prepares the patient to undergo the following investigations ordered by the doctor to enable him to confirm the diagnosis of ulcerative colitis.

Investigation	Abnormal findings		
Sigmoidoscopy	Mucous lining of rectum and sigmoid colon superficially ulcerated with contact bleeding and excessive mucus secretion		
Blood tests for:			
Haemoglobin	8 g/100 ml	(normal 14 g/100 ml)	
Electrolytes:			
potassium	3.4 mm/l	(normal 3.8–5.0 mm/l)	
sodium	136 mm/l	(normal 136–148 mm/l)	
Plasma proteins	60g/l	(normal 62·83 g/l)	
White cells	13.0×10^9/l	(normal 4.0×10^9/l–11.0×10^9/l)	

1. Devise a care plan for Susan's first 12 hours following admission.

Question 1
Care plan should include:
(a) Reduction of anxiety by explanation and reassurance.
(b) Care before, during and after investigations and attention to the following: general hygiene, skin, especially the anal region.
(c) Observation of frequency and consistency of bowel actions.
(d) Testing for blood in stools.
(e) Coping with odours.
(f) Fluid balance record.
(g) Preservation of dignity.
(h) Adequate rest.
(i) Encouragement of diet.
(j) Management of infusion and drug therapy.
(k) Observation of wanted, unwanted effects of (j).
(l) Observations of general condition.
(m) Management of relatives.

2. Give a physiological explanation of the abnormal findings in the blood in this condition.

3. Briefly explain the action and side-effects of medicines prescribed.

4. (a) Describe how you could encourage Susan to take an adequate diet.

   (b) Explain the current thinking regarding the benefits of high/low residue diet in this condition.

5. Identify the important considerations that the nurse needs to make in preparing Susan for return home.

6. List the possible complications in this condition during an acute exacerbation.

7. List the possible long-term complications of this condition.

Question 2
Your answer should include the effects of chronic blood loss, infection, loss of extracellular fluid, intestinal hurry, diminished absorption by the large intestine.

Question 3
Refer to your pharmacology textbook.

Question 4
Give small attractive meals containing her personal preferences. High protein and calories, drinks if reluctant to eat. Attention to personal hygiene and odours before each meal. Encourage mixing with other patients at mealtimes. Promote relaxed unhurried mealtime.

Refer to the dietician.

Question 5
Your answer should include involvement of parents and daughter with attention to the following:
- Continuing medicine and diet therapy.
- Issuing a steroid card.
- Continuing care of skin and general hygiene.
- Adequate rest.
- Resumption of schooling.
- Monitoring weight.
- Seeking medical advice if symptoms return.
- Follow-up appointment to see the doctor.

Question 6
Your list should include dehydration, anaemia, weight loss, fluid and electrolyte imbalance, haemorrhage, toxic dilation, perforation, abscess formation and peritonitis.

Question 7
Your answer should include the effects of chronic ill health, in two main ways: socially and physiologically.
Social effects
(a) Reduces opportunity for the making of friendships and activities outside the home.
(b) Increases social demands on family and can increase stress on the family members.
(c) Affects attendance at school and job prospects.
(d) Slows personal, emotional and social development.
Effects on physiology
(a) Development of a 'drain pipe' colon, adhesions, stenosis, anaemia; malignant change which may lead to surgery, e.g., colectomy and permanent ileostomy.
(b) Swollen ankles and development of perianal sepsis including fistula and abscesses.
(c) Iritis.
(d) Arthritis.

An adult with Crohn's disease

John Masters, aged 25 years, is married with a wife and 10-month-old son. He is a commercial traveller for a local firm and lives on a new housing estate. Interests include improving his own home and establishing the garden. He and his wife belong to the local social club but activities have been curtailed since the birth of the baby.

Past medical history includes removal of appendix when aged 16 years, following which the wound was slow to heal with discharging sinus present for almost two months. Pathology of the removed appendix revealed evidence of Crohn's disease. Since this time John Masters has never felt completely fit and well, i.e., he has been having difficulty in maintaining his weight, with episodes of abdominal pain and diarrhoea. His GP prescribed iron tablets when symptoms of anaemia recurred. Over the last year he has become increasingly anxious about absence from work and loss of earnings. Mr Masters eventually revisited his GP for advice. He examined Mr Masters and arranged for his admission to hospital for reassessment and improvement of nutritional state.

On admission his immediate assessment reveals the following:

- Appearance: slimly built, pale, worried looking; an unsightly appendicectomy scar on the abdomen.
- Lethargy.
- History of diarrhoea for several days accompanied by abdominal colic pain and weight loss.
- Appetite poor, history of reluctance to eat.
- Temperature 38°C.
- Pulse 100 beats per minute.
- Blood pressure 129/70 mmHg.

Following examination by the doctor the following investigations were arranged.

Investigation	Abnormal findings
Barium meal and follow through	Stomach, duodenum and jejunum normal but alternating portions of narrowing and normal ileum (string sign in narrow portion)

Blood tests
  Plasma protein
  Haemoglobin
	Diminished (normal 62.82 g/l)
	7 g/100 ml blood (normal 14g/100 ml)

Following the investigations the doctor prescribes the following treatment:

1. Prednisolone tablets, dose 10 mg three times daily.
2. Codeine phosphate tablets, dose 30 mg four times daily.
3. Intravenous whole blood followed by parenteral feeding (including Aminosol, Intralipid, Parentrovite).
4. Increased fluid intake to correct fluid and electrolyte loss due to diarrhoea.
5. High protein and calorie diet with vitamin supplement.

SELF-TESTING QUESTIONS

BRIEF ANALYSIS AND GUIDELINES TO SUITABLE ANSWERS

1. Devise a care plan for this patient while receiving intravenous parenteral feeding.

Question 1
Your care plan should include the following:
(a) Explanation of the procedure to the patient and his wife.
(b) Comfort and reassurance to patient.
(c) Fluid balance record.
(d) Management of apparatus:
  - Observation of cannulation site.
  - Preventive measures against sepsis of site.
  - Observation and management of rate of infusions.
  - Observation of abnormal response to substance infused and to the presence of cannula in vein.
(e) Arrangement of clothing.
(f) Assistance in daily activities.
(g) Special precautions in the use of drug additives.

2. Describe how a 24-hour intravenous regime can maintain the nutritional requirements of an adult.

Question 2
Refer to your teacher for up-to-date information on parenteral feeding regimes.

3. Briefly describe the pathological changes in the intestinal tract in Crohn's disease.

Question 3
Refer to J. Macleod (Ed.), *Davidson's Principles and Practice of Medicine,* 14th edition, Churchill Livingstone, London, 1984.

4. (a) List the possible complications of this condition and (b) describe why it is necessary to avoid surgical intervention in the long-term management.

Question 4

(a) Possible complications:
- Stenosis.
- Adhesions.
- Fistula and abscess formation.
- Perforation.
- Peritonitis.
- Malabsorbtion.
- Fluid and electrolyte imbalance.
- Anaemia.

(b) The avoidance of surgery is needed to prevent delayed wound healing and fistula formation.

5. Identify the possible social problems that could arise with this young family.

Question 5

For Mr Masters: loss of earnings, possible loss of job, reduced activity in the house and garden. Anxiety regarding support of wife and young son.

For Mrs Masters: anxiety regarding her husband's illness and its prognosis and its effects.

For family: change in life style, reduced social interaction, reduced financial resources, desires to increase family may need rethinking.

6. Identify supporting services available for this family.

Question 6

Your answer should include the following supporting services and personnel:
- Medical social worker.
- Social services.
- GP.
- Dietician.
- Health visitor.
- Family planning clinic.

In addition, discussion concerning wife's possible need for employment and child minder may be useful.

An adult with carcinoma of the oesophagus

Mrs Large, aged 68 years, lives with her retired husband in a small country town. Both their son and daughter are married with young families and they live 50 miles away in the major city of the region.

Past medical history consists of one previous admission to the local hospital eight years ago for repair of vaginal wall for uterine prolapse. She made a complete recovery from this and resumed her interest in the local branch of the Women's Royal Voluntary Service, which includes helping in the shop at the nearby hospital for mentally handicapped patients. She also takes orders for icing wedding and anniversary cakes.

For the past month Mrs Large found it an increasing effort to maintain her social interests, which seemed to make her feel more tired, and she needed to go to bed earlier than usual. Her interest in food diminished and some weight loss became apparent. She realised that on some occasions she hadn't completed a meal and seemed to need to drink more while eating. She became worried about herself after regurgitating food during a meal and sought advice from her local doctor. On questioning, she revealed that she had been experiencing a feeling of food 'getting stuck' although fluids caused no difficulty. Her GP referred her to the nearest district general hospital to be seen by a consultant surgeon.

After examining Mrs Large and discussing her symptoms the consultant surgeon advises admission to hospital in approximately two weeks' time for investigations to be made. Both Mr and Mrs Large are worried because hospital admission is considered necessary and they return home distressed. They decide to contact their son and daughter and Mrs Large makes arrangements for someone to take over her immediate commitments.

On admission Mrs Large seems almost pleased to be coming into hospital for some relief of her now increasing difficulty with swallowing. The nurse admitting Mrs Large assesses her present condition and obtains the following information:
- Increasing disinterest in food.
- Tolerates small helpings of a soft diet and requires fluid with all meals.
- Conscious of taking a long time to eat her meal.
- Constipation for the past week.

- Occasionally notices excess saliva which she has difficulty in swallowing.
- Pale skin and evidence of weight loss.
- Lacking in energy.

The nurse prepares the patient to undergo the following investigations which the doctor has ordered to confirm the diagnosis of carcinoma of oesophagus.

Investigation	Abnormal findings

Blood tests for:
  Haemoglobin
  Electrolytes
	Haemoglobin 9 g/100ml
	Normal

Fibre-optic endoscopy and biopsy	Abnormal mucous lining in middle third of oesophagus with evidence of infiltration to muscle layer causing stenosis Biopsy: infiltrating carcinoma
Chest x-ray	No abnormal findings

On confirmation of the diagnosis, Mrs Large is referred to the local consultant radiotherapist.

SELF-TESTING QUESTIONS

BRIEF ANALYSIS AND GUIDELINES TO SUITABLE ANSWERS

1. Describe and illustrate the mechanism of swallowing, and recall the related and specific anatomy of the oesophagus.

Question 1
See page 2 of this chapter and for pathology textbook refer to your teacher for guidance.

2. Devise a care plan for Mrs Large for use during the period of time while the investigations are being completed.

Question 2
Particular reference should be made to the following three types of care:
(a) Psychological care:
- Explanation and reassurance about immediate and later events.
- Support and sensitive management of difficulties such as slowness in eating, fear of regurgitation, tendency to avoid contact with other patients.
(b) Physical care:
- Adequate nutrition and hydration.
- Monitoring for the above, including weighing, measuring fluid intake and output, amount of food eaten and bowel actions.
- Management of difficulty in swallowing saliva and teaching oral hygiene.
- Positioning to avoid regurgitation.
(c) Social and spiritual care:
- Explanation and support of relatives and Mrs Large if she desires.

3. What advice will the dietician give Mrs Large when she is no longer able to tolerate a soft diet? Discuss the advantages and disadvantages of liquidised normal diet and commercially available preparations.

Question 3
Your answer should include:
- Normal daily nutritional requirements.
- Identification of high-protein, high-calorie preparations available.
- Difficulties that could be encountered at home.

4. Devise a care plan for Mrs Large before and after fibre-optic endoscopy.

Question 4
Your plan should include care in two stages.
(a) Before investigation:
- Physical preparation, i.e., clothing, hygiene, withholding food and drink, identification, obtaining consent, light sedation and local anaesthetic in form of throat lozenge.
(b) After investigation:
- Withholding food and drink until directed by the doctor.
- Observation for swallowing, bleeding, rupture of oesophagus, inhalation of vomit/saliva.
- Knowledge of result of investigation and opportunity for follow-up discussion.

5. Discuss how you would ensure effective communications with Mrs Large's family during her stay.

6. How would you prepare Mrs Large and her relatives for the prescribed radiotherapy?

7. Discuss the possible outcomes of carcinoma of the oesophagus, for example, the need for insertion of Celestin or Mousseau Barbin tube, insertion of gastrostomy feeding tube or resection of the oesophagus.

8. Discuss how Mrs Large's fluid, electrolyte and nutritional balance is monitored during the period of hospitalisation.

Question 5

Consideration should be given to:
- Patient allocation during span of duty.
- Nurse initiating a 'welcoming' contact with visiting relatives.
- Availability of trained nursing and medical staff to talk/listen to relatives.
- Contact telephone numbers.
- Ensuring that appropriate assistance is given to relatives and checking that this has been effective.

Question 6

You need to include:
- Possible transfer to another hospital.
- Explanation regarding nature and duration of treatment.
- Possible outcomes of treatment during early stages and when treatment complete.

Question 7

Refer to medical/surgical staff for information and to your teacher for guidance and suitable surgical textbook.

Question 8

Consideration should be given to observation of patient for weight loss, dehydration, electrolyte imbalance.

An adult with Addisonian crisis

Mr John Little, aged 55 years, has been receiving cortico-steroid therapy for the past 3 years for rheumatoid arthritis. During a recent bout of influenza he forgot to take his daily dose of cortico-steroids for a period of two days. Instead of starting to feel better after the influenza he began to vomit and feel increasingly weaker. As the vomiting continued overnight Mrs Little became concerned and rang the doctor. The doctor examined Mr Little and noted dehydration, gastric dilation, low blood pressure, rapid pulse and some mental confusion. He arranged for urgent admission to hospital. While awaiting the arrival of the ambulance Mr Little became semi-conscious.

On admission to the accident and emergency department, the nurse notices the following:
- The patient is semi-conscious.
- Blood pressure 90/60 mmHg.
- Pulse rate 120 beats per minute and weak.
- Skin dry and inelastic.
- Mucous membranes and tongue dry.

Mrs Little, who accompanies her husband, is distressed but she has remembered to bring his steroid therapy card.

SELF-TESTING QUESTIONS

BRIEF ANALYSIS AND GUIDELINES TO SUITABLE ANSWERS

1. Recall the normal physiology of the adrenal hormones on fluid and electrolyte balance and the effect of giving systemic steroid therapy.

Question 1

Refer to pages 11–14 for the effect of adrenal hormones on fluid and electrolyte balance and to a suitable pharmacology textbook recommended by your teacher.

2. What immediate care will be prescribed for Mr Little in the accident and emergency department? Explain the rationale for these decisions.

Question 2
Your answer should include:
(a) Prescription of intravenous fluids and drugs, including normal saline and hydrocortisone (refer to your answer to question 1).
(b) Management of semi-conscious patient.
(c) Observation for rehydration, and return of normal blood pressure, fluid balance and full consciousness.
(d) Management of intravenous apparatus.
(e) Support of Mrs Little.
For rationale refer to question 1.

3. How would you ensure that appropriate information is given to the staff in the ward to which Mr Little is to be admitted.

Question 3
Consideration of the following should be made:
(a) Written records of events in accident and emergency department and clear written instructions for management in the ward.
(b) Nurse allocated to Mr Little to be responsible for verbal information to ward staff.
(c) Nurse allocated to be aware of information regarding relatives and patient's property.

4. What future management will be needed for steroid therapy to be continued?

Question 4
This should include:
(a) Management while receiving intravenous hydrocortisone.
(b) Regime for return to oral therapy.
(c) Education regarding ongoing therapy at home for both Mr and Mrs Little.

(b) Fluid and electrolyte disturbances in patients with conditions of the kidney

1 Patient study and care plan for an adult with acute renal failure

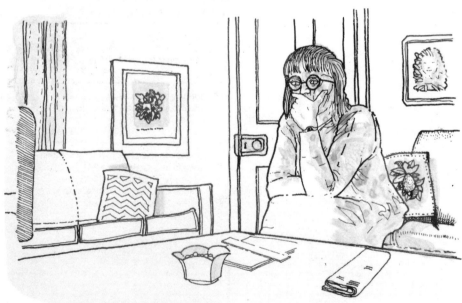

Figure 1.26   Mrs Jones

History of social, psychological and physical events leading to the present condition

The patient chosen for this section to illustrate fluid and electrolyte disturbance has acute renal failure following abdominal surgery for a ruptured ectopic pregnancy.

Mrs Jones, aged 30 years (Figure 1.26), lives on a new housing estate with her husband, who is a long-distance lorry driver. They have been married for 5 years and have no children. Over the past year Mrs Jones has been attending the infertility clinic as both she and her husband want a family.

While Mr Jones was away at work his wife developed severe lower abdominal pain. She contacted her GP, who visited her and arranged for her immediate admission to hospital with a suspected ruptured ectopic pregnancy.

By the time Mrs Jones arrives at the accident and emergency department she is profoundly shocked, with low blood pressure, rapid weak pulse and cold clammy skin.

In the accident and emergency department Mrs Jones's condition is assessed, including urinalysis, and a possible diagnosis made. Management includes the following:

- Restoration of blood volume by intravenous infusion.
- Emergency laparotomy.
- Contacting Mr Jones.

At operation the right fallopian tube is found to be ruptured and is removed. Recovery from the anaesthetic and surgical procedure is uneventful although Mrs Jones requires the transfusion of four units of blood to maintain her blood pressure and circulating blood volume.

Mrs Jones returns to the ward at 5 pm still slightly drowsy but able to be seen by her husband. At 9 pm the nurses looking after Mrs Jones report to the night nurse that Mrs Jones has not passed urine since her operation. During the night the intravenous infusion is continued, all general care is given and Mrs Jones spends a restful night.

The next morning the night nurse reports that Mrs Jones has still not passed urine and does not appear to have a palpable bladder. The doctor is informed. He examines Mrs Jones and diagnoses acute renal failure, after the insertion of an indwelling urinary catheter confirms the absence of urine in the bladder. He takes samples of blood for estimation of urea and electrolytes, and arranges for an emergency intravenous pyelogram.

Explanation of abnormal physiology and pathology

It is advised that you revise the normal structure and function of the urinary system and normal nutrition needs of the adult, and see Table 1.5.

Refer to *Manual of Nutrition*, 9th edition, Ministry of Agriculture, Fisheries and Foods, HMSO, London, 1985.

Table 1.5

Related normal physiology	Abnormal physiology
(a) Cardiac output: 25% to the kidneys necessary for normal filtration in the glomerulus	Cardiac output is reduced during period of profound hypotension from blood loss before surgical intervention, resulting in insufficient pressure for filtration in the glomerulus
(b) Filtrate contains water, glucose, electrolytes, urea, creatinine and uric acids	Filtrate contains protein due to ischaemic damage to glomerulus and a small amount of water, glucose, electrolytes, urea, creatinine and uric acids
(c) Secretion and selective reabsorption results in formation of a 24 hour total value of urine of approximately 1500 ml, containing urea, creatinine, uric acids, water and electrolytes, with a specific gravity of 1.010–1.020	Renal ischaemia results in oliguria (volume less than 500 ml/24 hours) or anuria and consequent retention in the blood stream of water, urea, creatinine, uric acids and electrolytes (potassium and sodium). Increased fluid volume in the blood stream results in rising blood pressure, oedema and weight gain. Retention of sodium increases oedema, including pulmonary oedema. Retention of potassium causes mental confusion and cardiac arrest. Retention of urea causes apathy, anorexia, nausea and vomiting followed by mental confusion and later muscular twitching, fits, drowsiness and coma. Bleeding episodes can occur
(d) Approximate normal blood level in an adult: Urea 2.5–6.6 mmol/l Sodium 136–148 mmol/l Potassium 3.8–5.0 mmol/l Chloride 95–105 mmol/l	Levels of urea and electrolytes are raised above normal

Care plan

This plan (see Table 1.6) is for Mrs Jones following the diagnosis of acute renal failure and does not include the care she would also need following surgery for ruptured ectopic pregnancy.

Table 1.6 Care plan for Mrs Jones's acute renal failure

Problem	Objective	Plan of care	Rationale
1. Patient and husband anxious because of complications affecting recovery	Reduce anxiety of patient and husband	(a) Explanation and reassurance to be given to both (b) Give opportunity for both to see medical staff and senior nursing staff	(a) Reduce problem (b) Assist in maintaining confidence, communications and relations with staff
2. Fluid imbalance	Prevent over-hydration until diuresis occurs and restoration of kidney function	(a) Restrict fluid intake to 500 ml plus volume equivalent to previous day's output (b) Record fluid output on fluid balance chart (c) Observe for signs of generalised oedema and weigh patient daily at the same time of day	(a) 500 ml to replace insensible loss, i.e. loss in urea, sweating and respiration. Previous day's output includes urine, vomit, wound drainage, diarrhoea, if any (b) Monitors fluid loss to enable correct prescription of fluid intake (c) Retention of fluid causes increase in tissue fluid and increase in weight. (NB 1 litre of water weighs 1 kilogram)
3. Patient reluctant to cooperate with her restricted fluid intake	Obtain patient's cooperation	Full explanation and patient involvement required in this section of the care plan	Aids patient's difficulty in coping with severe reduction in fluid intake
4. Dry mouth	Relieve discomfort and detect early signs of the complications of a dry mouth	(a) Inspect mouth and offer antiseptic mouthwashes (b) Suggest sweets to suck and also chewing gum	(a) and (b) Relieves discomfort and reduces tendency to abrasions and infections
5. Electrolyte imbalance (Refer to: J. Macleod (Ed.), *Davidson's Principles and Practice of Medicine*, 14th edition, Churchill Livingstone, London, 1984)	Prevent potassium and sodium retention until diuresis occurs and restoration of kidney function	(a) Low sodium and low potassium diet (b) Explain to patient and relatives foods to avoid	(a) Kidneys unable to secrete sodium and potassium, leading to retention in bloodstream (b) Ensures cooperation of Mrs Jones and maintenance of this diet
6. Accumulation of urea in the bloodstream (uraemia)	Minimise further uraemia	(a) Low protein diet as prescribed and monitored by the doctor – usually below 30 grams/ 24 hours (b) High carbohydrate diet (c) Explain to patient and relatives which foods can be eaten	(a) Urea is the end product of protein metabolism and is normally excreted via the kidneys (b) Minimises utilisation of patient's own body protein and promotes adequate nutrition (c) Ensures cooperation of Mrs Jones and maintenance of this diet
7. Oliguria or anuria	Monitor urine output: amount and constituents	(a) Catheterise and obtain specimen (if any) for microscopy, culture and chemical analysis (b) Hourly estimation and record made of urine passed/not passed	(a) and (b) Monitors kidney function
8. Urinary catheter	(a) Ensure comfort of patient (b) Prevent ascending infection	(a) Fix tubing to prevent dragging on catheter (b) (i) Maintain closed drainage system (ii) Aseptic procedures for obtaining urine specimens, changing drainage bag (iii) Vulval hygiene and catheter care 6-hourly or as necessary	(a) Catheter balloon can cause pain at bladder outlet (b) (i) – (ii) Minimises entry of pathogenic organisms

Table 1.6 (cont.)

Problem	Objective	Plan of care	Rationale
9. Patient being maintained on intensive and artificial regime until normal function returns	Monitor patient's general condition	(a) Temperature, pulse, respiration and blood pressure	(a) Temperature and pulse rise if infection present. Respirations rise if pulmonary oedema occurs. Blood pressure rises due to increased cardiac output and blood volume. Pulse rises and blood pressure falls if bleeding occurs. Pulse rises in potassium intoxication. Absent pulse in cardiac arrest
		(b) Observe for apathy, anorexia, nausea, vomiting, mental confusion, muscular twitching, fits, drowsiness and coma	(b) Refer to abnormal physiology section
10. Patient prone to infection	Minimise infection risks	(a) Nurse in single room if available	(a) Minimise airborne infection and contact
		(b) Give single dose of prescribed antibiotic	(b) Prophylactic, kidney not excreting antibiotics so no need for regular administration

Mrs Jones is maintained on this regime for a week and her general condition remains satisfactory. She and her husband accept the present situation and remain optimistic for the future. On the eighth day after her operation Mrs Jones produces increasing amounts of dilute urine of low specific gravity (see Table 1.7).

Table 1.7   Care plan for Mrs Jones during diuretic phase

Problem	Objective	Plan of care	Rationale
1. Excess fluid loss as diuresis starts	Maintain adequate hydration	Increase fluid intake by the equivalent volume of the previous day's urine output	Ensures adequate hydration
2. Excess loss of sodium due to failure of selective reabsorption by kidney tubules	Monitor sodium balance	Re-introduce salt into diet and give prescribed supplements while output is excessive	Takes several days for kidneys to restore selective reabsorption
3. Excess loss of potassium	Monitor potassium balance	Re-introduce potassium into diet and give supplements while urine output is excessive in form of either fruit and/or prescribed potassium chloride	Takes several days for kidneys to restore selective reabsorption
4. Inability of kidney to excrete urea during recovery phase (diuresis period)	Gradual increase of intake of protein to normal dietary requirements	Give increasing amounts of daily protein according to doctor's prescription and blood urea results	Allows kidney to return to normal function
5. Indwelling urinary catheter	Remove and allow patient to pass urine normally	(a) Remove and monitor return to normal micturition	(a) Reduces infection risk
		(b) Record urine output and amount and frequency	(b) and (c) Monitors return to normal function
		(c) Observe for evidence of bladder emptying and/or retention	
		(d) Observe for signs and symptoms of urinary tract infection	(d) Enables prompt treatment if required
6. Large amounts of dilute urine with low specific gravity being passed	Monitor return to normal concentration and volume	(a) Record an accurate fluid balance chart	(a) Monitors amount of urine passed each 24 hours
		(b) Test all urine specimens for specific gravity and albumin and record results	(b) and (c) Monitors recovery of kidneys
		(c) Send daily specimens of urine to laboratories for chemical analysis	

EVALUATION OF CARE AND SUGGESTED RECORD OF PROGRESS

Patient's Name ..Mrs Jones..

Date ..12.12.86..   Time ..1600 hours...

QUESTIONS TO HELP YOU WITH EVALUATING CARE AND PROGRESS

Nursing actions relating to patient comfort, safety and well-being

- What is the patient's response to his/her condition?
- Are the present nursing actions still required?
- Is the patient, and his/her family, informed?

Mrs Jones is very relieved that she is now producing urine but she has been told that it will be several days before it can be confirmed that normal function can be re-established. Is getting tired, sleep and rest disturbed by frequency of micturition. Is now feeling she needs to discuss the planning of future pregnancies. Needs to be assisted to increase mobility and be encouraged to participate in meeting her individual needs.

Nursing actions pertaining to observations and measurements

- What is the patient's response to the observations and measurements being made?
- Are the present measurements/observations still required?
- Have results been seen or relayed to the appropriate practitioner/carer?
- Has the patient been informed of the changes?

Mrs Jones is cooperating with measurements and observations required and she is recording her own fluid intake and saving her own specimens of urine for testing. All measurements still required to be continued; the doctor will receive test results tomorrow morning.

Nursing actions relating to diagnosis and treatment

- What is the patient's response to diagnosis and treatment?
- Are the patient's treatments still required?
- Have the course/s of treatment been completed or discontinued?
- Has the patient been informed?

Is enjoying reintroduction to normal diet but is having a problem remembering to drink the prescribed amount of fluid. She is worried about recurrence of kidney failure in the future and possible long-term effects of this episode. All treatment to continue pending review of laboratory results.
    Mrs Jones is to see the doctor when results are known.

* * * * * * *

- Who has visited the patient?
- What information has been given to relatives/visitors?

Mr Jones (husband) and Mrs Black (mother).
Informed of current situation but Mr Jones coming tomorrow afternoon to discuss long-term prognosis with his wife and doctor.

* * * * * * *

- Has the care plan been updated?
- Are the objectives/goals of care still relevant?

No change required.

Signature of
Reporting Nurse   ....

Designation   ....

Signature of
Supervising Nurse   ....

Designation   ....

RECOVERY AND DISCHARGE

After 5 days Mrs Jones's general condition is good; she feels well and her appetite is returning to normal. She is able to tolerate a normal diet and is maintaining an adequate fluid balance. Urea and blood test results are within normal limits and plans are being made for her discharge from hospital.

2 Patient histories illustrating further problems related to fluid and electrolyte disturbances in patients with conditions of the kidney

A child with acute glomerulonephritis

Abdul, aged 13 years, is admitted to hospital with acute glomerulonephritis. The nurse admitting Abdul obtains the following information from him and his parents:
- History of *sore throat* three weeks ago.
- Two days ago Abdul became unwell with headache, nausea and diminished urinary output which was darker than normal and cloudy.

On assessment the nurse records the following:

- Blood pressure 110/80 mmHg.
- Temperature within normal limits.
- Pulse normal rate/rhythm.
- Respirations 24 per minute.
- Urinalysis—albumin and blood present, specific gravity 1020.
- Disinterest in surroundings.
- Generally unwell and nauseated.
- Mouth and tongue dry.

In view of the diagnosis the doctor orders the following treatment:

1. Rest in bed.
2. Reduction of fluid intake.
3. Low-protein, high-carbohydrate and low-salt diet.
4. Mid-stream specimen of urine to be sent to the laboratory for microscopy.
5. Blood tests for urea, electrolytes and white cell count.
6. Daily monitoring of blood pressure, fluid balance and urinalysis.
7. Antibiotic therapy.

SELF-TESTING QUESTIONS

1. Describe (a) the abnormal physiology resulting from acute glomerulonephritis, and (b) the significance of the history of sore throat.

2. Explain the rationale for the orders given by the doctor for Abdul's management, taking each item in turn and explaining its significance.

3. Devise a care plan for Abdul during the oliguric phase and diuretic phase.

4. Discuss how you propose giving a 13-year-old boy the prescribed diet?

5. Identify potential problems in caring for a 13-year-old boy in a paediatric ward. Discuss how they could be overcome.

6. Discuss the achievement of effective communication between Abdul, the staff, the parents and siblings.

BRIEF ANALYSIS AND GUIDELINES TO SUITABLE ANSWERS

Question 1
Refer to normal physiology of kidney and to pathology textbook.

Question 2
Your answer should include the following, taking each of the doctor's orders in turn:
1. To ensure comfort of acutely ill child.
2. To prevent overloading of circulation during oliguric phase.
3. Low protein to minimise production of urea; high carbohydrate to prevent utilisation of own body protein; low salt to minimise retention of water leading to oedema.
4. To identify the presence of red cells due to damaged glomerular membrane.
5. To monitor those blood levels which will indicate progress of disease and treatment.
6. To give indication of ending of oliguric phase and beginning of diuretic phase.
7. To prevent further production of toxins from haemolytic streptococcus.

Question 3
Refer to care plan for Mrs Jones's acute renal failure (pages 37–38).

Question 4
Consideration should be given to the following aspects:
- His age (13 years).
- Personal likes/dislikes.
- Religious and family wishes and habits.
- His present physical state.

Question 5
Your answer should include reference to the selection of age groups, the various degrees of dependency of the sick children, the presence of parents, lack of stimulus and appropriate occupation during the recovery period; Abdul's reaction to being in this environment. You may find it useful to discuss each of these points with your colleagues in the paediatric ward.

Question 6
See previous patient history of Mrs Large (carcinoma of oesophagus), page 34, question 5. Communication can be helped by encouraging the parents to participate in Abdul's care and by allowing free visiting for parents and siblings.

7. It is expected that Abdul will make a complete recovery from acute glomerulonephritis but you are advised to find out possible complications which can occur as a result of this condition.

Question 7
Refer to J. Macleod (Ed.), *Davidson's Principles and Practice of Medicine*, 14th edition, Churchill Livingstone, London, 1984.

A child with nephrotic syndrome

Ten-year-old James is admitted to hospital with nephrotic syndrome following repeated attacks of acute glomerulonephritis. On admission, the nurse records the following:

- A fretful, ill-looking boy with oedema of the ankles and face.
- Temperature within normal limits.
- Pulse 100 beats per minute.
- Respirations 24 per minute.
- Blood pressure within normal limits.
- Urinalysis—albumin present, specific gravity raised.

The doctor orders the following treatment:

1. Bed rest.
2. Normal/reduced fluid intake.
3. High-protein, reduced-salt diet.
4. Monitor albumin content of urine, daily.
5. Blood tests for plasma proteins, urea and electrolytes, daily.
6. Monitor weight daily.
7. Observe for development of pulmonary oedema, ascites, pulmonary or pericardial effusions.

SELF-TESTING QUESTIONS

1. Describe the significance of albumin in the urine and explain what gross physiological effects result from this.

2. Explain the rationale for the orders given by the doctor for James's management. Take each item in turn and explain the significance of each.

3. Devise a care plan for James.

4. Identify the potential problems in giving this diet to James. Discuss how they could be overcome as this may be a long-term problem.

5. What questions are James's parents likely to ask regarding his immediate and future needs and life style?

BRIEF ANALYSIS AND GUIDELINES TO SUITABLE ANSWERS

Question 1
Presence of albumin in the urine is due to deterioration in glomerular basement membrane. Prolonged loss of albumin in the urine results in a reduction in plasma protein levels. Low plasma protein will cause reduction in the osmotic pressure of the blood, resulting in accumulation of fluid in the tissue spaces, i.e., oedema.

Question 2
1. To ensure comfort of acutely ill child.
2. Dependent on degree of oedema.
3. High protein is to replace loss in urine and to correct plasma protein level, which will relieve oedema. Reduced salt is to prevent water retention.
4. To monitor the progress of the disease and treatment.
5. To give indication of progress of disease and treatment.
6. An increase in weight could indicate retention of fluid.
7. To be aware of possible complications and instigate appropriate treatment.

Question 3
It is important to include careful measurement of daily albumin loss and method of giving this diet to James.

Question 4
Consideration should be given to the following aspects:
- His age (10 years).
- Personal likes/dislikes.
- Family and religious wishes and habits.
- His present physical state.

Question 5
Refer to your teacher for guidance and a suitable paediatric textbook.

41

Young adult with chronic renal failure

Mr Gibson, aged 30 years, a foreman in a car factory, is married with a wife and two children aged 6 and 8 years. They live in a council house on a large estate within five miles of the nearest district hospital.

Past medical history includes acute glomerulonephritis at the age of 7 years with persistant proteinuria. During a routine medical examination two years ago at work, his blood pressure was found to be raised and albumin was present in his urine.

Recently Mr Gibson visited his GP complaining of the following symptoms:

- Polyuria.
- Thirst.
- Loss of energy, weakness.
- Nausea, vomiting, diarrhoea.

On examination the doctor found Mr Gibson's skin to be sallow with a yellow-brown discoloration; and his skin and tongue were dry. Following discussion with Mr Gibson and his wife the doctor advised immediate hospital admission.

Mr Gibson is admitted to the local district hospital where investigations undertaken reveal the following:

1. Blood
   - (a) urea raised
   - (b) sodium depletion
   - (c) creatinine raised
   - (d) phosphates raised
   - (e) acid–base imbalance
   - (f) potassium raised.
2. Urine
   - (a) protein present
   - (b) red blood cells present
   - (c) specific gravity 1010.
3. Intravenous pyelogram shows abnormally small kidneys with poor function.

SELF-TESTING QUESTIONS

1. The doctor has recently explained to Mr Gibson that his kidneys are permanently damaged as a result of his history of acute glomerulonephritis and hypertension. Describe the possible effects this news could have on Mr Gibson and his family.

2. Describe a care plan for Mr Gibson's management during his stay in hospital.

3. Describe the progress of this condition and its effects.

4. Discuss some of the difficulties Mr Gibson and his family could encounter when he is referred for a dialysis programme.

5. Discuss (a) the indications for renal transplant and (b) its implications to society.

BRIEF ANALYSIS AND GUIDELINES TO SUITABLE ANSWERS

Question 1
Consideration should be given to Mr Gibson's immediate response, which could include a wide range of emotional reactions. He and his family will be subsequently concerned and affected by the following: effects on his job and social life; follow-up of personal queries regarding immediate and later care; involvement of paramedical staff, for example social worker, technician.

Question 2
This care plan should be directed towards his discharge home and self-care, including the following:
(a) Low-protein diet to keep blood urea within normal limits.
(b) Fluid and sodium intake increased to maintain adequate hydration and salt balance.
(c) Advice regarding prompt attention to early signs of infection.
(d) Importance of regular follow-up clinics for monitoring of kidney function.

Question 3
Refer to J. Macleod (Ed.), *Davidson's Principles and Practice of Medicine*, 14th edition, Churchill Livingstone, London, 1984.

Question 4
This should include:
(a) Effects of this programme at commencement and long term on his physical, psychological and social well-being.
(b) Resources available to assist the above, for instance, renal dialysis units, adaptation of home for home dialysis, support and training to patient and family.

Question 5
(a) Indications should include discussion of age group, dependents and any associated and other medical conditions.
(b) Implications to society should include discussion on current legislation, public opinion and advances in medical science.

6. Describe how tissue rejection is minimised following kidney transplant.

Revise immune response and discuss immunosuppressive therapy.

Chapter 2 Nursing patients with problems of oxygenation

Normal maintenance of respiration

(a) The respiratory system

Oxygen (O_2) is required continuously by all body tissues for normal metabolism, during which carbon dioxide (CO_2) is produced and, as a waste product, must be excreted. Before birth, this gas exchange is performed by the placenta, and exchange is between the blood of the mother and that of the

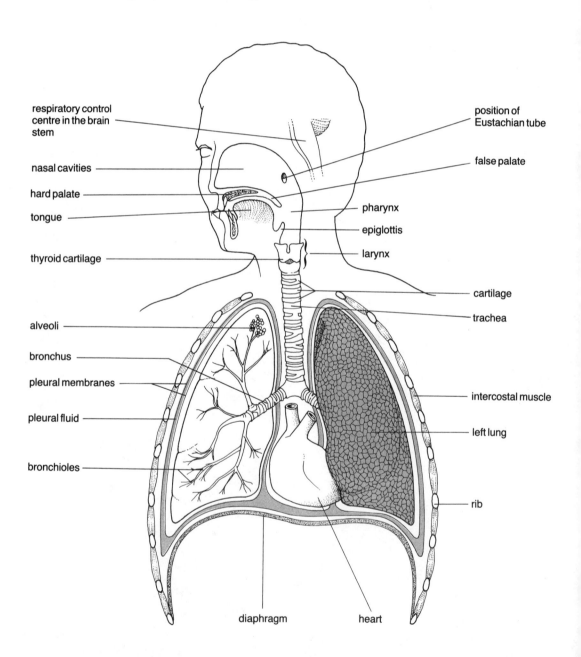

Figure 2.1   Respiratory system

foetus. After birth, this function becomes a gaseous exchange between blood and air and is taken over by the lungs, whose alveoli are so constructed that there is only a very thin barrier between blood and air, which facilitates the movement of O_2 and CO_2 between them.

The human respiratory system is shown in Figure 2.1 and consists of the following parts.

1. *The upper respiratory tract*   This comprises all the airways from the nostrils as far as the alveoli.
2. *The alveoli*   These form the gas exchange areas in each lung.
3. *The ribs, intercostal muscles and diaphragm*   Together these provide the mechanical apparatus for ventilation of the lungs.
4. *The respiratory centre*   This is the control centre in the brain stem which provides the nervous impulses required to regulate respiratory activity.

1   The upper respiratory tract

This series of branching airways is ventilated with each breath. Inspired air passes through the upper part of the tree, which is described in more detail in Figure 2.2.

The trachea branches to form the *left* and *right bronchi*, which supply each of the two lungs. Each bronchus divides to form *lobar bronchi*, which supply the two or three lobes of each lung. These divide further to form the *segmental bronchi*, which supply the broncho-pulmonary segments of each lung. These segments are self-contained and functionally independent units of lung tissue, each surrounded by a *septum* of connective tissue.

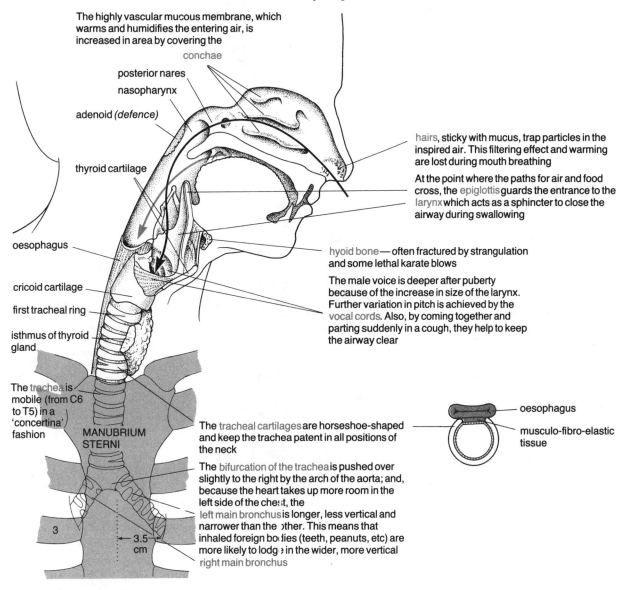

The highly vascular mucous membrane, which warms and humidifies the entering air, is increased in area by covering the conchae

posterior nares
nasopharynx
adenoid *(defence)*
thyroid cartilage

hairs, sticky with mucus, trap particles in the inspired air. This filtering effect and warming are lost during mouth breathing

At the point where the paths for air and food cross, the epiglottis guards the entrance to the larynx which acts as a sphincter to close the airway during swallowing

oesophagus

hyoid bone—often fractured by strangulation and some lethal karate blows

cricoid cartilage
first tracheal ring
isthmus of thyroid gland

The male voice is deeper after puberty because of the increase in size of the larynx. Further variation in pitch is achieved by the vocal cords. Also, by coming together and parting suddenly in a cough, they help to keep the airway clear

The trachea is mobile (from C6 to T5) in a 'concertina' fashion

MANUBRIUM STERNI

The tracheal cartilages are horseshoe-shaped and keep the trachea patent in all positions of the neck

oesophagus
musculo-fibro-elastic tissue

The bifurcation of the trachea is pushed over slightly to the right by the arch of the aorta; and, because the heart takes up more room in the left side of the chest, the left main bronchus is longer, less vertical and narrower than the other. This means that inhaled foreign bodies (teeth, peanuts, etc) are more likely to lodge in the wider, more vertical right main bronchus

3

3.5 cm

Figure 2.2   Upper respiratory tract

45

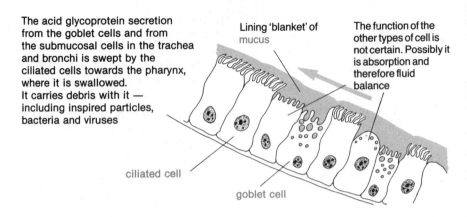

The acid glycoprotein secretion from the goblet cells and from the submucosal cells in the trachea and bronchi is swept by the ciliated cells towards the pharynx, where it is swallowed. It carries debris with it — including inspired particles, bacteria and viruses

Lining 'blanket' of mucus

The function of the other types of cell is not certain. Possibly it is absorption and therefore fluid balance

ciliated cell

goblet cell

Figure 2.3   Ciliated epithelium

The bronchial tree continues to branch, to form several 'generations' of bronchi, all of which have walls that contain plates of cartilage to support their structure. As the branches become finer, the cartilage support is replaced by a *myoelastic* coat (i.e., one consisting of muscle and elastin fibres). The ten generations of tubules with this structure are called *bronchioles*. The airways are lined with ciliated epithelium (Figure 2.3) which produces and carries a blanket of *mucus* (a glycoprotein) to transport debris, including inspired particles, bacteria and viruses, towards the pharynx. Mucus also contains lysosyme, antibodies and interferon, which are all anti-infective agents. Both functions are important defence mechanisms.

Little gas exchange between blood and air occurs in the upper respiratory tract, which simply conducts gases to and from the alveoli, where gas exchange does occur. Some gas exchange does happen across the walls of the finest alveolar ducts and the respiratory ducts, which have a non-ciliated epithelium.

Blood supply of lungs

The lungs have a double blood supply (Figure 2.4).

VENTILATION

On entering the hilum, the main bronchi divide into lobar bronchi (two to supply the two lobes of the left lung; three for the three lobes of the right.) They then divide into segmental bronchi. These supply the broncho-pulmonary segments, which are self-contained, functionally independent units of lung tissue

Each segment is enclosed by connective tissue called septa continuous with the inner pleural layer covering the lungs

As the bronchial tree continues to branch, the segmental bronchi are counted as the first generation, and so on

The branches are called *bronchi* as long as their walls contain cartilage (arranged in plates rather than in rings)

PERFUSION

The lungs have a *double* blood supply

The pulmonary arteries carry de-oxygenated blood from the right side of the heart. These subdivide, following the bronchial tree, to form capillary networks surrounding the alveoli. Reoxygenated blood is returned via the pulmonary veins to the left side of the heart for distribution to the body tissues by the aorta.

These tissues include those of the bronchi, lungs and pleura which are supplied by the bronchial arteries (BA) with capillary networks in the walls of the tubes, between the aveoli and under the pleura. Blood is returned either by the pulmonary veins or by the azygos vein (AV)

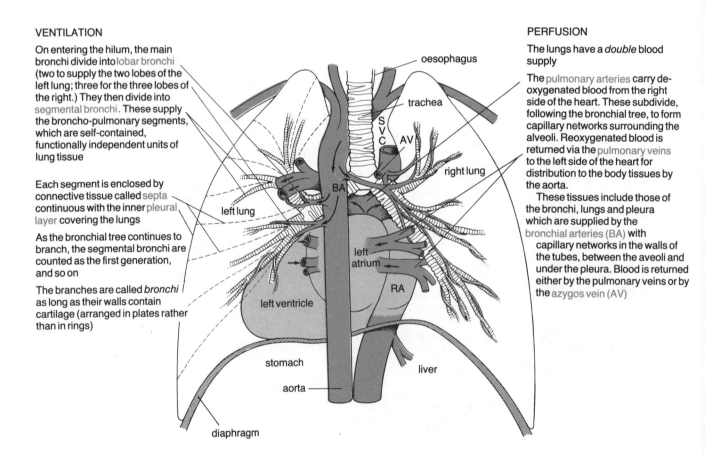

Figure 2.4   Double blood supply of the lungs (viewed from behind)

1. The *pulmonary arteries* carry deoxygenated blood (i.e., blood which has released much of its oxygen to the body tissues in the course of its passage around the body) from the right side of the heart. These subdivide, following the bronchial tree, to form the close network of capillaries surrounding the alveoli. Reoxygenated blood is returned via the *pulmonary veins* to the left side of the heart, for distribution to the body tissues via the aorta.
2. These body tissues include those of the bronchi, lungs and pleura, which are supplied by the *bronchial arteries* with capillary networks in the walls of the tubes, between the alveoli and under the pleura. Blood is returned either by the pulmonary veins or by the *azygos vein*.

Lymphatic drainage from the lungs

There are no lymphatics in the alveolar walls but many are found in the pleura, the septa and the blood vessel and airway walls. They drain from the periphery to the hilum of the lung, and into the tracheo-bronchial lymph nodes. These become blackened in town-dwellers by the particles from polluted air which are carried into the lung.

2 The alveoli

These are the air sacs whose thin walls are composed of a basement membrane and two types of pneumocyte. Groups of alveoli are positioned together around the atria, which are each supplied by an alveolar duct at the finer end of the respiratory tract, as shown in Figure 2.5.

The alveoli are closely surrounded by a network of capillaries and the places at which these capillaries and the alveoli touch form the sites for gas exchange (Figure 2.6).

The respiratory tract is developed in the foetus by the 16th week of intra-uterine life, but the number and size of alveoli increase after birth. More alveoli develop until the child is about eight weeks old and, after the age of three, they also increase in size and continue to grow as the chest expands until the lungs reach adult volume.

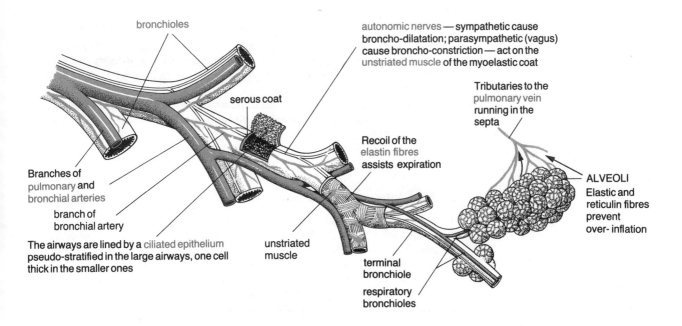

Figure 2.5 Gas conduction to and from the alveoli

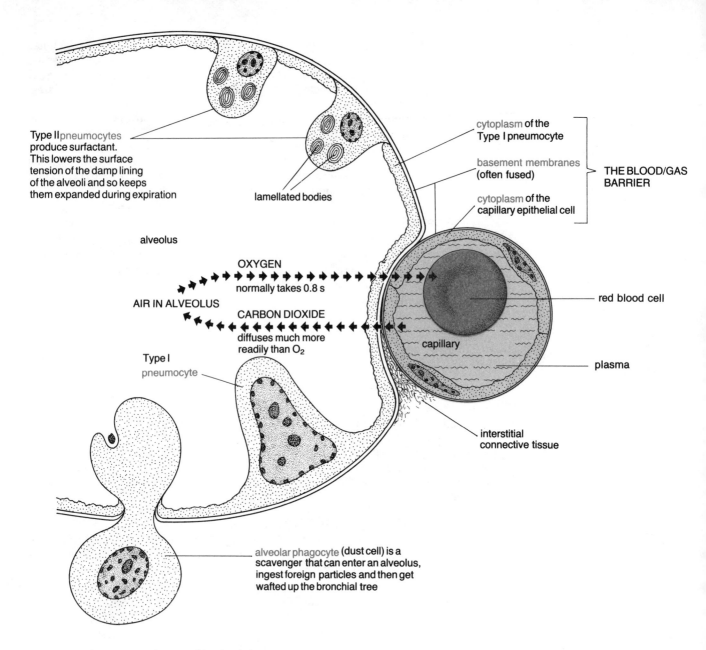

Type II pneumocytes produce surfactant. This lowers the surface tension of the damp lining of the alveoli and so keeps them expanded during expiration

lamellated bodies

cytoplasm of the Type I pneumocyte

basement membranes (often fused)

cytoplasm of the capillary epithelial cell

THE BLOOD/GAS BARRIER

alveolus

OXYGEN
normally takes 0.8 s

AIR IN ALVEOLUS

CARBON DIOXIDE
diffuses much more readily than O_2

Type I pneumocyte

red blood cell

capillary

plasma

interstitial connective tissue

alveolar phagocyte (dust cell) is a scavenger that can enter an alveolus, ingest foreign particles and then get wafted up the bronchial tree

Figure 2.6   Gas exchange between blood and air

The efficiency of respiration can be measured by estimating the amounts of O_2 and CO_2 in arterial blood. The blood is usually taken from the femoral artery using a sharp needle in a well-lubricated heparinised glass syringe, positioning the stab over the pulse.

Digital pressure should be maintained on the puncture wound for 5 minutes to prevent haemorrhage. Normal blood gas partial pressures are as follows:
pO_2: 100 mmHg (13.5 kPa)
pCO_2: 40 mmHg (5 kPa)

3   Ribs, intercostal muscles and diaphragm

Ventilation of the lungs is the mechanical process by which air is drawn into them and subsequently expelled after gas exchange has taken place in the alveoli. Ventilation is effected by movement of the ribs and the diaphragm which results in an alteration of the volume of the thoracic cavity.

Immediately surrounding each lung is a membrane called the *visceral pleura,* and lining the thoracic wall is the *parietal pleura.* The two pleura cannot part from each other because they are held together by the capillary attraction of the thin film of pleural fluid which is present between them. This fluid enables the surface of the lung to slide relative to the neighbouring thoracic wall, but ensures that the lung surface cannot move away from it.

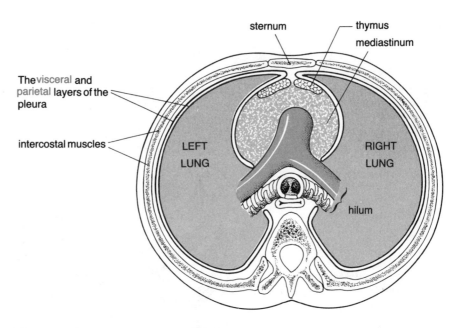

Figure 2.7   Transverse section through the lungs

Figure 2.7 shows the position of the pleural membranes. The lungs lie within the thoracic cavity as shown in Figure 2.8a, and their inner surfaces are shaped to accommodate the organs (heart, thymus, viscera, bronchi) found in the *mediastinum*, which is the space between the lungs (Figure 2.8b).

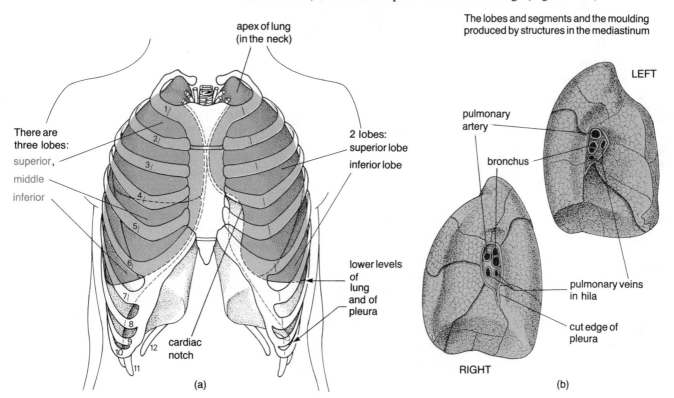

Figure 2.8   The lungs. (a) Surface anatomy and (b) medial aspects

Inspiration

The most important muscle of inspiration is the *diaphragm,* a dome-shaped sheet of muscle separating the thoracic and abdominal cavities. The diaphragm muscle fibres are arranged so that they radiate out from a central tendon to the circumference of the lower parts of the thoracic wall. When the muscles of the diaphragm contract, the central tendon is pulled down, pressing on the contents of the abdomen, which in turn push out the abdominal wall. The flattening of the diaphragm increases the vertical capacity of the thorax. Simultaneously, the lower ribs are forced to rise, as the flattened position of the

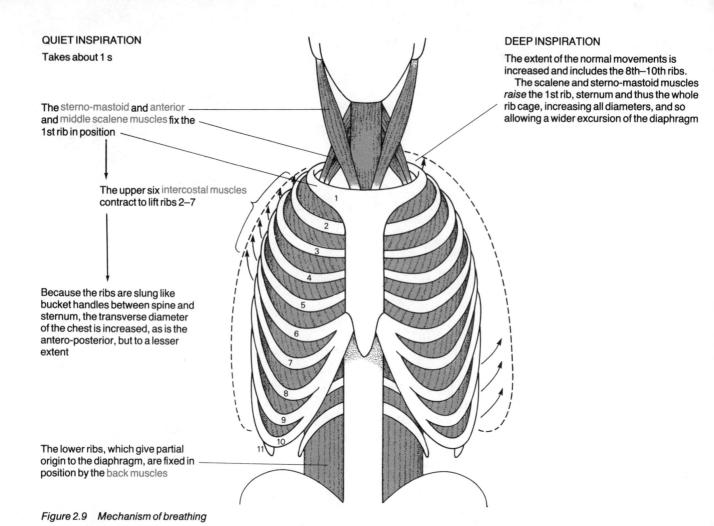

QUIET INSPIRATION
Takes about 1 s

DEEP INSPIRATION

The extent of the normal movements is
increased and includes the 8th–10th ribs.
The scalene and sterno-mastoid muscles
raise the 1st rib, sternum and thus the whole
rib cage, increasing all diameters, and so
allowing a wider excursion of the diaphragm

The sterno-mastoid and anterior
and middle scalene muscles fix the
1st rib in position

The upper six intercostal muscles
contract to lift ribs 2–7

Because the ribs are slung like
bucket handles between spine and
sternum, the transverse diameter
of the chest is increased, as is the
antero-posterior, but to a lesser
extent

The lower ribs, which give partial
origin to the diaphragm, are fixed in
position by the back muscles

Figure 2.9   Mechanism of breathing

diaphragm gives it a larger diameter. This upward and outward ('bucket handle') movement of the lower ribs increases the transverse diameter of the chest, also increasing the volume of the thoracic cavity.

The enlargement of the thoracic cavity, acting via the pleura, creates a negative pressure in the lungs and so air is drawn into them.

In quiet inspiration (Figure 2.9), the diaphragm may be the only respiratory muscle in action. In deeper inspiration, the intercostal muscles which lie between the ribs contract and so lift all the ribs upwards and outwards. This increases the chest diameter throughout its length, which results in a greater thoracic volume (and hence lung volume) than that created by the movement of the diaphragm alone.

In deep inspiration (Figure 2.9), the scalene and sterno-mastoid muscles raise the first rib and sternum and thus the whole rib cage, increasing the chest diameter and allowing a wider excursion of the diaphragm, resulting in the maximum possible increase in the volume of the lungs.

The diaphragm and the abdominal muscles play major roles in laughing, crying, coughing, sneezing, vomiting and the expulsion from the abdomen of babies, urine and faeces. Hiccups are caused by spasmodic contractions of the diaphragm.

Expiration

Quiet expiration is essentially a passive process, depending on the elastic recoil of the lungs, bronchial tree and chest wall. The respiratory muscles are gradually restored to their relaxed condition by the contraction of opposing muscles. In deep or forced expiration, the muscles of the abdominal wall contract, raising the intra-abdominal pressure and thus forcing the diaphragm up and the lower ribs down.

The respiratory cycle

A healthy person breathing normally at rest takes in, and expels, approximately half a litre of air during each respiratory cycle. This is the *tidal volume* and it can be measured by using a *spirometer*. The *ventilation rate* is the volume of air breathed per minute and is calculated as tidal volume × frequency of inspirations. At rest, the normal frequency of inspiration is about 14–18 per minute in adults and faster in children. The ventilation rate changes according to the body's needs. In exercise, for example, both the frequency and the tidal volume increase. The lungs have a much greater potential than is apparent from their resting condition, so that the respiratory apparatus can adapt to changing body requirements (Figure 2.10).

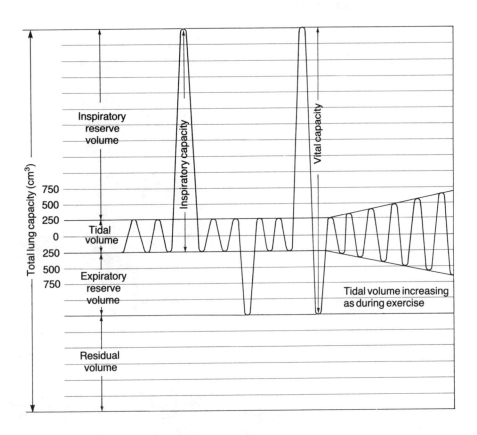

Figure 2.10   *Different lung volumes in an adult man*

A deep inspiration can draw into the lung approximately 3 litres of air in addition to the tidal volume. This is the *inspiratory reserve volume*. At the end of a normal expiration, a further 1 litre of air can be expelled; this is the *expiratory reserve volume*. The total amount of air which can be expired after a maximum inspiration is known as the *vital capacity,* and is between 4 and 5 litres in an average man, but can be increased by training, as by athletes or singers. It decreases during pregnancy, in the elderly, and in respiratory diseases which interfere with the volume of the lungs, or movement of the diaphragm.

Even after maximum expiration, some air (about 1.5 litres) remains in the lungs, and this is known as the *residual volume.*

4   The respiratory centre: control of respiration

Normal rhythmic respiration is controlled by a group of nerve cells in the pons and upper medulla of the brain called the *respiratory centre* (Figure 2.11).

These cells are directly sensitive to the concentration of CO_2 (pCO_2) in the blood perfusing the respiratory centre. As the pCO_2 rises, the respiratory centre is stimulated and initiates nerve impulses which travel down the *phrenic nerves* to the diaphragm, and down the *thoracic nerves* to the intercostal muscles. This results in inspiration.

The respiratory centre is also indirectly sensitive to the level of oxygen in the blood (pO_2). It receives stimuli via the *vagus* and *glossopharyngeal nerves* from chemoreceptors in the *carotid body* and in the *aortic bodies* which are stimulated when the pO_2 drops. On receipt of these stimuli, the respiratory

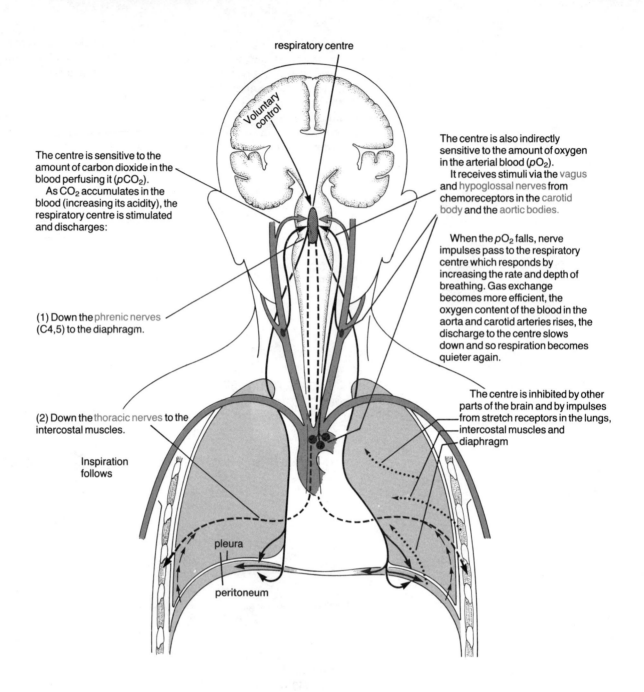

respiratory centre

Voluntary control

The centre is sensitive to the amount of carbon dioxide in the blood perfusing it (pCO_2).
As CO_2 accumulates in the blood (increasing its acidity), the respiratory centre is stimulated and discharges:

The centre is also indirectly sensitive to the amount of oxygen in the arterial blood (pO_2).
It receives stimuli via the vagus and hypoglossal nerves from chemoreceptors in the carotid body and the aortic bodies.

When the pO_2 falls, nerve impulses pass to the respiratory centre which responds by increasing the rate and depth of breathing. Gas exchange becomes more efficient, the oxygen content of the blood in the aorta and carotid arteries rises, the discharge to the centre slows down and so respiration becomes quieter again.

(1) Down the phrenic nerves (C4,5) to the diaphragm.

(2) Down the thoracic nerves to the intercostal muscles.

The centre is inhibited by other parts of the brain and by impulses from stretch receptors in the lungs, intercostal muscles and diaphragm

Inspiration follows

pleura

peritoneum

Figure 2.11   Control of respiration

centre responds by increasing the rate and depth of breathing. However, anoxia also depresses the respiratory centre and, if severe, the chemoreceptor response may not be able to stimulate breathing. When the pO_2 of the blood rises, and pCO_2 falls, the stimulation of the respiratory centre is reduced, and so respiration becomes quieter again. The centre is inhibited by other parts of the brain, and by stretch receptors in the lungs, intercostal muscles and diaphragm.

The effects of changes in pO_2 and pCO_2 on breathing are not merely additive; the response to a given pCO_2 is much greater when the pO_2 is low than when it is normal.

(b) The vascular system

The vascular system consists of the network of blood vessels which conduct blood to and from all parts of the body, bringing blood close enough to individual cells so that the local cellular environment can be kept constant by diffusion between blood plasma and extracellular fluid.

Figure 2.12 shows a simplified pattern of the vascular system, and the differing structures of the various blood vessels except for the capillaries, which

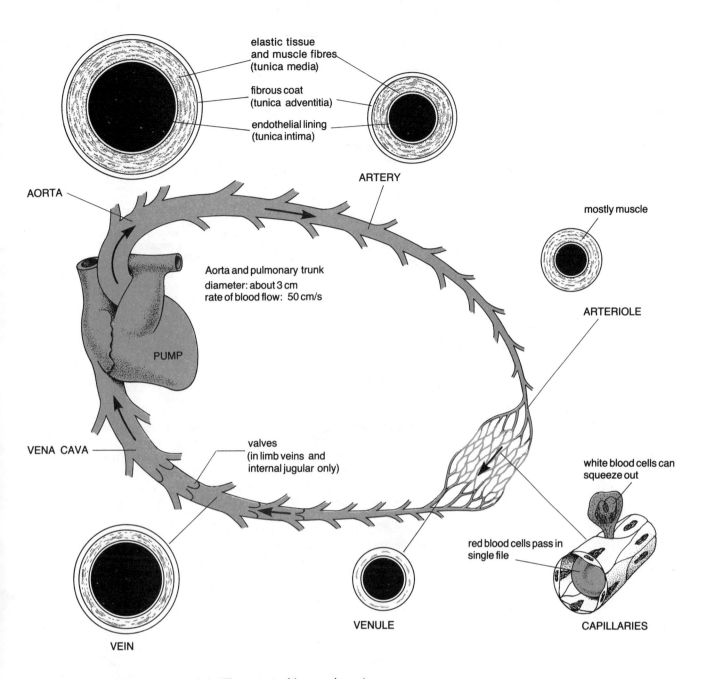

Figure 2.12   Structure of blood vessels in different parts of the vascular system

consist of a simple layer of endothelial cells only. All other blood vessels have a three-layered structure, which varies in composition.

1   Arteries and arterioles

The *aorta* and the *pulmonary artery* conduct blood immediately from the heart (the latter taking blood to the lungs). The middle layer (tunica media) of the aortic wall contains more elastic tissue than muscle fibres, and acts as the primary blood pressure regulator, although the arteries also share this function. The elastic tissue stretches as blood is pumped into the aorta from the heart, so limiting the rise in the systolic arterial blood pressure (the systolic pressure is that during the contraction of the heart). If the walls were rigid, the systolic pressure would be much higher. During diastole (relaxation and filling of the heart) the elastic recoil of the aorta and artery walls returns the energy stored in the wall to the blood and this tends to limit the fall in arterial pressure. In this way the blood is maintained at a more uniform pressure, as the effects of the pumping of the heart are evened out. The pulsating movements of the artery walls which do remain are the basis of the *pulse*, which can be monitored at convenient points, including the wrist (see Figure 2.13).

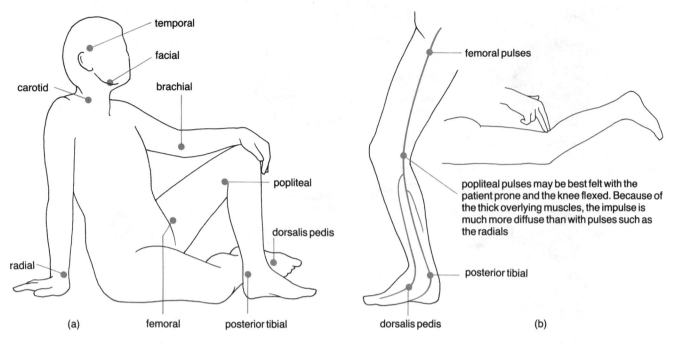

Figure 2.13 Pulse points. (a) Around the body and (b) in the leg and foot

The tunica media of the *arteries* has more muscle than elastic tissue. The involuntary (smooth) muscle fibres are arranged circularly and an artery can go into spasm as a life-saving device to reduce blood loss during haemorrhage.

The middle layer of the walls of *arterioles* consists mostly of muscle and these regulate the distribution of blood to different tissues according to demand. During exercise, blood supply is increased to the voluntary muscles; during digestion it is increased to the gut.

Capillaries consist of a single layer only of endothelial cells, and this forms a semi-permeable membrane allowing free passage of gases and solutes. White blood cells can squeeze out by a process known as *diapedesis*, but red blood cells cannot normally leave capillaries, and pass along them in single file.

2 Veins

Usually *veins* run alongside their corresponding artery, but they may follow a different route. As blood flow in the veins is slower, they are larger and more numerous than arteries. They have thinner walls and less elastic tissue, and can be more easily distended. The veins of the limbs possess valves, made from folds of internal endothelium, and these prevent reverse-flow of blood. Veins do not pulsate, but modification of the tone of the smooth muscle of their walls adjusts their capacity and regulates the flow of blood back to the heart.

3 The regulation of blood flow through arteries and arterioles

The vasomotor centre of the brain is sensitive to several influences, most important of which is the pressure gauge (baroreceptor) of the carotid body. A rise in blood pressure is detected by the carotid body and nervous impulses sent from it to the vasomotor centre (VMC) *inhibit* VMC activity, so fewer impulses are sent to the arterioles. As a result, the muscles in the arteriole wall relax, the arterioles dilate, and blood pressure drops.

The brain and the kidneys have a system of autoregulation not dependent on the carotid body.

(c) Oxygen and carbon dioxide carrying functions of the blood

The normal total blood volume is approximately 3.5 litres in women and 5 litres in men. Of this total volume, 55% is blood plasma and 45% consists of the various blood cells.

The blood plasma (Figure 2.14) is a fluid composed of inorganic salts, e.g., chloride, bicarbonate, sodium, potassium, calcium and plasma proteins,

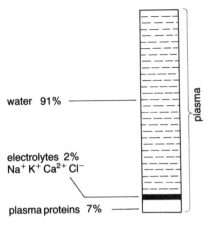

water 91%

electrolytes 2%
Na$^+$ K$^+$ Ca^{2+} Cl$^-$

plasma proteins 7%

plasma

Figure 2.14   Blood plasma composition

including fibrinogen, globulin and albumin, which are too big to pass through capillary walls under normal circumstances.

There are three main types of blood cells (Figure 2.15):

1. *Thrombocytes* (platelets), which are involved with blood clotting.
2. *Leucocytes* (white blood cells), which have an important role in defence against infection.
3. *Erythrocytes* (red blood cells), which are circular bi-concave discs with no nuclei, and which are responsible for the transportation of oxygen and carbon dioxide.

1   Erythrocytes

The main constituent of erythrocytes is *haemoglobin,* a protein molecule (globin) which possesses a porphyrin ring containing an iron atom (haem). One molecule of haemoglobin comprises a group of four polypeptide chains (globin) each containing one haem group. The haem group is the site of oxygen transport, and the chemical properties of it are such that O_2 is readily released where the pO_2 is low (e.g., in the tissues) and readily accepted where pO_2 is high (in the lungs).

Carbon dioxide is also largely transported within the erythrocytes, in the form of the bicarbonate ion, and the resultant acidity of the cell cytoplasm is 'buffered' (kept at a constant pH) by the haemoglobin. CO_2 combines with water only slowly under normal conditions, but this reaction is greatly accelerated by the presence of an enzyme, carbonic anhydrase, in the red blood cells.

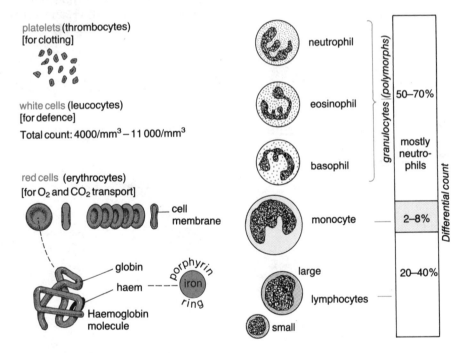

Figure 2.15   Blood cells

2   Erythropoiesis

Erythropoiesis (Figure 2.16) is the formation of the erythrocytes (red blood cells), and occurs in the red bone marrow of the adult. In the foetus and the infant, all bone marrow is actively producing red blood cells.

The concentration of erythrocytes remains remarkably constant in health, as the destruction of old cells is exactly balanced by the production of new. To achieve this, there is a delicately controlled feedback mechanism, the details of which are far from clear.

The production of red blood cells requires a supply of minerals including iron, copper and cobalt, amino acids and vitamins B12, folate, riboflavin, E, B6

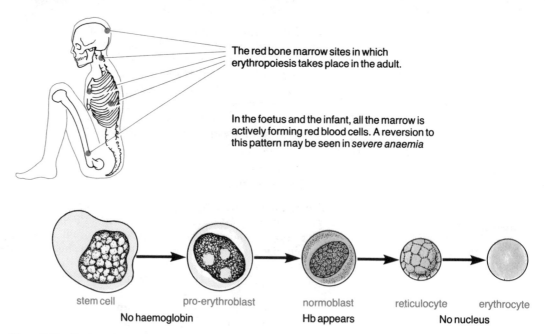

The red bone marrow sites in which erythropoiesis takes place in the adult.

In the foetus and the infant, all the marrow is actively forming red blood cells. A reversion to this pattern may be seen in *severe anaemia*

stem cell	pro-erythroblast	normoblast	reticulocyte	erythrocyte
	No haemoglobin	Hb appears		No nucleus

Figure 2.16   Erythropoiesis

and probably C to the red bone marrow. Also required is stimulation of the red bone marrow by a hormone called *erythropoietin,* a glycoprotein which is produced by the kidney. Production of erythropoietin is itself stimulated by the hormones thyroxine, ACTH and testosterone, and the fundamental stimulus is *hypoxia* (low pO_2 in the blood).

The patients with problems of oxygenation

(a) Oxygen want in patients with impairment of respiratory function

1 Patient study and care plan for an adult with chronic bronchitis

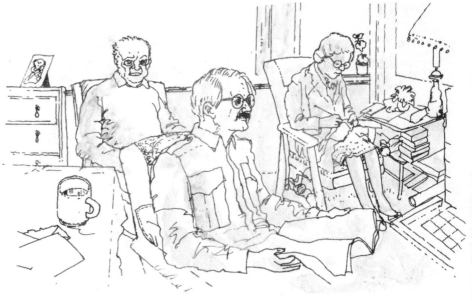

Figure 2.17   Mr Jones and family

History of social, psychological and physical events leading to the present condition

The patient chosen for this section to illustrate oxygen want has an acute exacerbation of chronic bronchitis.

Mr Jones, aged 58 years (Figure 2.17), lives with his wife and his 80-year-old father in a small mining community. Their two children are married and live nearby. Mr Jones enjoys going regularly to the local social club and is a member of the miners' choir. He has worked in the mine all his life and for the past 10 years has been a surface worker. He gave up smoking at that time due to repeated episodes of acute bronchitis. Since then he has complained of a productive cough both winter and summer and difficulty in breathing on exertion. During the past year these symptoms have worsened and he has found difficulty in singing in the choir. During a recent spell of cold weather he suffered from influenza which persisted for several days, leaving him feeling generally unwell.

Yesterday he was unable to go to work as he was having difficulty in breathing and had a raised temperature, so he stayed in bed and his wife called the GP to see him. The doctor advised Mr Jones to stay in a warm room, drink extra fluids and take the prescribed antibiotics. Mr Jones spent a restless night because of a persistent cough and feeling hot and sweaty. Mrs Jones became concerned when she noticed that her husband was weaker and his colour was greyish. He also became rather agitated and aggressive when she tried to give him his tablets in the morning. She contacted the doctor again. He explained that her husband had an acute exacerbation of his chronic bronchitis and needed to be admitted to hospital. As Mr Jones was suffering respiratory embarrassment, the doctor administered an intravenous injection of aminophylline prior to his transfer to hospital by ambulance.

Explanation of abnormal physiology and pathology

It is advisable to revise the physiology of normal respiration (see Table 2.1).

Table 2.1

Related normal physiology	Abnormal physiology
(a) Air passages lined with ciliated epithelium to trap and waft debris away from the lungs up to the pharynx	Ciliated epithelium damaged due to repeated episodes of acute bronchitis, atmospheric pollution and cold air entry, resulting in colonisation by pathogenic organisms
(b) Goblet cells in the epithelium produce clear mucus to warm and moisten air entering the lungs	Long-term irritation due to inhalation of coal dust results in proliferation of goblet cells and excessive manufacture of mucus. Pathogenic organisms cause the mucus to alter in consistency and colour to a thick, yellowish-green, offensive-smelling sputum
(c) Alveoli provide a large surface area for the exchange of gases between inspired air and the blood	Alveoli progressively destroyed, leading to emphysema and reduced surface area for exchange of gases
(d) Arterial blood gas partial pressures: pO_2—100 mmHg (13.5 kPa) pCO_2—40 mmHg (5 kPA)	pO_2—reduced pCO_2—raised
(e) Tissue and organs require adequate oxygen perfusion to maintain function	Skin loses normal pink colour and becomes cyanosed. Lack of oxygen to brain results in cerebral confusion and disorientation
(f) Respiration is dependent on chemical and nervous sensitivity to oxygen and carbon dioxide arterial blood levels	Reduced sensitivity and raised carbon dioxide arterial blood level results in respiration depending on a reduced oxygen arterial blood level

Care plan

PREPARATION FOR PATIENT WITH CHRONIC BRONCHITIS

This plan is for Mr Jones following his admission to the medical ward of the local hospital.

Nursing history and assessment
From the detailed history of Mr Jones, complete the nursing history and assessment sheet (Table 2.2).

Table 2.2   Blank nursing history and assessment sheet for Mr Jones, to be completed

NURSING HISTORY AND ASSESSMENT SHEET
Record No. _____

PATIENT LABEL

Mr/Mrs/Miss _____

Address _____

Male/Female   Age _____

Date of Birth _____

Date of admission/first visit

_____

Time _____

Type: ☐ Routine   ☐ Emergency

   Transfer from: _____

Religion _____

Practising/baptised _____

Minister _____

Telephone number _____

Next of kin (name) _____

Relationship to patient _____

Address _____

_____

Telephone numbers _____

Contact at night/in emergency   YES/NO

Occupation (or father) _____

Marital status _____

Children (or place in family) _____

Other dependants _____

Pets _____

School (children only) _____

Hobbies _____

Clubs _____

Favourite pastime _____

Does patient smoke?   YES/NO

Speech difficulty/language barrier

Dysphasia   Dysarthria

Accommodation

Lives alone   YES/NO

Part III/EMI/Old People's Homes/Rented

Other _____

Consultant _____

House officer _____

Presenting condition _____

_____

History of present complaint and reason for admission

_____
_____
_____
_____
_____

Past medical history

_____
_____

Allergies

Current medication

_____

What patient says is the reason for admission and attitude to admission

_____

Patient's expectations

Any problems at home while/because patient is in hospital?

Relevant home conditions (e.g. stairs)

_____
_____

Visiting problems

_____

Care at home

Community nurse _____

No. _____

Name of GP _____

Address _____

Other services involved

Home help _____   Day hospital _____

Laundry _____   Day centre/club _____

Inco supplies _____   Health visitor _____

Aids _____   Social worker _____

Meals on wheels _____   Voluntary worker _____

Daily living

Diet

Special _____

Food or drink dislikes _____

Appetite: ☐ GOOD   ☐ POOR

Remarks _____

Sleep

How many hours normally? _____

Sedation _____

What else helps? _____

Elimination

Bowels: Continent/Incontinent

How often opened? _____

Any medication? _____

Urinary: Continent/Incontinent

If incontinent; Day/Night/If not taken, how frequently? _____

Nocturia/Dysuria/Frequency/Urgency

Remarks _____

Female patients — Menstruation

Post-menopausal   Taking the pill

Regular   Irregular

Amenorrhoea   Dysmenorrhoea

Next period due: _____

Uses: STs Tampons

Hearing

Hearing aid: YES/NO

Remarks _____

Vision

Glasses/Contact lens: YES/NO

Remarks _____

Oral

Dentures or crowns: YES/NO

Any problems with mouth or teeth?

_____

Mobility

Help needed with:

Walking/Standing/In/Out of bed/Bathing/Dressing

In/Out of chair/

Feeding/Other: _____

Remarks _____

Prosthesis/appliance

Type of appliance _____

Help needed _____

General appearance

Normal   Dehydrated   Acutely ill

Obese   Thin   Emaciated

Remarks _____

Skin

Satisfactory   Broken areas   Dehydrated

Rash   Oedematous   Jaundiced

Pallor   Other _____
                  (including bruising)

Remarks _____

Level of consciousness

Orientated   Semi-conscious

Confused   Unconscious

Remarks _____

Mental assessment (if appropriate)

Mood

Elated   Irritable   Agitated

Cheerful   Anxious   Aggressive

Miserable   Withdrawn   Suspicious

Apathetic

Thought content

Hallucinations/Delusions/Paranoid Ideas

_____

Orientation

Time/Place/Person

Very confused   Slightly confused

Any particular time of day? _____

Confabulation _____

Remarks _____

Surveillance   Physical/Emotional

Information obtained from _____

Relationship to patient _____

By _____

Position/level of training _____

Date _____

Time _____

TREATMENT

In addition to the antibiotics already prescribed the doctor orders:
1. Chest x-ray.
2. Specimen of sputum to the bacteriology laboratory.
3. Intensive physiotherapy to include postural drainage, breathing exercises, percussion and vibration.
4. Broncho-dilator therapy via inhaler and orally.
5. Humidified oxygen in prescribed concentration, for example, 24%.

Table 2.3 shows the care plan for Mr Jones.

Table 2.3 Care plan for Mr Jones in medical ward

Problem	Objective	Plan of care	Rationale
1. Emergency admission of an anxious patient accompanied by wife	Reduce anxiety of patient and relative	(a) Explanation and reassurance to be given to both	(a) Reduces problem
		(b) Give wife opportunity to see medical staff and senior nursing staff	(b) Develops relationships and communications Increases confidence in staff
		(c) Exchange information (including telephone numbers)	(c) Ensures later communications
2. Breathlessness	Re-establish normal ventilation	(a) Position upright with adequate pillows and provide bed table to lean forward on and rest (i.e. orthopnoeic position)	(a) Allows expansion of rib cage and reduces pressure of abdominal contents on diaphragm. Facilitates use of accessory muscles of respiration
		(b) Administer humidified oxygen at 24% via face mask	(b) Improves arterial blood oxygen level without depressing the reflex stimulus to respiration which is caused by reduced blood oxygen levels
		(c) Administer prescribed bronchodilator, salbutamol (Ventolin) orally and by inhalation	(c) Reduces broncho-spasm at the terminal bronchioles to increase the vital capacity
3. Breathlessness due to excessive sputum	Enable expectoration of sputum	(a) Physiotherapy: (i) Breathing exercises (ii) Vibration of chest wall and percussion (iii) Assisted breathing including positioning and postural drainage	(a) (i) Breathing exercises expand chest capacity and improve vital capacity of lungs, and improve venous return (ii) Vibration and percussion frees sticky sputum from wall lining in air passages (iii) Positioning and postural drainage permits drainage of sputum with use of gravity
		(b) Provide clean sputum container, tissues and disposal bag as required. Leave within patient's reach and teach him how to use them	(b) Prevents cross-infection and ensures safe disposal of infected material
		(c) Observe and record the amount, nature, consistency and colour of sputum	(c) Monitors progress of disease and effects of treatment (see abnormal physiology, page 57)
		(d) Observe and report patient's ability to cough and expectorate	(d) Monitors progress of disease, effects of treatment and early detection of complications
		(e) Offer antiseptic mouth washes	(e) Prevents oral and pharyngeal sepsis
		(f) Obtain specimen of sputum for laboratory examination, culture sensitivity and cytology	(f) Identifies causative organism and its sensitivity to antibiotics. Checks for presence of abnormal pathology, e.g., malignant cells or tuberculosis
4. Potential development of respiratory failure	To detect early signs of respiratory failure	(a) Monitor respiration rate, depth, rhythm, difficulty	(a) Any alteration could indicate interference with gas exchange and mechanical and chemical stimulation of respiratory centre
		(b) Monitor mental function	(b) Cerebral anoxia produces confusion, drowsiness and eventually coma
5. Acutely ill patient receiving humidified oxygen therapy	Ensure safe administration and reduce discomfort	(a) Check regularly that prescribed concentration is being administered	(a) Refer to section on abnormal physiology
		(b) Gain cooperation of patient by ensuring mask fits comfortably and by explaining its use	(b) Reduces anxiety and ensures oxygen is being inhaled
		(c) Give frequent mouth washes	(c) Oxygen is drying to mucous membranes

Table 2.3 (cont.)

Problem	Objective	Plan of care	Rationale
		(d) Change face mask and ensure face is washed and dried as necessary	(d) Skin becomes sweaty and moist from humidification
		(e) Explain to patient and relative the precautions required when oxygen therapy is being given	(e) Oxygen supports combustion
		(f) Ensure adequate supply of oxygen for the next 24 hours	(f) Treatment will probably be continued for at least 24 hours
6. Acutely ill patient receiving bronchodilator and antibiotic therapy	To monitor desired and unwanted effects	(a) Measure and record temperature, pulse and respirations 1–2-hourly	(a) Improvement would be indicated by return of temperature, pulse and respirations to within normal limits
		(b) Observe for side-effects of medications (refer to pharmacology textbook)	(b) To ensure prompt withdrawal
7. Patient potentially dehydrated	Maintain hydration	(a) (i) Monitor fluid balance, using fluid balance chart (ii) Record amount of sputum (iii) Estimate insensible fluid loss, i.e. sweat and expired water vapour	(a) (i) Shows discrepancy in fluid intake and urinary output (ii) and (iii) Patient losing increased amounts of fluid from sweating due to pyrexia, sputum due to infection, water vapour due to increased respiration rate
		(b) Replace excessive fluid loss and maintain electrolyte balance by giving fluids intravenously	(b) (i) Patient unable to maintain balance by oral fluids due to breathlessness and difficulty in drinking (ii) Reduces viscosity of sputum
8. Sweating due to pyrexia	Reduce patient's discomfort and prevent maceration of skin folds	Cool bedclothes, frequent hands and face wash	Reduces discomfort and the likely sites for the growth of micro-organisms
9. Reluctance to move due to orthopnoea	To reduce risk of venous stasis, pressure sores and urinary stasis	(a) Reposition patient 2–3-hourly	(a) Relieves pressure and ensures adequate blood flow bringing oxygen and nutrients to the tissues
		(b) Inspect pressure sites for discoloration or abrasion	(b) Ensures early detection and change of care plan
		(c) Use appropriate aids such as ripple mattress, sheepskin foam or polystyrene cushions, bed cradle	(c) Relieves pressure on specific sites when patient is at particular risk due to immobility with an acute illness
		(d) Teach leg exercises and explain their importance	(d) Muscle pump aids venous return and prevents deep vein thrombosis
10. Anorexia due to febrile illness	To ensure adequate nutrition	(a) Give extra high-protein drinks and added vitamins	(a) Promotes healing of damaged lung tissue and maintains protein balance
		(b) Offer small easily digestible meals	(b) Patient unable to tolerate normal diet due to breathlessness and acute illness

EVALUATION OF CARE AND SUGGESTED RECORD OF PROGRESS

Patient's Name   Mr Jones

Date   3 days after admission   Time   0900 hours

QUESTIONS TO HELP YOU WITH EVALUATING CARE AND PROGRESS

Nursing actions relating to patient comfort, safety and well-being

- What is the patient's response to his/her condition?
- Are the present nursing actions still required?
- Is the patient, and his/her family, informed?

Mr Jones is feeling much better, he can breathe more easily and has more energy to look after himself. His appetite has returned and he feels less dependent on others. He can now tolerate sitting out in chair for short periods, can change and maintain his position in bed and can eat and drink unaided. Mr Jones is fully aware of the long-term implications of his chronic bronchitis and the possible length of stay in hospital.

Nursing actions pertaining to observations and measurements

- What is the patient's response to the observations and measurements being made?
- Are the present measurements/observations still required?
- Have results been seen or relayed to the appropriate practitioner/carer?
- Has the patient been informed of the changes?

Has wanted to sleep and has been disturbed by frequent monitoring of his condition. His temperature is normal, and pulse and respirations are slowing to within normal limits. Sputum is still copious but he has stopped sweating. Frequency of measuring temperature, pulse and respirations can be reduced to 4-hourly, observation of sputum and fluid balance to remain unchanged. Improvement in vital signs and laboratory results on sputum have been reported to the medical officer. Patient is not yet aware of possible changes in observations and that the vital capacity and peak flow readings are showing irreversible lung disease.

Nursing actions relating to diagnosis and treatment

- What is the patient's response to diagnosis and treatment?
- Are the patient's treatments still required?
- Have the course/s of treatment been completed or discontinued?
- Has the patient been informed?

Mr Jones is concerned about his discharge home and the facilities available at home to reduce the demands on his wife. The doctor has prescribed a reduction in the amount of oxygen administered and a reduction in the dose of bronchial dilation drug. Physiotherapy is now to be given less frequently. Doctor has explained the changes in medication and oxygen therapy to Mr Jones.

* * * * * * *

- Who has visited the patient?
- What information has been given to relatives/visitors?

Wife is unable to visit today and has rung to ask whether she can have any assistance with travelling to the hospital.

* * * * * * *

- Has the care plan been updated?
- Are the objectives/goals of care still relevant?

Yes — objectives remain unchanged but frequency of nursing actions and observations has been reduced.

Signature of Reporting Nurse   _J. Smith_

Designation   _Student Nurse_

Signature of Supervising Nurse   _E. Evans_

Designation   _Sister_

PREPARATION FOR MR JONES'S DISCHARGE

Progress is maintained and the possibility of Mr Jones being discharged home is now being considered. The following care plan (Table 2.4) is to prepare for his discharge.

2 Patient histories illustrating further problems related to problems of oxygenation

This part of the chapter consists of five patient histories followed by self-testing questions and guidelines for suggested answers.

A young person in an asthma attack

Susan, aged 16 years, recently left school and is due to start work in the local supermarket next week. She lives with her parents and younger sister in a block

Table 2.4 Care plan for preparation of Mr Jones's discharge

Problem	Objective	Plan of care	Rationale
1. Patient with long-term respiratory difficulty having to return home	Ensure sufficient facilities are available for Mr and Mrs Jones to enable Mr Jones to live at home	Arrangement and explanation to Mr and Mrs Jones regarding the following:	
		(a) Medical social worker contacted to discuss the need for home assessment, financial aid, contact with welfare services at the local mine, his present employers and home care assistant	(a) Ensures appropriate choice of facilities to enable Mr Jones to stay at home
		(b) District nurse contacted to discuss need for on-going oxygen therapy, commode, urinal, assistance with daily living activities, and monitoring of continuing treatment	(b) Ensures continuation of therapy, assistance to Mrs Jones in maintaining Mr Jones's daily living activities and early detection of complications
		(c) Arrange follow-up outpatient appointment and attendance at the physiotherapy department	(c) Provides opportunity for further medical and physiotherapy assessment and management
		(d) Arrange sitting stretcher transport for the patient to return home and to attend the appointments listed above	(d) Enables an incapacitated patient to attend appointments mentioned above
		(e) Arrange for prescription of medicines and oxygen cylinders	(e) Ensures continuation of treatment immediately after discharge
		(f) Arrange for Mrs Jones to meet physiotherapist for explanation of on-going therapy	(f) Enlists Mrs Jones's active participation in continuing physiotherapy to Mr Jones's chest

of high-rise flats in a city suburb. Her interests include going to a disco at weekends with her friends. She learnt to play the flute on advice from the physiotherapist to improve her breathing when she was first diagnosed as having asthma at the age of seven.

Halfway through an evening at the disco, Susan became distressed at her sudden difficulty in breathing. Her friends took her outside and sat her down but she became increasingly breathless, frightened and sweaty. Her friends became concerned as her breathing was noisy with an obvious 'wheeze'. With the help of the disco manager an ambulance was summoned and Susan was admitted to the accident and emergency department.

The nurse admitting Susan observes the following:
- Dyspnoeic with noisy respirations.
- Skin pale and sweaty.
- Agitated and not fully aware of her surroundings but complaining of a feeling of suffocation.
- Pulse rate raised to 140 beats per minute.
- Respirations laboured and rapid with noticeable difficulty in expiration.
- No cough or sputum apparent.
- Temperature raised.

The doctor examines Susan and obtains a past medical history from Susan's parents, who have been summoned. They reveal that Susan has had no asthma attacks since the age of seven years and is not receiving any medication. The doctor prescribes the following:
1. Humidified oxygen therapy in high concentration.
2. Intravenous aminophylline.
3. Intravenous hydrocortisone.
4. Intravenous infusion of normal saline.

Susan is monitored by the doctor and nurse for the effects of this treatment before being moved from the accident and emergency department. She becomes less distressed as her respiration becomes less laboured and quieter so that the doctor then authorises her admission to a medical ward. She continues the oxygen therapy and intravenous infusion and is prescribed salbutamol orally and as an inhalant. In addition, a dose of diazepam is prescribed if she is unable to go to sleep.

SELF-TESTING QUESTIONS

1. Describe the abnormal physiology related to Susan's acute asthma attack with special reference to:
   (a) Difficulty with expiratory phase of respiration.
   (b) Retention of sputum.
   (c) Dehydration.

2. Explain the rationale for the treatment ordered in the accident and emergency department.

BRIEF ANALYSIS AND GUIDELINES TO SUITABLE ANSWERS

Question 1
Refer to your teacher for guidance and a suitable textbook or journal.

Question 2
Your answer should include the following:

Treatment	Rationale
(a) High concentration of oxygen	Patient suffering from acute oxygen lack, and has *no* past history of chronic lung disease
(b) Intravenous aminophylline	This acts quickly on smooth muscle of bronchioles, relieving broncho-spasm and allowing air in and out of alveoli
(c) Intravenous hydrocortisone	This has an anti-inflammatory effect on mucosal lining of bronchioles so reducing oedema and increasing the lumen of the bronchioles
(d) Intravenous normal saline	Corrects dehydration induced by rapid respirations and sweating. Liquefies the tenacious sputum

Question 3

3. Devise a care plan for Susan after her admission to the ward.

Your answer should include:
(a) Reassurance of a frightened patient.
(b) Management of a breathless patient to re-establish normal ventilation (refer to care plan for Mr Jones, page 63).
(c) Observations for early detection of complications.
(d) Care during administration of intravenous infusion and oxygen therapy.

Question 4

4. Identify the factors that could precipitate an asthma attack.

Refer to appropriate medical textbooks and describe intrinsic and extrinsic factors.

Question 5

5. How could Susan be advised to avoid or minimise future attacks?

Your answer should include:
- Investigation of cause.
- Avoidance of precipitating factors.
- Long-term medication if required.
- Breathing exercises.

Question 6

6. Give a definition of each of the following terms:
   - Status asthmaticus.
   - Cardiac asthma.
   - Forced expiratory volume.

Refer to W.A.R. Thompson (Ed.), *Black's Medical Dictionary*, 34th edition, A. and C. Black, London, 1984.

An adult with pneumonia

Mrs Parker, aged 70 years, lives alone in a basement flat. She is described by her neighbours as a 'recluse' who is reluctant to mix with the local community. Her neighbours informed the police when they realised that they had not seen her for several days and were unable to get any reply. Mrs Parker was found in neglected surroundings, obviously ill, and was admitted to hospital.

She is examined by the doctor, who diagnoses broncho-pneumonia. He orders bed rest, an intravenous infusion, antibiotics, physiotherapy (to chest) and oxygen therapy. Investigations include:

- Chest x-ray.
- Electrocardiograph.
- Sputum specimen for culture and sensitivity.
- Full blood count.
- Urea and electrolyte estimation.

Mrs Parker is transferred to a medical ward.

SELF-TESTING QUESTIONS

BRIEF ANALYSIS AND GUIDELINES TO SUITABLE ANSWERS

1. List the possible findings of the nurse admitting Mrs Parker when she takes a nursing history and assessment.

Question 1
Your answer should include:
(a) Anxious and confused due to cerebral anoxia.
(b) Peripheral cyanosis due to inadequate ventilation and poor tissue perfusion.
(c) Dyspnoea due to obstruction of air passages and alveoli by inflammation and excessive exudate; and accumulation of fluid in pleural cavity.
(d) Pyrexia due to presence of infection.
(e) Oliguria due to inadequate intake over previous 48 hours and sweating due to pyrexia.
(f) Discoloration of skin over sacrum and heels.
(g) Productive cough and pleuritic pain on inspiration.

2. Discuss the physiology of pleuritic pain and pleural effusion.

Question 2
Refer to J. Macleod (Ed.), *Davidson's Principles and Practice of Medicine*, 14th edition, Churchill Livingstone, London, 1984.

3. Mrs Parker is to have a chest aspiration to remove a pleural effusion. Describe the nurse's reponsibilities before, during and after this procedure.

Question 3
Refer to Nurses Procedures Manual.

4. Describe how the total management of this condition will correct this patient's oxygen lack.

Question 4
Your answer should include:

Patient care	Rationale
(a) Bed rest	Reduces oxygen demand
(b) Intravenous infusion	Increases blood circulating volume and therefore tissue perfusion
(c) Physiotherapy to chest	Improves ventilation and expectoration to permit exchange of gases
(d) Antibiotic therapy	Combats infecting organism and permits resolution of inflammatory responses
(e) Oxygen therapy	Improves arterial oxygen partial pressure and relieves cerebral and tissue anoxia

5. Discuss the possible outcomes of this patient's period of hospitalisation.

Question 5
Your answer should include discussion of the following:
(a) Return to her home with social and health service support.
(b) Possibility of convalescing with relatives.
(c) Provision of part III accommodation.

Patient with a spontaneous pneumothorax

Stephen Hall, aged 20 years, is admitted to the accident and emergency department with a spontaneous pneumothorax. Treatment consists of the insertion of an apical drainage tube connected to an underwater seal drainage apparatus.

His parents have been informed of his admission to hospital but they live 100 miles away and will be unable to reach the hospital for several hours. Stephen is currently a student in his final year at University, reading mathematics. He normally has good health but is not particularly involved in athletic activities. He is of slight build and 1.8 metres tall. He was working late preparing for his examinations when he suddenly felt breathless, became frightened and summoned help from his flatmates.

Following treatment in the accident and emergency department Stephen is transferred to a medical ward for further observation.

SELF-TESTING QUESTIONS

1. Define pneumothorax and explain the effects of a spontaneous pneumothorax on the normal physiology of respiration.

2. Devise a care plan for Stephen for the first 48 hours after insertion of the apical drainage tube.

3. Identify hazards associated with underwater seal drainage and discuss their prevention.

BRIEF ANALYSIS AND GUIDELINES TO SUITABLE ANSWERS

Question 1
Refer to medical dictionary, e.g., W.A.R. Thompson (Ed.), *Black's Medical Dictionary*, 34th edition, A. and C. Black, London, 1984 (page 42).

Question 2
Your answer should include care of patient's physical, social and psychological needs with particular reference to:
(a) Monitoring of respiratory function.
(b) Management of underwater seal apparatus.
(c) Positioning of patient.
(d) Physiotherapy.
(e) Care and explanation to parents.

Question 3
Your answer should include discussion of the *hazards* illustrated in Figure 2.18.

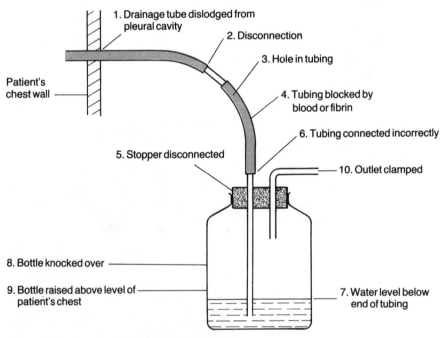

Figure 2.18   Hazards of an apical drainage system

4. Discuss the following:
   (a) The rationale for inserting an apical drainage tube.
   (b) The effects of Stephen's anxiety on his progress.

Question 4
(a) This is because air is less dense than lung tissue and will collect at the apex of the pleural cavity when the patient is positioned upright.
(b) Anxiety due to loss of study time will cause low morale; it will lower pain threshold, reduce mobility and cause reluctance to cooperate in treatment and rehabilitation. In addition, anxiety will tend to affect measurement of pulse and respiration rates and blood pressure.

(c) The function of the pleura and its involvement in the mechanics of respiration.

(d) The usual outcome of spontaneous pneumothorax.

(c) Refer to pages 46–47.

(d) Refer to J. Macleod (Ed.), *Davidson's Principles and Practice of Medicine*, 14th edition, Churchill Livingstone, London, 1984.

An adult with carcinoma of the bronchus

Mr James Bradshawe, aged 55 years, has a nine-month history of carcinoma of the bronchus. He is one of the managing directors of a hypermarket and has a wife and two sons, both of whom are in the armed forces. He had smoked heavily for many years and was fully investigated following a haemoptysis nine months ago. Following diagnosis of carcinoma of the bronchus he was given a course of radiotherapy and on completion of this he improved and was able to take a holiday abroad with his wife. He was fully aware of his diagnosis and prognosis. He resumed work for a short period but his general condition rapidly deteriorated. He becomes weak and unable to visit his GP so a home visit is arranged.

The doctor examines Mr Bradshawe and finds him emaciated, lethargic and anaemic. He has orthopnoea and a productive cough which causes discomfort. The doctor discusses with Mr and Mrs Bradshawe whether Mr Bradshawe should be admitted to hospital. They decide that Mr Bradshawe should remain at home with supporting services. The doctor prescribes the following medication to be given when necessary:

- An expectorant and a linctus.
- A broncho-dilator orally.
- An analgesic orally (to be kept under review).
- An aperient.
- Oxygen.

He also advises Mr Bradshawe to do as much as he feels able and to try to manage small, easily digestible, high-protein meals and/or drinks. He explains to Mr and Mrs Bradshawe that he will be contacting the district nurse and arranging for her to call and discuss future nursing management.

SELF-TESTING QUESTIONS

1. Describe the complications that can occur from *local* spread of carcinoma of bronchus.

2. Describe what would lead you to suspect that each of the above complications had occurred.

3. Discuss the role of the district nurse in supporting this family.

BRIEF ANALYSIS AND GUIDELINES TO SUITABLE ANSWERS

Question 1
Complications from local spread for carcinoma of bronchus include:
- Haemoptysis.
- Pleural effusion.
- Pulmonary collapse and infection.
- Superior vena cava obstruction.
- Damage to recurrent laryngeal nerve.
- Dysphagia due to spread to oesophagus.
- Pericarditis and aortic obstruction.
- Horner's syndrome.

Question 2
Haemoptysis: blood-stained sputum, breathlessness with rising pulse and falling blood pressure.
Pleural effusion: sharp pain on inspiration and increasing dyspnoea.
Pulmonary collapse and infection: dyspnoea, cyanosis and pyrexia; sputum infected.
Superior vena cava obstruction: discoloration of face, neck and shoulders; engorged jugular veins; oedema of face and neck; feeling of 'fullness' in head.
Damage to recurrent laryngeal nerve: hoarseness.
Dysphagia: increasing difficulty in swallowing solid food.
Pericarditis and aortic obstruction: irregular pulse, reduced cardiac output and blood pressure.
Horner's syndrome: stimulation of sympathetic cervical fibres causing dilation of pupil, protrusion of eyeball and elevation of upper eyelid *or* paralysis causing constriction of pupil, exophthalmos and ptosis.

Question 3
Your answer should cover attention to physical, psychological, social and spiritual needs of Mr Bradshawe and his family. You should also discuss how you would assess, plan, implement and evaluate Mr Bradshawe's care.

4. What other services may the district nurse call upon to care for this family?

Question 4
Other services include:
(a) Social services: home care assistant; laundry service; aids such as bed cradle, commode, oxygen apparatus; disposable equipment including oxygen face masks, incontinence sheets, syringes, catheters.
(b) Visitors from local hospice.
(c) Night sitting service.

5. What alternatives are there if it becomes no longer possible to care for Mr Bradshawe at home?

Question 5
Your answer should include discussion on possible transfer to hospital, hospice, nursing home.

6. Describe how Mrs Bradshawe may react to her husband's death and how she may be assisted during this period.

Question 6
Relate your answer to the grieving process. See G. Garrett, *Health Needs of the Elderly*, in The Macmillan Nursing Series.

An adult with pharyngeal obstruction requiring a tracheostomy

Mrs James, aged 25 years, is admitted to the accident and emergency department for a tracheostomy under local anaesthetic with insertion of a cuffed tracheostomy tube.

A few hours ago Mrs James was enjoying a picnic with her family when she was stung by a bee at the back of the throat. Within a short period of time she became alarmed and frightened as the swelling in her throat increased causing difficulty in swallowing and breathing.

Her family bring her to the accident and emergency department where examination reveals gross pharyngeal obstruction. The following observations are made:
- Respirations laboured.
- Pulse rapid.
- Blood pressure raised.
- Pupils dilated.
- Skin pale and sweating.

SELF-TESTING QUESTIONS

BRIEF ANALYSIS AND GUIDELINES TO SUITABLE ANSWERS

1. You are working in the accident and emergency department and you are informed that a patient is coming in with acute pharyngeal obstruction.
(a) Describe what preparations you would make prior to Mrs James's arrival and (b) state how you would assess Mrs James's condition on arrival.

Question 1
(a) Your preparations should include:
- Preparation of a resuscitation room including the following equipment and medicines: oxygen and suction apparatus; emergency sterile tracheostomy set with selection of tracheostomy tubes; pharyngeal examination mirrors; emergency medicines including hydrocortisone, adrenaline; intravenous infusion apparatus; equipment for neck support.
- Allocation of one nurse to receive the patient.
- Ensure appropriate theatre staff are aware of the expected admission.
(b) Method of assessment should include:
- Measuring and recording respiration rate, depth and difficulty, chest movement on inspiration.
- Observation for presence of central cyanosis, signs of cerebral anoxia.
- Signs of increase of sympathetic activity—raised pulse, raised blood pressure, dilated pupils, sweaty skin.
- Degree of difficulty in swallowing saliva.
- Signs of anaphylactic shock, i.e., severe bronchospasm, marked drop in the blood pressure, pulse disappearing, loss of consciousness.

2. Describe the senior nurse's role in the management of Mrs James and her family while in this department.

Question 2
The senior nurse should act in the following ways:
(a) Ensure that a nurse is allocated to care for Mrs James before, during and after tracheostomy.
(b) Ensure that the relatives are informed of progress of Mrs James and given the opportunity to discuss their immediate fears and give consent if Mrs James is unable to do so.
(c) Following Mrs James's tracheostomy, give explanation to the relatives of the treatment carried out and further management.
(d) Alert the receiving ward to Mrs James's expected transfer once her condition is stable.

3. Describe how you would obtain the patient's cooperation (a) during and (b) after performance of the tracheostomy.

Question 3

Your answer should include the following explanations and support.

(a) During procedure:
- Inform Mrs James of what is to happen.
- Position and support during the procedure.
- Offer an eye shield or advise Mrs James to keep her eyes closed during the operation.
- Staying close to the patient, holding her hand and talking reassuringly.
- Ensure that the environment is calm and quiet.

(b) After procedure:
- Explain the effects of the presence of a tracheostomy tube, including difficulty in coughing and expectoration, and in speaking.
- Explain further management and possible outcome.

4. Write a care plan for Mrs James for the first forty-eight hours.

Question 4

Your answer should include:

(a) Management of the airway, with adequate supervision and education of staff in management of tubes, suction apparatus, humidifier.

(b) Need for emergency anti-inflammatory medicines, hydrocortisone and antihistamines.

(c) Patient/staff communications with use of visual aids, writing material, all within reach.

(d) Explanation and support for relatives.

(e) Offering of emotional and psychological support to Mrs James.

(f) Management of hygiene, nutrition and elimination.

(g) Management as oedema subsides and removal of tube.

5. (a) Explain the term anaphylactic shock and briefly describe why Mrs James is at risk. (b) Describe the management of this form of shock should it occur.

Question 5

(a) Anaphylactic shock is an immune reaction causing release of histamine from the mast cells following injection of an antigen. Mrs James is at risk because, in this case, the antigen is an insect sting.

(b) Treatment includes the giving of antihistamines, adrenaline and hydrocortisone.

(b) Oxygen want in patients with impairment of peripheral vascular function

1   Patient study and care plan for peripheral vascular disease causing intermittent claudication and rest pain

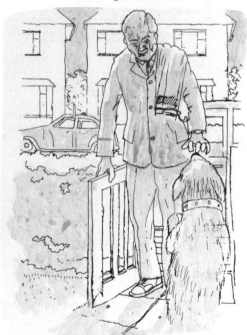

Figure 2.19   Mr Brittain

History of social, psychological and physical events leading to the present condition

The patient chosen for this section to illustrate oxygen want has impairment of peripheral vascular function causing intermittent claudication and rest pain.

Mr Brittain (Figure 2.19), aged 50 years, is employed as a postman and lives in a city suburb with his wife and his dog. His interests include supporting the local football club and tending his allotment. He smokes 30 cigarettes a day.

As a postman Mr Brittain has been used to walking in his work, making two delivery rounds each day. At the beginning of this year he was aware of heaviness in his left leg towards the end of his rounds. For the past two months he has been woken up at night with severe pain in his left foot, finding relief only when he hung his leg out of the bed. During the past two weeks he found he had to stop two or three times during his post round because of severe cramping pain in his left calf. After resting for five minutes he was able to continue and finish his post round. Up to this time he had been in good health and was concerned that his leg pain was hindering him in his work, so he attended his GP's surgery.

The GP examined Mr Brittain and found the following:

- Skin pale, dry and flaky.
- Diminished hair growth.
- Opaque ridged nails.
- Absence of sweating in the foot.
- Leg cold to the touch.
- Diminished popliteal and anterior and posterior tibial pulses.

He discussed with Mr Brittain his findings and the possibility of reduced blood flow to his left leg, and arranged for an outpatient appointment for further investigation. He gave Mr Brittain advice on how to care for his feet and avoid unnecessary trauma to skin or nails. The GP prescribed Dihydrocodeine tablets (60 mg 4-hourly) as necessary for relief of pain.

In the outpatient department the consultant who examined Mr Brittain advised urgent admission to hospital for femoral arteriogram and possible vascular surgery.

Explanation of abnormal physiology and pathology

You are advised to revise the normal arterial circulation to the lower limbs and see Table 2.5.

Table 2.5

Related normal physiology	Abnormal physiology
(a) Adequate arterial blood supply ensures oxygen and nutrients to skin, nails, hair, sweat glands of periphery	Any reduction in arterial blood reduces oxygen and nutrient supply to the tissues, giving cold, pale, dry skin with reduced sweating, loss of hair, opaque nails
(b) Whether the lower limbs are active or not, adequate blood supply is maintained by healthy heart, blood vessels and autonomic nervous system affecting smooth muscle of arterioles	Arterial blood flow to lower limbs with obstructed arteries becomes dependent on gravity and development of collateral circulation
(c) Oxygen demand is satisfied by increased blood flow	During activity obstructed arteries are unable to deliver sufficient oxygen demanded by the muscles. Obstruction of an artery can be due to atheroma and/or vasoconstricting substances, e.g., nicotine due to smoking
(d) (i) To give an increased blood flow there is a need for blood vessels that are capable of dilating to increase the amount of blood flow	(i) Metabolites resulting from metabolic activities of the tissues are vasodilator substances, but have *no* effect on diseased blood vessels
(ii) Vasodilatation is initiated by vasomotor centre and local metabolites which are released during muscle activity	(ii) Accumulation of metabolites resulting from an obstruction to blood flow to a contracting muscle causes ischaemic pain. The pain disappears within a few minutes of the circulation being restored (intermittent claudication)

Care Plan

PREPARATION FOR PATIENT WITH PERIPHERAL VASCULAR DISEASE

Nursing history and assessment
Following his admission to the surgical ward, a nursing history assessment (Table 2.6) is made and the doctor orders various investigations.

Table 2.6   Nursing history and assessment sheet for Mr Brittain

NURSING HISTORY AND ASSESSMENT SHEET

Record No. ____999999____

PATIENT LABEL

Mr/~~Mrs/Miss~~ ____Charles BRITTAIN____

Address ____11 Turnover Close, London____

Male/Female   Age ____50____

Date of Birth ____2.4.36____

Date of admission/first visit

____1.9.86____

Time ____

Type: ☐ Routine ☑ Emergency

Transfer from: ____

Religion ____C/E____

Practising/baptised ____Non-practising____

Minister ____

Telephone number ____

Next of kin (name) ____Mrs Brittain____

Relationship to patient ____Wife____

Address ____Same address____

____

Telephone numbers ____1234____

Contact at night/in emergency   YES/~~NO~~

Occupation (or father) ____Postman (full-time)____

Marital status ____Married____

Children (or place in family) ____—____

Other dependants ____—____

Pets ____Dog____

School (children only) ____

Hobbies ____Gardening (allotment)____

Clubs ____Football____

Favourite pastime ____—____

Does patient smoke?   YES/~~NO~~ 30 cigarettes a day

Speech difficulty/language barrier

Dysphasia   Dysarthria

Accommodation

Lives alone   YES/__NO__

Part III/EMI/Old People's Homes/Rented

Other ____Ground floor flat____

Consultant ____Mr Brown____

House officer ____Dr Jones____

Presenting condition ____Intermittent claudication____

History of present complaint and reason for admission

Ischaemic left leg. Severe pain in left foot and severe cramping pain in leg for past 2 months.
Urgent admission for femoral arteriogram and possible vascular surgery

Past medical history

____None____

Allergies

Current medication   4-hourly
Dihydrocodeine orally 60mg, if nec.

What patient says is the reason for admission and attitude to admission

Severe pain in left foot

Patient's expectations _Possible vascular surgery._
Optimistic of satisfactory outcome

Any problems at home while/because patient is in hospital?

_N/a_

Relevant home conditions (e.g. stairs)

____—____

Visiting problems

____—____

Care at home

Community nurse ____

No. ____

Name of GP ____Dr Smith____

Address ____The Health Centre, Turnover Road, London____

Other services involved

Home help ____   Day hospital ____

Laundry ____   Day centre/club ____

Inco supplies ____   Health visitor ____

Aids ____   Social worker ____

Meals on wheels ____   Voluntary worker ____

Daily living

Diet

Special ____—____

Food or drink dislikes ____—____

Appetite: ☑ GOOD ☐ POOR

Remarks ____

71

Sleep

How many hours normally? ___6___

Sedation _____

What else helps? _____

Elimination

Bowels: Continent/Incontinent

How often opened? ___Daily___

Any medication? _____

Urinary: Continent/Incontinent

If incontinent; Day/Night/If not taken, how frequently? _____

Nocturia/Dysuria/Frequency/Urgency

Remarks _____

Female patients — Menstruation

Post-menopausal   Taking the pill

Regular   Irregular

Amenorrhoea   Dysmenorrhoea

Next period due: _____

Uses: STs Tampons

Hearing

Hearing aid: YES/NO

Remarks _____

Vision

Glasses/Contact lens: YES/NO

Remarks _____

Oral

Dentures or crowns: YES/NO

Any problems with mouth or teeth?

_____No_____

Mobility

Help needed with:

Walking/Standing/In/Out of bed/Bathing/Dressing

In/Out of chair/

Feeding/Other: _____

Remarks ___Claudication at 800m (½ mile)___

Prosthesis/appliance

Type of appliance ___N/a___

Help needed _____

General appearance

| Normal | Dehydrated | Acutely ill |
| Obese | Thin | Emaciated |

Skin

Satisfactory	Broken areas	Dehydrated
Rash	Oedematous	Jaundiced
Pallor	Other *Left foot pale, cold,*
	(including bruising) *pressure sore*

Remarks _____

Level of consciousness

| Orientated | Semi-conscious |
| Confused | Unconscious |

Remarks _____

Mental assessment (if appropriate)

Mood

Elated	Irritable	Agitated
Cheerful	Anxious	Aggressive
Miserable	Withdrawn	Suspicious
Apathetic		

Thought content

Hallucinations/Delusions/Paranoid Ideas *N/a*

_____

Orientation

Time/Place/Person *Yes*

Very confused   Slightly confused

Any particular time of day? _____

Confabulation _____

Remarks _____

Surveillance Physical/Emotional

Information obtained from ___Patient and wife___

Relationship to patient _____

By ___A.JC___

Position/level of training _____

Date ___1·9·86___

Time _____

INVESTIGATIONS AND RESULTS

Investigations
The doctor orders the following investigations:
- Left femoral arteriogram.
- Chest x-ray.
- Electrocardiogram.
- Blood count.
- Urea and electrolytes.
- Blood grouping and cross-matching.
- Check urine and sputum for evidence of infection.
- Blood clotting times.
- Intravenous urogram.

The care plan shown in Table 2.7 is put into action for Mr Brittain.

Table 2.7   Care plan for Mr Brittain

Problem	Objective	Plan of care	Rationale
1. Urgent admission of a patient to a surgical ward	To ensure adequate arrangements have been made for work and home	(a) Discuss arrangements with patient and his wife	(a) Ensures payment of sickness benefit and notification to place of work
		(b) Ensure both are seen by medical staff and senior nurse in charge for explanation of condition, investigations and treatment	(b) Relieves anxiety, ensures cooperation of patient and relative and enables Mrs Brittain to inform their son and make suitable arrangements for visiting
2. Ischaemic left leg	To alleviate symptoms of ischaemia (pain and claudication)	(a) Encourage him to mobilise as he is able	(a) Activity improves heart action and oxygenation of blood and peripheral performance
		(b) Use gravity to assist blood flow to feet by avoidance of elevation of lower limbs and by elevating head of bed	(b) Gravity assists arterial blood flow to the periphery
		(c) Reduce oxygen demand of the left lower leg by reducing the temperature: (i) Insertion of bed cradle (ii) Use of fan	(c) Use of bed cradle reduces weight of bed clothes on painful foot and encourages loss of heat from foot by convection
		(d) Offer oral analgesia as required	(d) To ensure good night's sleep prior to investigations and surgery
		(e) Give vasodilator medicines as required	(e) These medicines dilate the blood vessels of the collateral circulation
		(f) Stop his habit of smoking	(f) Nicotine causes vasoconstriction
		(g) Offer alcohol with night sedation	(g) Alcohol increases peripheral vasodilation and reduces sensitivity to pain, enhances effect of night sedation
	To relieve pressure and detect early signs of development of pressure sores	(a) Ensure patient has comfortable footwear	(a) Prevents development of blisters and abrasions
		(b) When in bed: (i) Alter position hourly (ii) Use of aids, e.g., sheepskin boots, foam or ripple mattress, sheepskin	(b) (i) and (ii) Relieves pressure between mattress and underlying bone and prevents total occlusion of a precarious circulation
		(c) Inspect limb for discoloration, abrasion, blisters and report in writing and verbally	(c) Detection of early signs of pressure sores and/or gangrene enables modification of care plan and treatment as necessary
	To monitor the effects of the ischaemia to leg	(a) Observe the temperature, colour, sensation, movement of the limb *hourly*	(a) Refer to abnormal physiology explanation (page 70)
		(b) Measure and record pulses of anterior and posterior tibial and popliteal	(b) Any further disappearance of pulses would indicate complete occlusion
		(c) Monitor pain levels	(c) Increased pain is an indication of further extension of the occlusion
3. Patient has to undergo the listed investigations before treatment can start	Sustain the patient while waiting for investigations and their results	(a) Arrange the investigations for the coming week	(a) Minimises disruption of daily living, physical and mental exhaustion
		(b) Ensure preparation for each investigation	(b) Preparation assists a successful investigation to take place
		(c) Keep patient fully informed of each procedure and its results	(c) Gives psychological and social support
		(d) Ensure safety and comfort following each procedure	(d) Assists in early detection of complications and maintenance of daily living and physical and mental health

Results of investigations

Investigations reveal the following:

1. Discrete occlusion of the left femoral artery due to atheroma.
2. Chest, heart and kidney function normal.
3. Haemoglobin 10 g/100 ml.
4. Clotting times, urea and electrolytes within normal limits.
5. No evidence of infection in urine and sputum.

EVALUATION OF CARE AND SUGGESTED RECORD OF PROGRESS

Patient's Name ....Mr Brittain...

Date ...3.9.86... Time ...1800 hours..

QUESTIONS TO HELP YOU WITH EVALUATING CARE AND PROGRESS

Nursing actions relating to patient comfort, safety and well-being

- What is the patient's response to his/her condition?
- Are the present nursing actions still required?
- Is the patient, and his/her family, informed?

Mr Brittain is very concerned about his leg, which is now too painful to stand on and the pain has kept him awake at night. He is getting impatient at the delay in reaching a decision regarding treatment and is going to be seen by the Consultant tomorrow for full discussion.

Nursing actions pertaining to observations and measurements

- What is the patient's response to the observations and measurements being made?
- Are the present measurements/observations still required?
- Have results been seen or relayed to the appropriate practitioner/carer?
- Has the patient been informed of the changes?

Mr Brittain is aware that his foot is getting worse. Skin of foot is cyanosed and pedal pulses are difficult to find; frequency of observation has been increased to 2-hourly and the doctor has been informed. Mr Brittain is aware that the doctor has been called to see him urgently.

Nursing actions relating to diagnosis and treatment

- What is the patient's response to diagnosis and treatment?
- Are the patient's treatments still required?
- Have the course/s of treatment been completed or discontinued?
- Has the patient been informed?

Mr Brittain has little idea of the implications of his condition and the need for surgical intervention. Oral analgesia is insufficient to control rest pain and the doctor will review the medication when he comes to see Mr Brittain.

* * * * * * *

- Who has visited the patient?
- What information has been given to relatives/visitors?

His wife this afternoon. The doctor will be seeing Mr Brittain later today and the Consultant will see him tomorrow morning. She has been asked to ring or visit later tomorrow morning.

* * * * * * *

- Has the care plan been updated?
- Are the objectives/goals of care still relevant?

Yes – increased frequency of observations of leg. Objectives/goals unchanged.

Signature of Reporting Nurse ......*Susan Andrews*......

Designation ......*Student Nurse*......

Signature of Supervising Nurse ......*Denny Stewart*......

Designation ......*Senior Nurse*......

TREATMENT

In view of the results and the clinical features of his left leg a decision is made to perform a femoro-popliteal bypass graft on Mr Brittain's leg using one of his own saphenous veins. The following day Mr Brittain is prepared for operation in the usual way—in addition to the shaving of the pubis, check the need for the shaving of the left leg and for the transfusion of three units of blood.

POST-OPERATIVE PROGRESS

By the end of the operation Mr Brittain's left foot is pink, warm, has all pulses present and, on recovery from anaesthetic, he is able to feel and move his toes normally.

Mr Brittain's post-operative recovery is uneventful and oxygenation to his lower limbs is maintained, leading to satisfactory wound healing, complete absence of foot pain and resolution of claudication with increase of mobility and exercise tolerance.

2 Patient histories illustrating further problems relating to impairment of peripheral vascular function

An adult with gangrene

Mrs Cummings, aged 60 years, has been a widow for ten years. Recently she arranged for her elderly parents to stay with her in her semi-detached house on the outskirts of the city. She has been a diabetic for eight years, controlled on oral hypoglaemic agents and diet. She attends her GP on a regular basis and her diabetes is well controlled. She was given advice on care of her feet and she attends the chiropodist every two months. Six months ago when she was helping her father out of bed he trod on her left foot. She forgot the incident but several days later her great toe became painful and discoloured; it became increasingly painful and skin blisters occurred. On her routine visit to the chiropodist she was advised to seek urgent medical attention.

The doctor's examination reveals the following:
- A purplish mottled great toe with a patch of black, necrotic tissue under the flexure surface, extending around under the nail.
- Blisters oozing and offensive-smelling.
- Urine indicates glycosuria.
- Blood test shows raised blood glucose levels.

The doctor advises urgent admission to hospital for assessment and possible local amputation.

SELF-TESTING QUESTIONS

BRIEF ANALYSIS AND GUIDELINES TO SUITABLE ANSWERS

1. Explain why a seemingly trivial injury to Mrs Cummings's toe caused such severe effects.

Question 1
Refer to Chapter 6 for explanation of abnormal physiology. Your answer should include explanation of the local effects of diabetic neuropathy and peripheral vascular disease, and the susceptibility to trauma and infection.

2. Is an *obvious* injury to the foot a necessary precursor to these effects? Give reasons for your answer.

Question 2
No. Generalised peripheral vascular disease could result in arterial occlusion and development of gangrene.

3. Give a brief definition of the term 'gangrene'.

Question 3
Gangrene is death of tissue due to sudden or gradual reduction in arterial blood supply leaving tissues deprived of oxygen and nutrients. The skin becomes cyanosed, then black. If sudden occlusion occurs the skin becomes macerated and infection may become quickly superimposed. Where gradual reduction of blood flow occurs the skin becomes dry and mummified with a clear line of demarcation between dead and living tissue.

4. Devise a care plan to admit and prepare Mrs Cummings for the investigations and surgery she is likely to need.

Question 4
Your answer should include:
(a) Relevant details as in Mr Brittain's nursing history and assessment sheet.
(b) Provision of support for elderly parents at home and ongoing liaison between hospital and community. Arrangements for visiting which could include use of voluntary agencies.
(c) Investigations as in Mr Brittain's care plan (pages 72 and 74) but with the following additions:
- Fasting blood glucose levels.
- Glucose tolerance test.
- Urinalysis 3-hourly.
- Swab from wound for culture and sensitivity.

(d) Care of gangrenous toe including wound toilet and protection from further injury.
(e) Monitoring and evaluating diabetes mellitus, in respect of diet and oral hypoglycaemic agents.
(f) Management of the diabetes prior to surgery which may include temporary change to soluble insulin and intravenous dextrose.
(g) Psychological care if amputation becomes necessary.

Question 5

5. If the great toe is amputated what possible complications could occur at the wound site?

Your answer should include reference to the possibility of generalised peripheral vascular disease which may continue to result in a low oxygen tension at the wound site, leading to breakdown of the wound edges and development of infection due to reduced white cells circulating to the area.

An adult with a femoral artery embolism

Mr Forbes, aged 50 years, an assistant bank manager, is recovering in hospital following a myocardial infarction which occurred some ten days ago. His wife visits him every day and is preparing for his return home as he is now able to take gentle exercise and has not experienced any more chest pain. He has required no medication since the first forty-eight hours after admission. Despite his understandable anxiety since knowing that he has had a myocardial infarction, he is optimistic about the future.

The day before he is due to go home he notices a sudden sensation of tingling pins and needles in his right leg and blotchiness of the skin. He tries to walk to relieve the discomfort but finds his leg heavy and difficult to use. He calls a nurse who observes that the whole limb is pale with blue blotches and the skin is cold with reduced sensitivity to touch. She assists Mr Forbes back to his bed and calls the doctor. On examination he finds signs of anaesthesia, paralysis and serious ischaemia with absent peripheral pulses. This leads him to suspect that Mr Forbes has a femoral artery embolism and needs urgent surgical intervention.

SELF-TESTING QUESTIONS

1. Explain the significance of Mr Forbes's femoral artery embolism following myocardial infarction.

BRIEF ANALYSIS AND GUIDELINES TO SUITABLE ANSWERS

Question 1
Your answer should include description of the formation of a mural thrombus on the lining of the wall on the left ventricle following myocardial infarction which then becomes detached, passes into the aorta and becomes lodged in the systemic circulation. This can occur 10 days after the infarction.

Question 2
The occlusion will be sudden, causing the features tabulated below.

2. Discuss the clinical features of arterial occlusion due to embolism.

Clinical features	Explanation of abnormal physiology
(a) Sudden skin pallor and blue blotchiness of the skin	Pallor due to sudden lack of arterial blood to the limb. Blue blotchiness due to stagnation of blood in the limb
(b) Absence of peripheral pulses	Complete occlusion of blood flow to periphery
(c) Limb remains blue and becomes cold	The oxygen is used up from the stagnant blood in the limb
(d) Limb becomes paraesthetic and eventually anaesthetic	The sensory nerves are deprived of oxygen
(e) Limb becomes paralysed	The motor nerves fail to transmit impulses to the muscle fibres due to lack of oxygen
(f) Limb becomes necrotic if blood supply not restored within maximum of 6 to 8 hours	All tissues deprived of oxygen and nutrients for a prolonged period will die

3. Identify the essential preparation for Mr Forbes and his wife prior to femoral embolectomy.

Question 3
Your answer should include the following:
(a) An opportunity for discussion and explanation, and obtaining consent for operation under local anaesthetic, if necessary, in view of recent history of myocardial infarction.
(b) Preparation for arteriogram possibly in operating theatre.
(c) Emptying of stomach.
(d) Establishment of intravenous infusion and estimation of prothrombin and clotting time.
(e) Monitoring and recording of the ischaemic effects.
(f) Protection of the limb from pressure and injury.
(g) Cooling of the limb to minimise oxygen demand.

4. Following successful embolectomy state what signs and symptoms would lead you to seek *immediate* medical aid.

Question 4
(a) Swelling under the incision or bleeding from the wound due to leakage from the sutured artery.
(b) Any sudden reversion to features described in answer to question 2 which could indicate thrombus in the operated artery or rupture of the suture line of the artery.

An adult with Raynaud's disease

Jane Williams, a 22-year-old typist, has suffered with hypersensitivity to cold, which affects both hands, for the past three years. In winter she experiences episodes when her fingers become white and painful. She was diagnosed as having Raynaud's disease last year and since then has found that the number of occasions when she has difficulty in typing is increasing despite avoiding putting her hands in cold water and exposing them to cold. The doctor has advised conservative measures only, such as wearing warm but loose fitting gloves to avoid exposure to cold. Now she notices that after a period when her fingers turn white they then go blue and after some minutes they become red, swollen and painful before returning to normal.

SELF-TESTING QUESTIONS

BRIEF ANALYSIS AND GUIDELINES TO SUITABLE ANSWERS

1. What is the basic clinical feature of Raynaud's disease?

Question 1
Raynaud's disease is the sudden constriction of the arterioles leading to the skin of the fingers.

2. What are the triggers for episodes of this condition?

Question 2
Commonly, (a) exposure to cold causing physiological constriction of blood vessels and (b) in some patients due to autonomic nervous system activity as a result of intense emotion.

3. Explain the sequence of physiological changes in the skin during episodes of this condition when oxygen deprivation occurs.

Question 3
Your answer should include the following features and physiological explanations. Hypersensitivity to cold causes vasoconstriction — fingers go white. Stagnation of blood — fingers go blue. Reactive hyperaemia — fingers go red, are swollen and painful.

4. Repeated attacks of vasoconstriction and ischaemia may result in permanent effects of atrophy of the skin and pulp of the fingers and eventually gangrene of the finger tips. What treatment is available for severe disability or threatening gangrene?

Question 4
Your answer should include:
(a) Explanation of sympathetic activity in relation to arterial constriction (refer to J. H. Green, *Basic Clinical Physiology,* Oxford University Press, 1979).
(b) Use of vasodilator medicines.
(c) Possibility of surgical operation of cervical sympathectomy (refer to R. E. Horton, *Vascular Surgery*, Unibooks, 1980).

(c) Oxygen want in patients with impairment of oxygen-carrying capacity of the blood

1 Patient study and care plan for pernicious anaemia

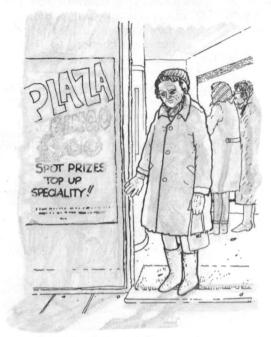

Figure 2.20 Mrs Browning

History of social, psychological and physical events leading to the present condition

The patient chosen for this section to illustrate impairment of oxygen-carrying capacity of the blood is an adult with pernicious anaemia.

Mrs Browning (Figure 2.20), aged 62 years, lives with her husband, a retired motor mechanic, in a terraced house in a city suburb. It is an established, closely knit community and her three married children and her grandchildren all live nearby. She is interested in weekly attendance at Bingo and activities at the local community centre. She has been physically fit and has only recently retired from her part-time job in the baker's shop. Over the past few weeks she began to feel tired and found it an effort to carry on with her usual activities. She became concerned when she found herself getting breathless on hurrying to catch the bus and when her daughter remarked that she looked pale and unwell. She decided to visit her GP after experiencing palpitations and dizziness during one of her visits to the Bingo hall.

On examination and discussion the doctor found the following:

- A history of recent anorexia and weight loss but despite this Mrs Browning was well-nourished.
- Skin and mucous membranes pale with a slight yellow tint.
- Tongue red and smooth.
- Some paraesthesia in fingers and toes but Mrs Browning hadn't noticed this until questioned.

She gave no history of dietary inadequacy, of any bleeding or of receiving any medication. A blood sample was taken and this revealed a macrocytic anaemia with reduction in white blood cells and platelets. The doctor suspected a diagnosis of vitamin B12 deficiency and arranged for Mrs Browning to be admitted to hospital for further investigations.

Explanation of abnormal physiology and pathology

You are advised to revise the factors necessary for the formation and function of the red blood cell, and for the absorption and utilisation of vitamin B12. Anaemia is a condition in which there is a reduced oxygen-carrying capacity of the blood (see Table 2.8).

Table 2.8

Normal physiology	Abnormal physiology
(a) The function of the red blood cell is to carry oxygen to all tissues of the body	If the oxygen-carrying capacity is reduced: (i) Reduced oxygen to tissues leads to lethargy and dizziness (ii) Compensatory mechanisms increase the heart rate in an attempt to deliver more blood/oxygen to the tissues. Patients often complain of palpitations (iii) Reduced oxygen in the blood results in pallor of the skin and mucous membrane
(b) Absorption and utilisation of vitamin B12 is necessary for the development of red blood cells, healthy peripheral nerves and healthy tongue. Vitamin B12 is found in wholemeal products, liver and meat extracts. For it to be absorbed the mucous lining of the stomach secretes the intrinsic factor which combines with vitamin B12 and both are absorbed in the terminal ileum and stored in the liver until required. The liver is able to store adequate supplies of vitamin B12 for up to two years	The gastric mucosa atrophies and fails to produce intrinsic factor and hydrochloric acid. Without intrinsic factor the absorption of vitamin B12 cannot take place. As stores of the vitamin in the liver diminish, the production of mature red blood cells is reduced, and immature red blood cells are released into the circulation. The peripheral nerves are affected, giving paraesthesia and, if untreated, subacute combined degeneration of the spinal cord. The tongue becomes smooth, red and painful
(c) Mature red blood cells are destroyed by the reticulo-endothelial system after approximately 120 days	Immature, abnormal red blood cells are destroyed earlier, resulting in excess urobilinogen in the urine and yellow tinge to the skin
(d) Gastric mucosa produces gastric juices to allow normal dietary intake	Atrophy of the gastric mucosa results in reduction in gastric juice and hydrochloric acid leading to dyspepsia, anorexia and weight loss

Care plan

PREPARATION FOR PATIENT WITH PERNICIOUS ANAEMIA

On admission to the medical ward of the local hospital, Mrs Browning is greeted by the nurse and both she and her husband are shown to her bed and given a brief explanation of the proposed investigations which are to be carried out. Mr Browning is given the telephone number of the ward and details concerning visiting.

Nursing history and assessment
The nurse responsible for Mrs Browning explains that she wishes to obtain some information from her in order to fill in the nursing history and assessment sheet which will help in planning Mrs Browning's care during her stay in hospital (see Table 2.9).

Table 2.9   Nursing history and assessment sheet for Mrs Browning

NURSING HISTORY AND ASSESSMENT SHEET
Record No. _____ *666666* _____

PATIENT LABEL	Type: ☑ Routine ☐ Emergency
Mr/Mrs/Miss *Elaine Browning*	Transfer from: _____
Address *6 Stanley Villas, Beaumont*	Religion *Methodist*
Male/Female Age *62*	Practising/baptised *Practising*
Date of Birth *8.12.24*	Minister _____
	Telephone number _____
Date of admission/first visit	
15.12.86	Next of kin (name) *Mr Browning*
Time _____	Relationship to patient *Husband*

Table 2.9 (cont.)

Address _____*Same address*_____

Telephone numbers _____*1234 (Neighbour - Mrs White)*_____
Contact at night/in emergency   YES/NO

Occupation (or father) _____*Retired shop assistant*_____
Marital status _____*Married*_____
Children (or place in family) _____*3 (all married)*_____
Other dependants _____
Pets _____
School (children only) _____
Hobbies _____*Bingo*_____
Clubs _____*Local community centre*_____
Favourite pastime _____
Does patient smoke?   YES/<u>NO</u>

Speech difficulty/language barrier

Dysphasia   Dysarthria

Accommodation

Lives alone   YES/<u>NO</u>

Part III/EMI/Old People's Homes/Rented
Other _____*Own terraced house*_____

Consultant _____*Mr Surrey*_____
House officer _____*Dr Green*_____
Presenting condition _____*Anaemia*_____

History of present complaint and reason for admission
_____*Recent anorexia and weight loss.*_____
_____*Pernicious anaemia*_____

Past medical history
_____*Past health good*_____

Allergies *None*

Current medication
_____*None*_____

What patient says is the reason for admission and attitude to admission
_____*Anaemia*_____

Patient's expectations

Any problems at home while/because patient is in hospital?

Relevant home conditions (e.g. stairs)
_____*Stairs*_____

Visiting problems

Care at home

Community nurse _____
No. _____
Name of GP _____*Dr White*_____
Address _____*The Health Centre, Beaumont*_____
Other services involved

Home help _____		Day hospital _____
Laundry _____		Day centre/club _____
Inco supplies _____		Health visitor _____
Aids _____		Social worker _____
Meals on wheels _____		Voluntary worker _____

Daily living

Diet

Special _____
Food or drink dislikes _____

Appetite: ☑GOOD ☐POOR
Remarks _____*Some pain, sore tongue and occasional dyspepsia*_____

Sleep

How many hours normally? _____*6-7*_____
Sedation _____*No*_____
What else helps? _____

Elimination

Bowels: Continent/~~Incontinent~~
How often opened? _____*Daily*_____
Any medication? _____*No*_____
Urinary: Continent/~~Incontinent~~
If incontinent; Day/Night/If not taken, how frequently? _____

Nocturia/Dysuria/Frequency/Urgency

Remarks _____

Female patients — Menstruation

<u>Post menopausal</u>	Taking the pill
Regular	Irregular
Amenorrhoea	Dysmenorrhoea

Next period due: _____
Uses: STs Tampons

Hearing

Hearing aid: YES/NO
Remarks _____

Vision

Glasses/Contact lens: YES/NO
Remarks _____*For reading/TV*_____

Oral

Dentures or crowns: YES/<u>NO</u>

Any problems with mouth or teeth?

_____

Mobility

Help needed with:

Walking/Standing/In/Out of bed/Bathing/Dressing

In/Out of chair/

Feeding/Other: _____

Remarks *Breathlessness on exertion*

Prosthesis/appliance

Type of appliance _____

Help needed _____

General appearance

Normal	Dehydrated	Acutely ill
Obese	Thin	Emaciated

Remarks *Recent weight loss*

Skin

Satisfactory	Broken areas	Dehydrated
Rash	Oedematous	Jaundiced
Pallor		

Other *Tongue red and*
(including bruising) *smooth*

Remarks _____

Level of consciousness

Orientated	Semi-conscious
Confused	Unconscious

Remarks _____

Mental assessment (if appropriate)

Mood

Elated	Irritable	Agitated
Cheerful	Anxious	Aggressive
Miserable	Withdrawn	Suspicious
Apathetic		

Thought content

Hallucinations/Delusions/Paranoid Ideas

_____

Orientation

Time/Place/Person *Yes*

Very confused   Slightly confused

Any particular time of day? _____

Confabulation _____

Remarks _____

Surveillance   Physical/Emotional
Information obtained from *Patient and Husband*

Relationship to patient _____

By _____ *P. Brown* _____

Position/level of training _____

Date _____ *15·12·86* _____

Time _____

INVESTIGATIONS AND RESULTS

Investigations

After examining Mrs Browning the doctor orders the following investigations:

1. Blood specimens for:
   - Full blood count and examination.
   - Serum vitamin B12.
   - Serum bilirubin.
   - Haemoglobin.
2. Bone marrow puncture.
3. Schilling test.

The care plan for Mrs Browning (Table 2.10) is implemented, including investigations listed above.

Table 2.10   Care plan for Mrs Browning

Problem	Objective	Plan of care	Rationale
1. Patient is suffering the effects of oxygen want due to anaemia	Minimise and relieve the effects of oxygen want	(a) Provide adequate rest and avoid over-exertion by assisting with hygiene and elimination and by anticipating her needs	(a) Reduces the demand for oxygen by the tissues
		(b) Position sitting upright	(b) Allows easier ventilation of lungs
		(c) Give oxygen therapy if necessary after unavoidable exertion	(c) Improves the oxygen uptake by the blood
		(d) Prepare patient and equipment for blood transfusion	(d) Raises haemoglobin level in the blood and improves oxygen-carrying capacity

Table 2.10 (cont.)

Problem	Objective	Plan of care	Rationale
		(e) Monitor patient during blood transfusion of packed cells: (i) Ensure correct blood group, rhesus factor, identity and that it is within expiry date	(i) Prevents transfusion of incompatible blood
		(ii) Observe and regulate rate of transfusion and record on fluid balance chart	(ii) Prevents overloading of the circulation by transfusion
		(iii) Observe patient for signs of over-transfusion—raised blood pressure, rapid pulse, difficulty in breathing. Frusemide may be given to reduce blood volume	(iii) Increased fluid volume in the circulation could result in heart failure
		(iv) Observe patient for signs of incompatible blood transfusion—raised temperature, loin pain, chest pain, jaundice, oliguria	(iv) Incompatible blood causes haemolysis and/or agglutination of the recipient's red blood cells
		(v) Observe the cannulation site for leakage into the tissues, inflammation and thrombophlebitis	(v) The cannula is a foreign body and is a direct route for infection into the blood circulation
2. Anorexia and dyspepsia	Relieve symptoms of anorexia and dyspepsia	Give small, light, easily digestible meals, high-protein drinks and multivitamin supplements	Minimises weight loss and encourages adequate nutrition
3. Investigations: (a) Involving venepuncture for various listed blood tests	Minimise discomfort	(a) Ensure that all tests are ordered and obtained at same time if possible	Minimises infection risk and trauma to patient
(b) Bone marrow biopsy	Minimise discomfort and ensure safety	(b) (i) Prepare patient by explanation and reassurance	(i) Relieves anxiety
		(ii) Prepare equipment and check sterility	(ii) Minimises introduction of infection
		(iii) Allocate a nurse to stay with the patient	(iii) Gives reassurance and confidence
		(iv) Apply pressure to puncture site on conclusion and maintain observations of site for leakage of blood during the two hours that follow	(iv) Stops bleeding and minimises bruising and risk of shock
(c) Schilling test	To ensure that patient knows what is required of her during this investigation	(c) (i) Explain to the patient that she will not be able to have anything to eat or drink on the evening before the test and until after the dose of radioactive B12 which will be given by mouth in the morning. She will be asked to empty her bladder prior to commencement of the test	(i) Empty stomach is necessary for estimation of production of intrinsic factor when radioactive B12 is given
		(ii) Give injection of 1000 micrograms non-radioactive B12 intramuscularly	(ii) Floods the body's stores and ensures excretion by the kidneys of any of the radioactive B12 absorbed
		(iii) Tell patient that all urine passed in the next 24 hours must be saved	(iii) Used for estimation of amount of radioactive B12 that is absorbed and excreted in the urine
			NB Normal persons eliminate 15-50% of the given dose in the urine but patients with pernicious anaemia eliminate less than 10%

Results of tests

The investigations carried out on admission show the following results:
1. Blood tests:
   - Full blood count and examination: macrocytic anaemia; larger than normal red blood cells, oval in shape; reduction in white blood cells; moderate reduction in platelets.
   - Serum B12: reduced.
   - Serum bilirubin: raised.
   - Haemoglobin: 6 g/100 ml of blood.
2. Bone marrow biopsy:
   - Megaloblasts present.
   - Reduced white cell and platelet production.
3. Schilling test: reduced excretion of administered radioactive B12.

TREATMENT

The tests confirm the diagnosis of pernicious anaemia and vitamin B12 replacement therapy is started immediately in the form of hydroxocobalamin, 1000 micrograms by intramuscular injection, twice in the first week and then to continue weekly until the blood count returns to normal.

Mrs Browning and her husband receive a full explanation regarding her condition and the necessity to continue treatment for life as she will never be able to absorb vitamin B12 in the normal way. She is told that eventually she will need monthly injections and yearly blood tests for estimation of red and white cells, platelets and haemoglobin levels. It is explained that she could return home and to normal activities after an initial quiet period. The nurse arranges for her to receive twice weekly injections of vitamin B12 and repeat blood test at her local health centre.

2 Patient histories illustrating further problems relating to impairment of oxygen-carrying capacity of the blood

An adult with iron-deficiency anaemia

Mr Old, aged 72 years, lives alone following the death of his wife one year ago. His only son and family live in Canada.

During the past year he has found difficulty in adjusting to life alone and is reluctant to shop and cook for himself, but remains very independent and reluctant to seek social contact. Over the last few weeks he seemed lacking in energy and found it difficult to get out of bed in the mornings. He found it an increasing effort to do his shopping and small amount of housework as he became breathless easily, and frequently needed to stop and rest. A neighbour became concerned about him as he seemed listless, pale and tired. She offered to make an appointment for him to see his GP, to which he reluctantly agreed.

After examination and discussion the doctor diagnoses iron-deficiency anaemia.

SELF-TESTING QUESTIONS

1. Discuss the possible causes of iron-deficiency anaemia.

2. Devise a care plan for Mr Old's management at home under the care of the community staff.

BRIEF ANALYSIS AND GUIDELINES TO SUITABLE ANSWERS

Question 1
Refer to your teacher for guidance to a suitable textbook.

Question 2
Your answer should include:
(a) Support of Mr Old while the doctor investigates the cause of the anaemia.
(b) Education and monitoring regarding diet and cooking.
(c) Consideration immediately regarding meals-on-wheels and/or attendance at a luncheon club.
(d) Assistance with social rehabilitation, for example, putting him in touch with local men's clubs.
(e) Offering financial advice if required.
(f) Arranging a home assessment by the occupational therapy department with reference to cooking facilities.
(g) Ensuring adequate supplies of iron supplements and monitoring his recovery.
(h) Monitoring unwanted effects of iron therapy.

3. Explain the complications which may occur in an elderly person with anaemia.

Your answer should include the fact that the reduced oxygen-carrying capacity of the blood can produce exacerbation of:

- Chronic heart failure.
- Peripheral vascular disease.
- Cerebral anoxia and dementia.
- Hypothermia.

An adult with sickle-cell anaemia (haemolytic anaemia)

Mr Joseph, a 30-year-old Nigerian businessman, lives with his wife and family in a flat in a large city. He went to his doctor complaining of sudden weakness, breathlessness and vomiting. He felt hot and feverish and had a feeling of fullness in the left side of his abdomen. The doctor examined him and found evidence of severe anaemia, with yellow-tinged sclera and an enlarged spleen. The doctor arranged for a blood test and, after seeing the results, diagnoses sickle-cell anaemia and advises admission to hospital for a blood transfusion.

SELF-TESTING QUESTIONS

1. What do you understand by the following terms: (a) sickle-cell anaemia, (b) haemolytic anaemia?

2. Explain why a patient with sickle-cell anaemia may be at risk during general anaesthesia.

3. Discuss other causes of haemolytic anaemia in all age groups and give an outline of the management of each cause.

4. Describe what advice should be given to Mr Joseph following this diagnosis.

BRIEF ANALYSIS AND GUIDELINES TO SUITABLE ANSWERS

Question 1
Refer to J. Macleod (Ed.), *Davidson's Principles and Practice of Medicine*, 14th edition, Churchill Livingstone, London, 1984.

Question 2
During general anaesthesia the oxygen tension may be lowered, precipitating an acute crisis. For further reading see J. H. Green, *Basic Clinical Physiology*, 3rd edition, Oxford University Press, London, 1979.

Question 3
Your answer should include:
Causes
(a) Hereditary causes:
- Hereditary spherocytosis.
- Thalassaemia.

(b) Acquired causes:
- Haemolytic disease of the newborn—rhesus incompatibility.
- ABO blood group incompatibility.
- For other acquired haemolytic anaemias refer to J. C. Houston, C. L. Joiner and J. R. Trounce, *A Short Textbook of Medicine*, Unibooks; 7th edition, Hodder and Stoughton, London, 1982.

Management
(a) Symptomatic treatment of the symptoms of oxygen 'want'.
(b) Specific treatment of the cause.

Question 4
Your answer should include explanation of the need to inform his dentist and any doctor giving emergency treatment and/or any admission to hospital.

An adult with aplastic anaemia

Miss Simpson, aged 45 years, has had rheumatoid arthritis for the past ten years. Her medication has recently been changed to include phenylbutazone as an anti-inflammatory agent. During this time Miss Simpson has developed the symptoms and signs of anaemia, as well as painful throat ulcers and a purpuric rash. Being the nurse in charge of a local geriatric hospital she realises the importance of these symptoms and the necessity to seek medical advice urgently.

Following discussion and examination, Miss Simpson's doctor advises her to discontinue phenylbutazone immediately and prescribes an alternative anti-inflammatory medicine. He arranges for her to be admitted to hospital as she is severely anaemic from the toxic effects of phenylbutazone. Blood tests reveal reduced haemoglobin, leucopenia and thrombocytopenia. She is prescribed a blood transfusion for the correction of the anaemia and antibiotics for the ulceration of her throat.

Soon after admission Miss Simpson experiences a severe epistaxis that requires local diathermy and a platelet transfusion. Bone marrow biopsy reveals a severe bone marrow depression and a course of steroid therapy is commenced in the form of prednisolone 60 mg orally daily to stimulate the bone marrow.

SELF-TESTING QUESTIONS

1. Devise a care plan for Miss Simpson for the first twenty-four hours.

BRIEF ANALYSIS AND GUIDELINES FOR SUITABLE ANSWERS

Question 1
Your answer should include:
(a) Relieving the effects of oxygen want (refer to care plan for Mrs Browning, pages 81–82).
(b) Minimising the risks of infection and detection of early signs of infection in a patient with leucopenia.
(c) Minimising the effects and detection of incidence of bleeding due to thrombocytopenia.
(d) Management of a patient receiving steroid therapy.
(e) Management of Miss Simpson's difficulties as a result of rheumatoid arthritis.

2. Describe briefly other possible causes of aplastic anaemia.

Question 2
Your answer should include idiopathic, toxic reaction to certain drugs, e.g., chloramphenicol, sulphonamides, indomethacin, carbimazole, heavy metals, gold, excessive exposure to x-rays or radioactive materials.

3. Discuss the possible outcomes of Miss Simpson's depressed bone marrow.

Question 3
Your answer should include:
(a) The possibility of recovery and return to normal function.
(b) The possibility of failure of the bone marrow to recover resulting in the need for repeated transfusions and prompt treatment of any infections.
(c) The discussion of a bone marrow transplant.

A child with acute lymphatic leukaemia

Wayne, aged 4 years, was taken to his doctor by his mother because she noticed that he seemed to be rather quiet and listless and had developed several large bruises. During the past 6 months, since joining the local playgroup, he has had repeated colds and upper respiratory infections.

On examination the doctor found the following:
- Mucous membranes pale.
- A few enlarged nodes in the neck.
- Enlarged spleen.

He arranged for a blood test, the results of which confirmed the diagnosis of acute leukaemia: red blood cells and platelets severely reduced in number; white blood cells increased in number but 90% approximately are immature blast cells.

The doctor advises Wayne's mother that he needs to be admitted to hospital for assessment and commencement of treatment. She is distressed at this news and is anxious about her son, and about his younger sister and elder brother, who are at home being cared for by a neighbour.

SELF-TESTING QUESTIONS

1. Devise a care plan for the problems listed below that will be encountered when nursing Wayne in hospital.

(a) Involvement of the mother in caring for Wayne.

(b) Small child with oxygen want.

(c) Risk of developing infection.

BRIEF ANALYSIS AND GUIDELINES TO SUITABLE ANSWERS

Question 1
Your answer should include:

(a) Involvement of mother in caring for Wayne by allowing her to participate in as many aspects of his care as possible. Sensitive explanation of procedures that are used.
(b) Small child with oxygen want:
- Consideration to the prevention of over-exertion.
- Use of oxygen tent.
- Blood transfusion.
- Choice of suitable play.
(c) Small child with risk of developing infection:
- Isolation in a cubicle and use of barrier nursing procedures.
- Observation for early signs of infections and prompt administration of antibiotics.
- Psychological care of a child in isolation.

(d) Risk of bleeding.

(e) Depletion of social contact of brother, sister, mother and grandparents.

(f) Choice of suitable play.

(g) Preparation and ongoing support for frightening investigations and treatment.

(d) Small child with risk of bleeding:
- Care in handling.
- Choice of safe toys.
- Reporting of new bruises or bleeding from gums when cleaning teeth or from the nose.

(e) Depletion of social contact:
- Encourage siblings to visit and play with Wayne.
- Involve mother and grandparents with his care.
- Allocate a particular nurse to enable relationships to develop.

(f) Refer to above problems and gain mother's cooperation and help.

(g) Preparation for frightening investigations and treatment which may include:
- Blood tests.
- Bone marrow puncture.
- X-rays.
- Blood transfusion.
- Intravenous infusion and lumbar puncture for giving cytotoxic drugs.
- Radiotherapy.

Preparation and after care requires involvement of Wayne's mother and his brother and sister by using appropriate play and a calm sensitive approach. Opportunity should be given for Wayne's mother to talk about her worries.

Question 2

Cytotoxic drugs aim to destroy the leukaemic cells and allow recovery of normal red and white cells and platelet production.

2. Explain the aims of drug treatment for Wayne's condition.

Question 3

Refer to your teacher for guidance to suitable pharmacology textbook.

3. Describe the possible unwanted effects of cytotoxic therapy.

Question 4

She may experience the following fears:

4. What possible fears may Wayne's mother have for the future?

(a) Whether Wayne will recover sufficiently to start school and be able to live a normal childhood.

(b) Effects of Wayne's illness on his brother and sister and whether they will develop leukaemia.

(c) Her ability to cope with the present and future demands.

(d) Lack of understanding of her friends and relatives and social isolation.

An adult with chronic myeloid leukaemia

Mr Alexander, aged 50 years, a local plumber, is married and lives with his wife in a council house. He has lately complained of progressive tiredness and dragging sensation in his abdomen. His wife becomes concerned because recently he has become anxious, lost weight and suffered from night sweats. She persuades him to visit his GP.

After examination, the GP makes a provisional diagnosis based on the symptoms described and from the grossly enlarged spleen. Blood count tests reveal severe anaemia and greatly increased white cell count. The GP arranges for Mr Alexander to be admitted to the local hospital for assessment and commencement of treatment.

SELF-TESTING QUESTIONS

BRIEF ANALYSIS AND GUIDELINES TO SUITABLE ANSWERS

Question 1

For answer see care plan for Mrs Browing (pages 81–82).

1. Recall the management of a patient with oxygen lack due to severe anaemia and risk of infection due to abnormal white cells.

Question 2

Your answer should include details of wanted and unwanted effects.

2. Mr Alexander may be prescribed radiotherapy to his enlarged spleen. What may be the effects of this treatment?

(a) Wanted effects:
- Reduction in spleen size.
- Fall in abnormal white cell count.
- Improvement of anaemia by reducing excessive destruction of red blood cells.

(b) Unwanted effects:
- Anorexia.
- Diarrhoea/constipation.
- Depression.
- General effects of radiotherapy.

Chapter 3

Nursing patients with hypovolaemic and cardiogenic shock

Normal maintenance of blood pressure and circulation

(a) The heart and circulation

The cardiovascular system consists of an enclosed tubular system comprising the *heart, arteries, veins* and *capillaries,* through which *blood* flows. Its function is the *transportation* around the body of oxygen, carbon dioxide, water, ions, nutrients, hormones, waste products of metabolism, and cells and molecules involved with the defence of the body against disease.

1 The action of the heart

The heart is the pump of the system and consists of four chambers: the right and left *atria (auricles)* and the right and left *ventricles,* as shown in Figure 3.1.

Deoxygenated blood returning from the body enters the right atrium from the *superior* and *inferior venae cavae*, and then passes into the right ventricle.

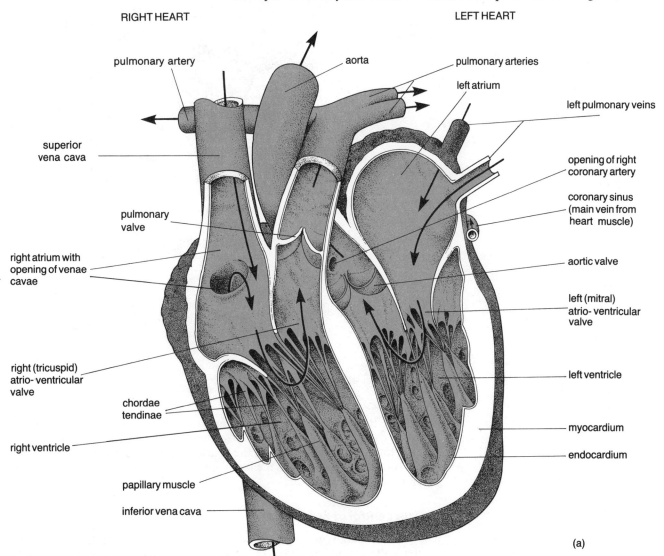

RIGHT HEART   LEFT HEART

pulmonary artery — aorta — pulmonary arteries — left atrium — left pulmonary veins — superior vena cava — opening of right coronary artery — coronary sinus (main vein from heart muscle) — pulmonary valve — right atrium with opening of venae cavae — aortic valve — left (mitral) atrio- ventricular valve — right (tricuspid) atrio- ventricular valve — chordae tendinae — left ventricle — right ventricle — myocardium — endocardium — papillary muscle — inferior vena cava

(a)

Figure 3.1   Anatomy of the heart. (a) Hinged open and with the interventricular wall removed

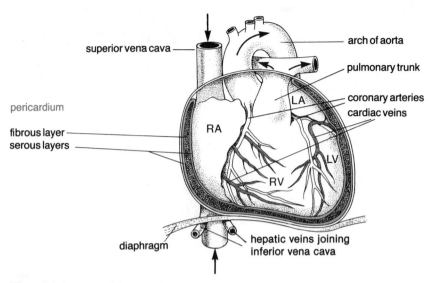

superior vena cava

arch of aorta

pulmonary trunk

coronary arteries

cardiac veins

pericardium

fibrous layer
serous layers

RA

LA

LV

RV

diaphragm

hepatic veins joining
inferior vena cava

Figure 3.1 Anatomy of the heart (continued). (b) The external appearance

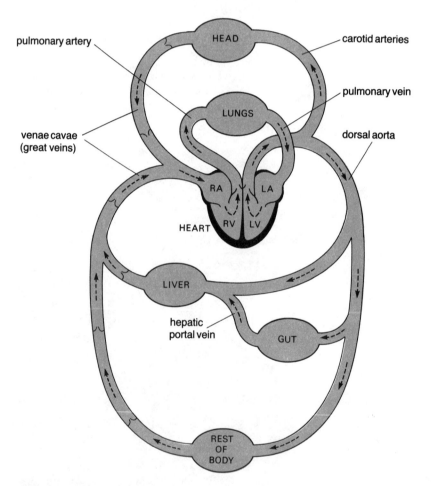

pulmonary artery

HEAD

carotid arteries

LUNGS

pulmonary vein

venae cavae
(great veins)

dorsal aorta

RA LA

HEART RV LV

LIVER

hepatic
portal vein

GUT

REST
OF
BODY

Figure 3.2   Circulation of the blood

From here it is pumped into the *pulmonary circulatory system* and the blood becomes oxygenated during its course through the lungs. This oxygenated blood returns to the left atrium of the heart, then passes into the left ventricle, which, on contraction, pumps the blood into the *aorta* on the start of its course around the body (Figure 3.2).

2   The control of heart beat

The heart undergoes contraction *(systole)* and relaxation *(diastole)* rhythmically throughout life. As blood returns (during diastole) to the right atrium the pressure of it in this chamber forces open the flaps of the *atrioventricular valve* (also called the *tricuspid* valve because it consists of three flaps), and blood flows into the right ventricle. When the atrium and ventricle are full of blood, the atrium suddenly contracts, forcing its remaining blood into the ventricle. The pulmonary valve is closed during this filling. The contraction (systole) spreads from the right atrium over the rest of the heart. The atrial systole is comparatively weak, but the ventricles, which have much thicker muscles (Figure 3.3), contract much more powerfully, and, as a result, blood is pumped from the right ventricle into the pulmonary artery. Blood is prevented from flowing back into the atrium by the flaps of the atrio-ventricular valve, which close tightly and are prevented from turning inside-out by tough strands of connective tissue, the *tendinous cords* or heart strings, running from the ventricle walls to the undersides of the valve flaps.

Simultaneous with this cycle of blood flow and pumping in the right heart, the blood returning from the lungs to the left atrium flows and is pumped into the left ventricle. The aortic valve is closed during ventricular filling but opens when the blood is pumped powerfully by the left ventricle into the aorta. The *mitral valve* is now closed. So, although systole starts in the right atrium, and the two sides of the heart are two distinct pumps, their action is simultaneous, and the whole heart contracts at the same time. Figure 3.4 summarises the cycle of one heart beat.

This pattern of blood movement is accompanied by electrical activity in the wall of the heart, and by 'heart sounds' which correspond to the closing of the various valves. Each ventricle contains the same volume of blood just before

The *thickness* of the muscle is related to the amount of work it has to do:

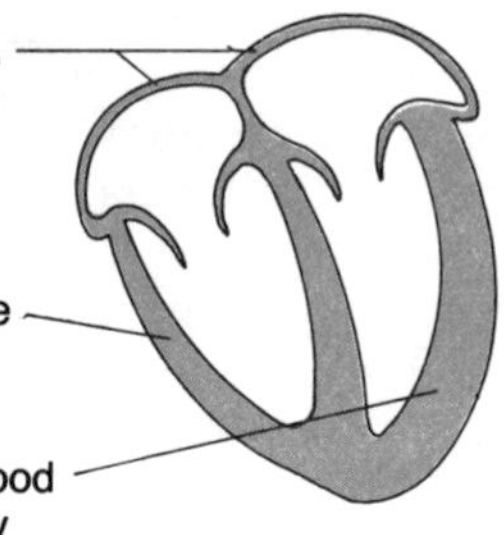

thinnest in the atria, enough to squeeze blood into the ventricles

thicker in the right ventricle to send the blood to the lungs

thickest in the left ventricle to send blood right round the body

Figure 3.3 Thickness of heart muscle

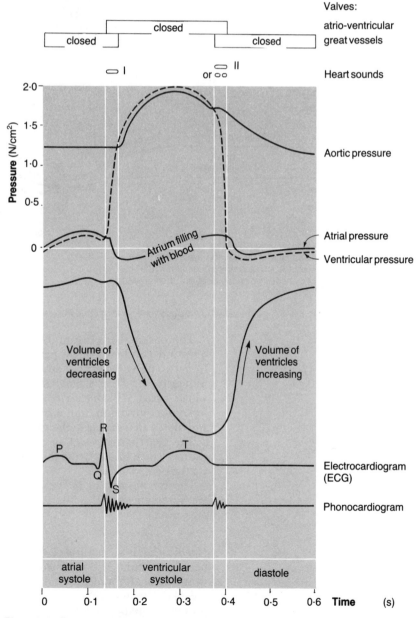

Figure 3.4 Pressure and volume changes during the cardiac cycle

systole, and so equal volumes of blood are pumped into the pulmonary system and into the systemic circulation. This volume is approximately 70 ml of blood pumped from each ventricle at each contraction, and this is described as the *stroke volume*. Stroke volume multiplied by heart rate (approximately 70 beats/minute at rest) is the *cardiac output*, which amounts to about 5 litres per minute when the body is at rest. This can increase to 30 litres per minute on exercise. The ventricles can only pump out blood which they receive, so that cardiac output is dependent upon venous return.

Cardiac muscle has the remarkable property of contracting rhythmically without fatigue. It consists of a network of muscle fibres interconnected by bridges which ensure a rapid and uniform spread of excitation throughout the heart wall, thus ensuring synchronous contraction. Cardiac muscle is *myogenic*, rhythmical contractions arising from within the muscle itself. A piece of living heart muscle, if excised, will beat on its own: atrial muscle at about 60 beats per minute, and ventricular muscle at about 25 beats per minute. However, there is a specialised plexus of fine cardiac muscle fibres embedded in the wall of the right atrium close to the point at which the great veins enter it. This will continue to beat at 70 beats per minute if excised, and is the *pacemaker* or sinu-atrial node of the heart. It produces electrical impulses, which spread out in all directions across the walls of both atria, causing them to contract. When the wave of impulses reaches the junction between the atria and the ventricles, it excites another specialised group of cardiac muscle fibres called the *atrioventricular node*. This is continuous with a bundle of modified muscle fibres called the *atrioventricular bundle* or *bundle of His*, which runs down the inter-ventricular septum and fans out over the ventricle walls, forming a sheet of fine fibres called the Purkinje tissue just below the endothelial lining of the heart. These carry excitation from the atrioventricular node and stimulate the muscular contraction of the ventricles.

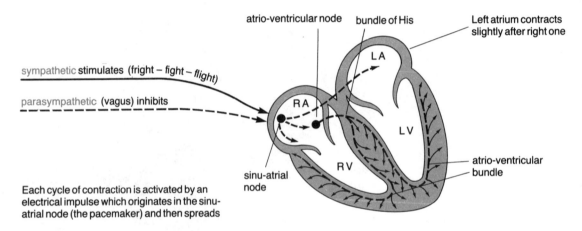

Figure 3.5   Innervation of the pacemaker and conduction of excitation throughout the heart

The pacemaker (Figure 3.5) *initiates* the rhythmical beating of the heart quite independently of any nervous control. However, it does receive impulses from two nerves which modify the activity of the pacemaker and hence the rate of heartbeat. The pacemaker has contact with a branch of the *vagus nerve,* which is part of the *parasympathetic* system and which slows down the rate and force of contraction, and a branch of the *sympathetic* nervous system, which stimulates an increase in the rate and force of heartbeat.

The heart muscle itself is supplied with oxygenated blood by the *coronary arteries* which branch from the aorta. This blood is returned to the right atrium via the *cardiac veins*.

The functioning of the heart and blood vessels can be monitored by the measurement of pulse, by listening to the heart, and by measuring blood pressure.

(b) Blood clotting

Haemostasis is the natural clotting or coagulation of the blood, and is important because without it even a slight injury could result in a person bleeding to death. In health, the blood within the circulatory system remains fluid because the platelets remain stable, and there is a small amount of anticoagulant present in the plasma. The smooth linings of the blood vessels also provide no points at which clots could form.

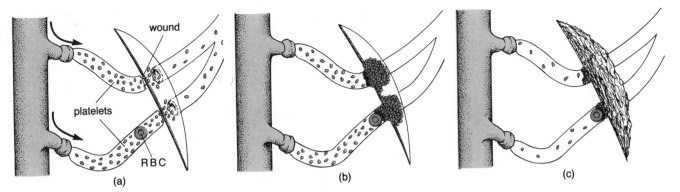

Figure 3.6　Haemostasis after injury. The three stages (a), (b) and (c) are discussed in the text

After injury, blood clotting occurs in the following way.

1. The precapillary sphincters contract and, in severe injury, the artery supplying the injured area also contracts. The pressure and rate of blood flow thus fall, but the small platelets and blood serum (containing clotting factors) get through to the site of the injury (Figure 3.6 a).
2. Platelets (also known as *thrombocytes*) stick to each other and to the damaged tissue, and, for a small wound, this action will prevent further blood loss (Figure 3.6 b).
3. If damage is severe, clotting proceeds further as *thromboplastin* or *Factor III* is released from broken platelets and the damaged tissue. This activates a chain of enzyme reactions in the blood plasma, resulting in the conversion of *fibrinogen* (a soluble protein in plasma) to the solid, non-soluble protein *fibrin*. This forms a fine meshwork which adheres to the platelet plug, and traps red blood cells and forms a clot, which then retracts, as it contains a contractile protein similar to the *actomyosin* of muscle cells (Figure 3.6 c).

Platelets are produced in the bone marrow by cells called *megakaryocytes*. Once released into the blood, platelets survive for between seven and fourteen days, and are then destroyed by the spleen.

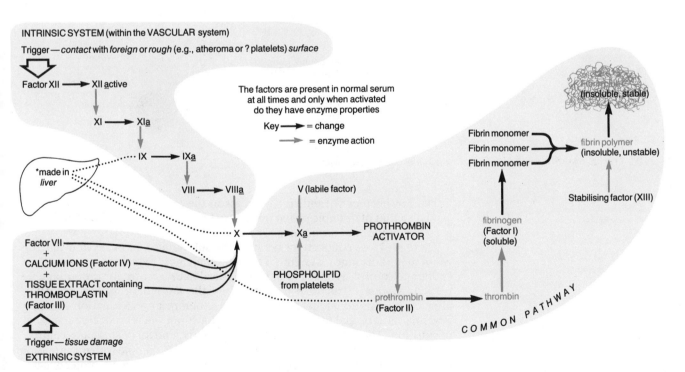

Figure 3.7　Clotting of blood

The complex process of clotting is summarised in Figure 3.7.

When wound healing is complete the fibrin threads are broken down to small peptides, resulting in the eventual disposal of the clot (Figure 3.8).

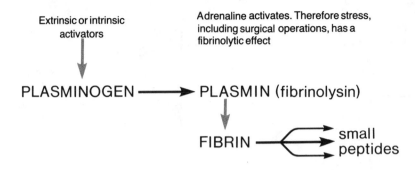

Figure 3.8   Fibrinolysis (disposal of a clot). This takes place when healing is complete

(c) The autonomic nervous system

This part of the nervous system is concerned with controlling the body's involuntary activities, such as heartbeat, movements of the gut and secretion of sweat. It supplies all smooth (or involuntary) muscle wherever it occurs (for example in the bronchioles, gut, blood vessels, uterus and bladder) and also supplies cardiac muscle and glands (including sweat, salivary and lacrimal glands). The system was originally called 'autonomic' because it appeared to be separate (autonomous) from the main sensory and motor systems of the central nervous system (CNS). Its *ganglia* (complex synapses or junctions between nerves) lie outside the CNS and, experimentally, structures innervated by it show some activity when isolated from the body. However, in the healthy person, all parts of the nervous system work closely together.

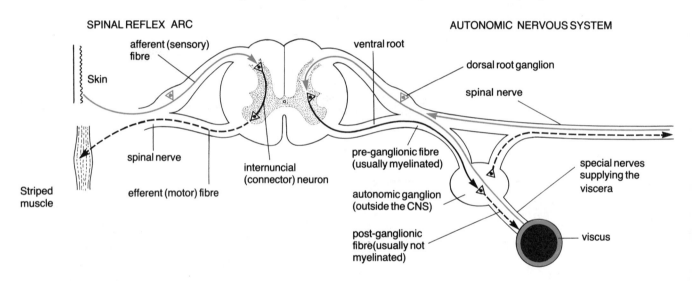

Figure 3.9   Comparison of a simple reflex arc with the autonomic nervous system

The arrangement of individual nerves in the autonomic nervous system is similar to that of a simple spinal reflex arc (Figure 3.9), but with the additional presence of the *autonomic ganglion* outside the CNS.

There are close connections between the autonomic nervous system and the *endocrine* (hormone) system. The hypothalamus, which is important in endocrine control, is believed to be the coordinating centre for the autonomic nervous system. Structures innervated by the autonomic system are often affected by emotional states: for example, before an examination one may develop sweaty palms, diarrhoea and have an increased frequency of micturition. The autonomic system is largely independent of conscious control, but some voluntary control can be learnt: for example, people with hypertension can learn to lower their blood pressure. This has been termed 'biofeedback'.

The autonomic system has two distinct systems: the *sympathetic* and the *parasympathetic*. The nerves of the sympathetic system leave the CNS between the first thoracic and the second lumbar segments of the spinal cord; the parasympathetic nerves leave the CNS alongside four of the cranial nerves, and from the second and third sacral segments of the spinal cord, as shown in Figure 3.10.

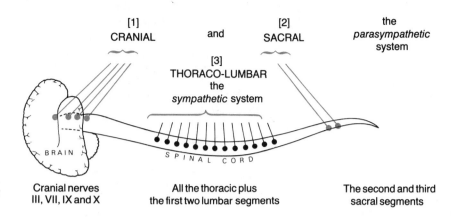

Figure 3.10   Arrangement of the autonomic nervous system relative to the central nervous system

[1] CRANIAL   and   [2] SACRAL   the *parasympathetic* system

[3] THORACO-LUMBAR the *sympathetic* system

Cranial nerves III, VII, IX and X

All the thoracic plus the first two lumbar segments

The second and third sacral segments

1   The sympathetic system

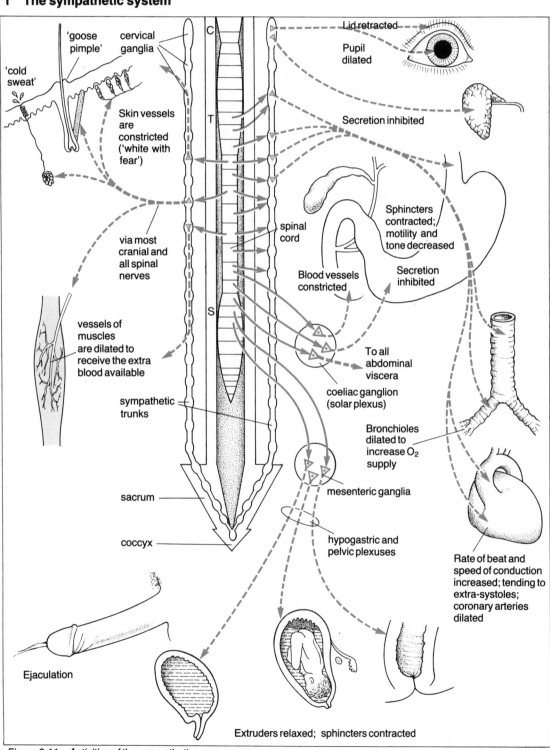

Figure 3.11   Activities of the sympathetic nervous system

The whole function of the sympathetic system is to prepare the body for emergency action. This is called the 'flight or fight' reaction and tends to be a whole body response, generally involving the body in the upright position. Throughout the nervous system, nerves make contact with each other by forming *synapses*. The two nerves do not touch, but one transmits neurochemicals across the small gap (synapse) which are detected by the other, and the nerve impulse is transmitted (and often modified) in this way. This will be discussed in more detail in Chapter 4, pages 113–115.

The neurotransmitter released by the post-ganglionic efferent nerve fibres of the sympathetic system is, with one exception, *noradrenaline*, which is similar chemically and in its action on the body to the hormone *adrenaline*. The activities of the sympathetic nervous system are summarised in Figure 3.11.

2 The parasympathetic system

This part of the autonomic nervous system tends to produce a localised response, and is involved with activities carried out while sitting or lying. The neurotransmitter released by the post-ganglionic fibres of the parasympathetic system is *acetylcholine*. This also acts at *all* autonomic ganglia, in the CNS, at neuromuscular junctions and in the sympathetic system at the sweat glands. (This is the one exception to the pattern of noradrenaline release by the sympathetic post-ganglionic fibres.) Once released, acetylcholine is rapidly destroyed by the enzyme *cholinesterase*, thus making the transmission sites available for re-use. The activities of the parasympathetic system are summarised in Figure 3.12. A comparison of sympathetic and parasympathetic systems is given in Figure 3.13.

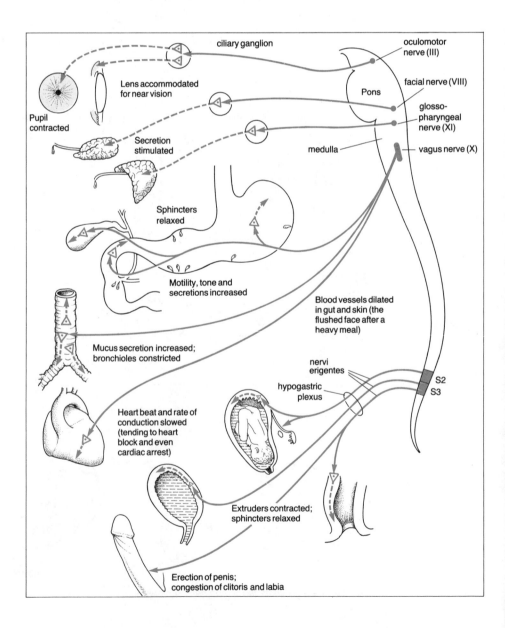

Figure 3.12   Activities of the parasympathetic nervous system

Sympathetic nervous system	Parasympathetic system

Overall effect:
    Fight, flight and fright
    Emergency action
	Normal physiological control of many body functions

Involvement of the body:
    Whole body response
    Person is usually standing
	Localised response
	Person is usually sitting or lying

Chemical transmitter used: Noradrenaline	Acetylcholine
Arrangement of nerve fibres: Pre-ganglionic fibres are short; post-ganglionic fibres are long	Pre-ganglionic fibres are long; post-ganglionic fibres are short

Figure 3.13 Comparison of sympathetic and parasympathetic systems

(d) The adrenal glands

The adrenal glands are located close to the kidneys and embryologically are formed from the same tissue as the nerve cells of the sympathetic nervous system.

The functional relationship between these two systems is so close that the secretory cells in the adrenal medulla can be thought of as post-ganglionic sympathetic neurons without axons, as illustrated in Figure 3.14.

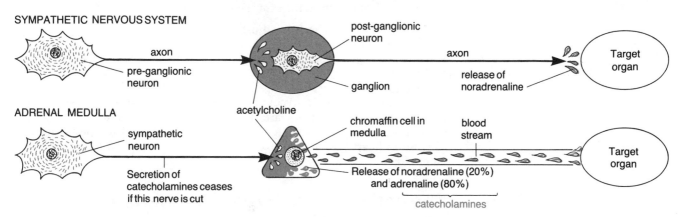

Figure 3.14 Comparison of the arrangement of nerve fibres in the sympathetic nervous system with the nervous control of the adrenal medulla

The adrenal medulla secretion (see Figure 3.15) consists of approximately 20% adrenaline and 80% noradrenaline which are together known as *catecholamines*. Secretion by the adrenal medulla is stimulated by acetylcholine released from the sympathetic nerve which supplies it. Sympathetic nerve stimulation of the adrenal medulla is initiated by the *hypothalamus* and *reticular formation* of the lower brain, in response to impulses from all over the body.

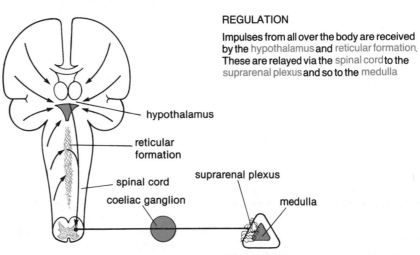

REGULATION

Impulses from all over the body are received by the hypothalamus and reticular formation. These are relayed via the spinal cord to the suprarenal plexus and so to the medulla

Fibres pass *through* the coeliac ganglion without synapsing

Figure 3.15 Regulation of secretion by the adrenal medulla

1 Functions of the adrenal medulla

Both the adrenal medulla and the sympathetic nervous system are concerned in the 'flight or fight' reaction but, because the adrenal medulla primarily produces adrenaline and the sympathetic nervous system releases noradrenaline, there are some differences. For instance, adrenaline increases heart beat rate; noradrenaline slows it down.

The catecholamines have the following effects.

1. They affect the *metabolism*. Their presence stimulates the breakdown of *glycogen* (a glucose compound) from the liver, and fat from adipose tissue, to provide glucose and free fatty acids which are sources of energy for heart and skeletal muscle. Catecholamines inhibit the production of insulin by the pancreas, and facilitate the manufacture of glucose from lactose (a sugar).
2. They stimulate sweating.
3. They stimulate dilation of the bronchi to facilitate ventilation.
4. Adrenaline increases heartbeat rate and cardiac output. Noradrenaline slows the heart and increases its force but, because it raises peripheral resistance more than adrenaline, the cardiac output falls. As the medullary secretion of adrenaline is four times that of noradrenaline, the overall effect is that of adrenaline.
5. They stimulate selective vasoconstriction so that blood is diverted from skin to gut and active muscles. Blood pressure is raised, and skin looks pale. Heat loss from the skin is thus reduced.

These actions help the body to adjust to:
- Physical exertion.
- Some emotions, including fright.
- Exposure to cold.
- Need for stored energy.

There are two basic types of receptor in the organs upon which catecholamines act. These are the alpha (α)- and beta (β)-receptors. Generally, α-receptors mediate vasoconstriction and the β-receptors mediate increase in heart rate and strength of contraction, although there are some other effects.

The patients with hypovolaemic and cardiogenic shock

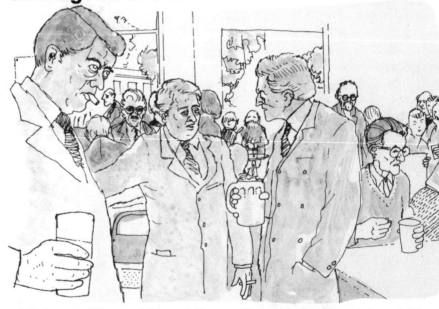

(a) Patients with hypovolaemic shock

1 Patient study and care plan for an adult with severe haematemesis

Figure 3.16   Mr Robinson

History of social, psychological and physical events leading to the present condition

The patient chosen for this section to illustrate hypovolaemic shock is an adult with severe haematemesis.

Mr Robinson (Figure 3.16), aged 40 years, lives with his wife and three children in a terraced house on a new housing estate on the outskirts of a major city. A year ago Mr Robinson was found to have a peptic ulcer which has since been treated conservatively. He works as a foreman in a local factory which for the past six months has been under threat of closure. Recently, Mr Robinson has become increasingly irritable at home and has spent more time at the local pub. He drinks and smokes moderately.

In the middle of one of his working shifts a fellow worker finds Mr Robinson collapsed in the toilet; he has vomited a large amount of blood and appears cold and clammy. The occupational health nurse is informed and an ambulance is summoned to take Mr Robinson to the accident and emergency department at the local hospital. The occupational health nurse informs Mrs Robinson of her husband's transfer to hospital.

On arrival at the accident and emergency department, an initial assessment of Mr Robinson reveals the following:

- Frightened, anxious, nauseated and not fully aware of his surroundings.
- Skin pale, cold and clammy.
- Deep sighing respirations.
- Pulse 110 beats per minute, weak and thready.
- Blood pressure 80/60 mmHg.

Explanation of abnormal physiology and pathology

It is advisable to revise the normal circulation, maintenance of blood pressure and tissue perfusion, and see Tables 3.1 and 3.2.

SHOCK

Shock is, in essence, a story of survival, a struggle by the organism in an adverse environment to preserve the life of its most vital functions. (Refer to A. P. Thal, *Shock: A Physiological Basis for Treatment,* Year Book Medical Publishers, Chicago, 1971.)

Table 3.1

Related normal physiology	Abnormal physiology
(a) The purpose of the cardio-vascular system is to supply oxygen and nutrients to the mitochrondria within individual cells	Shock is a condition where the circulation or perfusion of blood is inadequate to meet tissue metabolic demands, thereby leading to cellular anoxia and death
(b) *The normal physiological response to sudden blood loss is:*	*Related clinical features of Mr Robinson on arrival at accident and emergency department*
(i) Reduction in blood volume stimulates the vasomotor centre to increase peripheral resistance by constricting the peripheral blood vessels	(i) Low blood pressure, pulse of weak volume, skin pale, cold and clammy
(ii) The vasomotor centre also stimulates the sympathetic nervous system to increase the rate and force of contraction of the heart, which increases cardiac output	(ii) Pulse rate 110 beats per minute
(iii) Reduction of blood volume causes the adrenal medulla to secrete adrenaline and noradrenaline, which further increases sympathetic vasoconstriction	(iii) Skin remains pale, cold and clammy
The response described above results in: (iv) Increase in the central blood pressure ensuring perfusion of the brain and heart	(iv) Consciousness preserved but has episodes when he is barely responsive. Heart function preserved
(v) Decrease in blood flow from less vital centres such as muscle, skin, kidney, intestine and liver	(v) Skin remains pale and cold. Oliguria. Muscle tone reduced. Peristalsis reduced
(vi) Decreased perfusion to tissues results in metabolic acidosis	(vi) Deep sighing respirations in an attempt to restore blood pH by eliminating carbon dioxide
(vii) Movement of tissue fluid into the capillaries from the tissue spaces, so restoring the plasma volume (due to decrease in pressure) within the capillaries	(vii) Preserves a minimal blood pressure and circulating blood volume
(viii) *Other response* Posterior lobe of the pituitary gland secretes antidiuretic hormone and the adrenal gland secretes aldosterone. Both these hormones cause retention of water and sodium in the body, so conserving the plasma volume	(viii) Preserves a minimal blood pressure and circulating blood volume

This systemic response to shock sustains the vital functions of the body for a limited time until the underlying pathology can be corrected, i.e., restoration of blood volume by transfusion.

EXPLANATION OF IRREVERSIBLE SHOCK

When the body can no longer compensate for low blood volume it may be in a condition of irreversible shock. Until the blood volume is restored the prolonged under-perfusion of non-vital organs leads to cellular anoxia, and tissue death, which results in irreversible shock and ultimate death of the individual. The decreased tissue perfusion forces production of increased lactate levels, resulting in metabolic acidosis. The blood pressure may still be normal at this time. As tissue metabolites continue to accumulate they cause vasodilation which allows leakage of fluid back into the tissue spaces and reverses the normal compensatory mechanism. This results in decrease of venous return to the heart with reduction of cardiac output. Decrease in circulation of blood to brain and heart results in death of the individual.

Explanation of pathology of gastric ulceration

Table 3.2

Related normal physiology	Abnormal physiology
(a) Intact mucous lining of the stomach secretes gastric juices, hydrochloric acid and mucus	Break in mucous lining which exposes the submucosa and blood vessels to the gastric juices. Erosion of blood vessels causes haemorrhage into the stomach cavity
(b) Normally stomach contents pass by peristalsis into the duodenum, small and large intestine	A large volume of blood in the stomach is irritant to the mucosa and causes gastric dilation and vomiting. Some blood passes by peristalsis into the duodenum, small and large intestine, and is eliminated as melaena in the stool. (For further reading refer to pathology textbook)

Care plan

PREPARATION FOR PATIENT WITH SEVERE HAEMATEMESIS

The care plan for Mr Robinson is shown in Table 3.4, including the care required prior to emergency surgery.

Nursing history and assessment
Table 3.3 shows the nursing history and assessment for Mr Robinson.

Table 3.3   *Nursing history and assessment sheet for Mr Robinson*

NURSING HISTORY AND ASSESSMENT SHEET
Record No. __33333__

PATIENT LABEL
Mr/~~Mrs/Miss~~   *John Robinson*
Address   *150 Water Terrace, Newtown*
Male/~~Female~~   Age   *40 years*
Date of Birth   *6·7·46*
Date of admission/first visit
   8·10·86
Time _____
Type: ☐ Routine ☑ Emergency
   Transfer from: ___*C/E*___
Religion   *Non-practising*
Practising/baptised _____
Minister _____
Telephone number _____

Next of kin (name) __*Mrs Alice Robinson*__
Relationship to patient __*Wife*__
Address   *Same address*

Telephone numbers   *9876*
Contact at night/in emergency YES/~~NO~~

Occupation (or father)   *Factory Foreman*
Marital status   *Married*
Children (or place in family)   *3*
Other dependants _____
Pets _____
School (children only) _____
Hobbies _____
Clubs _____

Favourite pastime _____

Does patient smoke?   YES/NO

Speech difficulty/language barrier

Dysphasia   Dysarthria

Accommodation

Lives alone   YES/NO

Part III/EMI/Old People's Homes/Rented

Other _____ *Terraced House* _____

Consultant _____ *Mr Sussex* _____

House officer _____ *Dr Gray* _____

Presenting condition _____ *Haematemesis* _____

History of present complaint and reason for admission

Diagnosis of peptic ulcer 1 year ago,
treated conservatively.
Admitted in state of severe shock
and vomiting blood? bleeding
gastric ulcer

Past medical history

_____ *N/a* _____

Allergies

Current medication

_____ *Cimetidine* _____

What patient says is the reason for admission and attitude to admission

Patient's expectations

Any problems at home while/because patient is in hospital?
Factory under threat of closure.
          Possible loss of job
Relevant home conditions (e.g. stairs)
          Stairs

Visiting problems

_____

Care at home

Community nurse _____

No. _____

Name of GP _____ *Dr. Groom* _____

Address _____ *The Medical Centre, Mill Road,* _____
                            Newtown

Other services involved

Home help _____   Day hospital _____

Laundry _____   Day centre/club _____

Inco supplies _____   Health visitor _____

Aids _____   Social worker _____

Meals on wheels _____   Voluntary worker _____

Daily living

Diet

Special _____

Food or drink dislikes _____

Appetite: ☑GOOD   ☐POOR

Remarks _____

Sleep

How many hours normally?   *8*

Sedation _____

What else helps? _____

Elimination

Bowels: Continent/~~Incontinent~~

How often opened? _____ *Daily* _____

Any medication? _____ *No* _____

Urinary: Continent/~~Incontinent~~

If incontinent; Day/Night/If not taken, how frequently? _____

Nocturia/Dysuria/Frequency/Urgency

Remarks _____

Female patients — Menstruation

Post-menopausal   Taking the pill

Regular   Irregular

Amenorrhoea   Dysmenorrhoea

Next period due: _____

Uses: STs Tampons

Hearing

Hearing aid: YES/NO

Remarks _____

Vision

Glasses/Contact lens: YES/NO

Remarks _____

Oral

Dentures or crowns: YES/NO

Any problems with mouth or teeth?

_____

Mobility

Help needed with:

Walking/Standing/In/Out of bed/Bathing/Dressing

In/Out of chair/

Feeding/Other: _____

Remarks _____ *Normally fully active* _____

Prosthesis/appliance

Type of appliance _____

Help needed _____

Table 3.3 (cont.)

General appearance

| Normal | Dehydrated | Acutely ill |
| Obese | <u>Thin</u> | Emaciated |

Remarks _____

Skin

Satisfactory	Broken areas	Dehydrated
Rash	Oedematous	Jaundiced
<u>Pallor</u>	Other *Cold and clammy*	
	(including bruising)	

Remarks _____

Level of consciousness

| Orientated | Semi-conscious |
| <u>Confused</u> | Unconscious |

Remarks _____

Mental assessment (if appropriate)

Mood

Elated	<u>Irritable</u>	Agitated
Cheerful	<u>Anxious</u>	Aggressive
Miserable	<u>Withdrawn</u>	Suspicious
Apathetic		

Thought content

Hallucinations/Delusions/Paranoid Ideas

_____
_____

Orientation

Time/Place/Person

Very confused   Slightly confused

Any particular time of day? _____

Confabulation _____

Remarks _____

Surveillance   <u>Physical</u>/Emotional

Information obtained from _____ *Mrs Robinson* _____

Relationship to patient _____ *Wife* _____

By _____ *SMD* _____

Position/level of training _____

Date _____ 8·10·86 _____

Time _____

Table 3.4   Care plan for Mr Robinson

Problem	Objective	Plan of care	Rationale
1. Patient in severe shock	Preserve circulation to vital centres	(a) Elevate foot of trolley	(a) Ensures maximum blood to brain
		(b) Prepare equipment for immediate commencement of intravenous infusion and the taking of blood for grouping and cross-matching	(b) Restores circulating blood volume
		(c) Monitor and record intravenous flow rate, blood pressure, pulse and respirations	(c) Assesses patient's response to treatment
		(d) Give oxygen therapy	(d) Increases oxygen content of inspired air
2. Patient very frightened	Reduce fear	Inform patient and wife as procedures are undertaken	Receiving information reduces fear of the unknown, establishes confidence in hospital staff
3. Patient vomiting blood	Minimise the unpleasant aspects of vomiting	(a) Stay with patient	(a) Reassure patient
		(b) Provide clean vomit bowl promptly	(b) Reduces stimulus of unpleasant smells and sights
		(c) Provide mouthwash as appropriate	(c) Removes unpleasant taste of vomit
		(d) Support patient's head during vomiting	(d) Prevents choking and undue distress
		(e) Introduce nasogastric tube	(e) Aspirate stomach contents to reduce vomiting and give more accurate assessment of blood loss
		(f) Aspirate nasogastric tube as necessary	(f) As above

Table 3.4 (cont.)

Problem	Objective	Plan of care	Rationale
	Assess amount and nature of fluid and blood loss	(a) Measure and record all vomit/aspirate	(a) To estimate replacement requirements
		(b) Save vomit/aspirate for inspection	(b) Determines the continuation of bleeding
4. Potential problem of passing a melaena stool	Be alert to the significance of the passing of a melaena stool	Observe, measure and save stools if passed	Gives additional information of amount of blood loss
5. Patient has upper abdominal pain	Relieve pain	Prepare for the giving of prescribed analgesia intravenously	(a) Absorption from intramuscular route would be prolonged due to poor tissue perfusion so for rapid effect intravenous route is used
			(b) Giving of analgesia assists relaxation prior to surgery
6. Patient for emergency surgery	Ensure patient's safety	(a) Obtain consent	(a), (b), (c), (d) and (e) Complies with safe practice to ensure correct patient receives correct operation and prepares patient both physically and psychologically for surgery
		(b) Apply identification bracelet	
		(c) Empty bladder, record result of urine test	
		(d) Check skin and umbilicus	
		(e) Dress in operating gown	
		(f) Ensure all observations are recorded	(f) Gives doctor up-to-date information of condition of patient
		(g) Change infusion to prescribed blood as soon as it is available	(g) Maintains circulatory needs of patient
		NB For care of blood transfusion refer to Chapter 2	

EMERGENCY SURGERY

Within an hour and a half of admission, Mr. Robinson is transferred to the operating theatre for partial gastrectomy because of the large size of the ulcer and the fact that it would be unlikely to respond to further conservative treatment.

2 Patient histories illustrating further problems related to hypovolaemic shock

This part of the chapter comprises patient histories, self-testing questions and suggested answers.

An adult with hypovolaemic shock due to burns

Mrs Edith Cutler, aged 68 years, lives in a basement flat with her sister. Having prepared herself for bed she came into the sitting room to fetch a letter off the mantelpiece when her nightdress caught alight from a spark from the open fire. Her sister rushed to her aid from the bathroom when she heard her scream. She picked up a nearby rug from the sofa and wrapped her sister in it. She immediately dialled 999 to summon an ambulance and fire services.

Mrs Cutler is brought into the accident and emergency department having sustained burns to the front of her trunk, thighs, both arms, and her hair and eyebrows are singed.

Assessment in the accident and emergency department reveals the following:

- Partial skin loss to thighs, abdomen and superficial loss to arms, equivalent to approximately 25% loss of the skin surface area. The burnt tissue is either oozing serous fluid or forming large serum-filled blisters.
- Conscious and in severe pain, especially over superficial burns on arms.
- Raised pulse rate.
- Deep sighing respirations.
- Blood pressure impossible to take due to burns.

Mrs Cutler's condition deteriorates as she becomes increasingly shocked.

1. Discuss the *immediate* management of Mrs Cutler in the accident and emergency department.

Question 1

Your answer should include:

(a) Alert nearest burns units.

(b) Check that airway is intact.

(c) Support circulation, insert central venous pressure line and start intravenous fluids at a rate fast enough to establish a urine flow of 30–75 millilitres per hour.

(d) Catheterise and measure hourly urine output.

(e) Insert nasogastric tube to prevent gastric dilatation.

(f) Obtain blood samples for blood count, sugar, urea, plasma proteins, bilirubin, electrolytes, pH (arterial blood gases if necessary).

(g) Initial chest x-ray.

(h) Medical history.

(i) Small doses of intravenous morphine.

(j) Record area of burn on a burn chart and from this calculate fluid requirements using the following formula:

2–4 millilitres of intravenous fluid × percentage surface burned × kilogram body weight.

For Mrs Cutler this would be:

$4 \times 25 \times 50 = 5000$ millilitres

Add 2000 millilitres to this total (in an adult). 7000 millilitres is the amount estimated as a requirement for the first 24 hours. 3500 millilitres should be given in first 8 hours. The rest should be given in the remaining 16 hours.

(k) Commence monitoring the following:
  - Central venous pressure.
  - Respiratory rate.
  - Temperature.
  - Urinary output.

(l) Protect the burnt areas from any further injury.

Question 2

2. Discuss the *later* management of Mrs Cutler in the accident and emergency department.

Your answer should include:

(a) Cut away any clothes from the burnt area.

(b) Remove all blistered debris aseptically, leaving intact blisters.

(c) Wrap in sterile towels in preparation for transfer.

(d) Give tetanus toxoid and antibiotics.

(e) Transfer patient to burns unit or intensive care unit.

Question 3

3. Explain why Mrs Cutler is suffering from hypovolaemic shock.

Burn damages capillary walls allowing leakage of serum from the circulation on to the surface of the burn, which will continue for a period of up to 48 hours until a crust is formed. Minimal loss of cells occurs; therefore the viscosity of the blood increases as the volume rapidly reduces. Usual compensatory mechanism involving vasoconstriction is not possible over a large part of the surface area that is burned and this can result in profound shock.

Question 4

4. Draw a simple diagram to illustrate the estimation of percentage tissue loss in a patient with burns.

Refer to your teacher for guidance and suitable textbook and/or journal.

A young adult with hypovolaemic shock due to multiple injuries

John Kershaw, aged 18 years, lives with his parents and sister in a council house in a city suburb. He was admitted to the accident and emergency department having been involved in a road traffic accident in which he was knocked off his motorcycle.

On his arrival, John was examined and found to have an open fracture of his left femur, injury to his left upper abdomen and superficial lacerations to his face and hands. John was fully conscious and gave no history of having hit his head in the accident. The ambulance men had applied a pressure dressing to the bleeding left thigh wound and a splint to support his left leg. They estimated that he had lost 500 ml of blood at the scene of the accident. In addition, the following observations were made:

- Pulse 108 beats per minute.
- Blood pressure 90/60 mmHg.
- Skin cold, clammy and pale.

During x-ray examination John's blood pressure drops to 70/50 mmHg and his pulse becomes weak and almost imperceptible. The nurse summons medical aid. On further examination the doctor discovers a tense abdomen and in view of increasing shock suspects a ruptured spleen.

SELF-TESTING QUESTIONS

1. Discuss the immediate management of John in the accident and emergency department.

2. Discuss whether the ruptured spleen or the fractured femur should be treated first and give reasons for your choice.

BRIEF ANALYSIS AND GUIDELINES FOR SUGGESTED ANSWERS

Question 1
Your answer should include details covering the management of hypovolaemic shock (see page 100).

Question 2
The ruptured spleen requires immediate management because haemorrhage is continuing, the amount cannot be assessed and no first aid treatment is possible. The fractured femur is not life threatening and the pressure dressing can remain in place.

A young adult with hypovolaemic shock due to spontaneous abortion

Tracy Goddard, aged 17 years, is a student at the Polytechnic, living in the hall of residence. For the past 6 weeks she has been aware that she is pregnant and has been to see her GP, who confirmed her pregnancy. Her parents do not know of her pregnancy and she is planning to marry her boyfriend in a month's time. One night Tracy experiences severe abdominal pain and some vaginal bleeding. She becomes frightened and summons help from her friends, who drive her to the local accident and emergency department.

On arrival at the hospital Tracy feels faint, appears pale, cold and clammy, and has bled profusely.

SELF-TESTING QUESTIONS

1. Describe how you would make an initial assessment of Tracy's condition on her arrival at the hospital.

2. As a nurse, what could you do to minimise the effects of hypovolaemic shock?

3. It is decided that Tracy should have evacuation of retained products of conception under general anaesthetic as soon as her shock is under control. Describe the psychological preparation that is needed and discuss who else may need to be informed.

4. What further help and support could be offered to Tracy following her termination of pregnancy?

BRIEF ANALYSIS AND GUIDELINES TO SUITABLE ANSWERS

Question 1
Your answer should include assessment of Tracy's blood loss before and after arrival. Measurements should include:
● Temperature.
● Pulse rate.
● Respiration.
● Blood pressure.
Observations should include:
● Skin—temperature and colour.
● Pain site.
● Mental state and attitude to being pregnant.

Question 2
Position lying flat with foot of trolley raised. Prepare equipment for intravenous replacement therapy, and for taking blood samples for cross-matching.

Question 3
Psychological preparation needs to include clear simple explanation of what has happened to her and the reasons for planned surgery. If Tracy wishes, her parents and boyfriend may be informed, but if not, then her wishes need to be respected.

Question 4
Tracy could be offered help by the counsellor of the Polytechnic, local family planning clinic and/or her GP.

(b) Patients with cardiogenic shock

1 Patient study and care plan for an adult with myocardial infarction

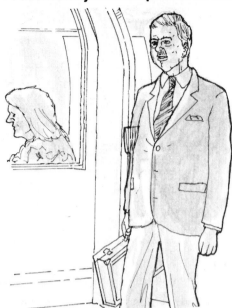

Figure 3.17   Mr Charles Fox

History of social, psychological and physical events leading to the present condition

The patient chosen for this section to illustrate cardiogenic shock is an adult with myocardial infarction.

Mr Charles Fox (Figure 3.17), aged 50 years, lives with his wife and youngest daughter in a semi-detached house in a city suburb. He is employed in the local inland revenue office, and is involved in the activities of the local church and is at present chairman of the parents/teachers association. Mr Fox has been fit and well, although slightly over-weight, and drinks and smokes moderately. In the last week he has complained to his wife that he has had 'indigestion' on occasions. One evening, while watching television, he complained of sudden severe chest pain, radiating down his left arm and up to his left jaw. He became ashen grey and vomited; his wife telephoned the GP who came immediately.

On discussion and examination of Mr Fox, the doctor makes the following observations:
- Severe central chest pain.
- Skin cold, clammy and pale.
- Pulse 100 beats per minute.
- Blood pressure 100/80 mmHg.
- Very frightened, shaky and with dilated pupils.
- Rapid respirations.
- Peripheral cyanosis.
- Weakness and feebleness.

Following his examination the doctor gives Mr Fox some intravenous diamorphine to relieve his pain and anxiety, prior to transferring him to hospital for treatment of suspected myocardial infarction and cardiogenic shock. The situation is explained to Mrs Fox who travels with him in the ambulance. On arrival in the accident and emergency department, Mr Fox's condition is worse, with further reduction in cardiac output. Observations reveal the following:
- Blood pressure lowered to 80/60 mmHg.
- Pulse 120 beats per minute, weak and possibly irregular.
- Respirations rapid and patient over-ventilating.
- Mentally unaware of his surroundings but responds to simple instructions.

Explanation of abnormal physiology and pathology

It is advisable that you revise the normal structure and function of the heart and circulation and see Table 3.5.

Table 3.5

Related normal physiology	Abnormal physiology
(a) Normally the heart receives blood from the venous circulation and delivers it via the lungs to the arterial circulation to the rest of the body	Damaged heart muscle is unable to deliver sufficient blood to the arterial circulation for the body's requirements. As the cardiac output falls, the central venous pressure rises because the heart fails to transfer blood to the arterial circulation

Table 3.5 (cont.)

(b)	The heart contracts at approximately 70 beats per minute and each contraction ejects 70 millilitres of blood into the circulation. This is the cardiac output, which equals approximately 5 litres of blood per minute while at rest	Due to weak irregular contractions the cardiac output is reduced. For example, if only 50 millilitres is ejected at 60 beats per minute, the cardiac output falls to 3 litres per minute
(c)	The heart muscle is stimulated by the electrical impulses initiated by the pacemaker in the right atrium. A wave of contraction spreads throughout the healthy myocardium	In damaged heart muscle, conduction of electrical impulses may be interrupted, resulting in irregular myocardial contractions
(d)	Heart muscle is dependent on receiving an adequate blood supply from the coronary arteries	In myocardial infarction a portion of the myocardium is deprived of its circulation by an occlusion of a coronary artery or one of its branches

OCCLUSION OF A CORONARY ARTERY

This may be caused by a plaque of atheroma on the lining of the vessel, a thrombus within the lumen or, more rarely, an embolus. The extent of damage to the heart muscle is dependent on the site of the occlusion. This may involve a large area of the wall of the ventricle, or may involve the septum of the heart or papillary muscles. The effect disturbs the conducting mechanism of the heart and its ability to contract. Massive infarction is incompatible with life.

The body attempts to compensate for cardiogenic shock as in hypovolaemic shock, described on page 97.

Components of hypovolaemic shock are:
- normal heart with
- reduced blood volume.

Components of cardiogenic shock are:
- damaged heart pump with
- normal blood volume.

Care plan

PREPARATION FOR PATIENT WITH MYOCARDIAL INFARCTION AND CARDIOGENIC SHOCK

Nursing history and assessment
Table 3.6 shows Mr Fox's assessment details.

Table 3.6   Nursing history and assessment sheet for Mr Fox

NURSING HISTORY AND ASSESSMENT SHEET
Record No. _____ *22220*

PATIENT LABEL
Mr/~~Mrs/Miss~~ _____ *Charles Fox*
Address _____ *12 Culcott Ave, Manchester*

Male/~~Female~~   Age _____ *50 years*
Date of Birth _____ *2·2·36*

Date of admission/~~first visit~~
_____ *6·7·86*

Time _____
Type: ☐ Routine ☑ Emergency
   Transfer from: _____

Religion _____ *Baptist*
Practising/baptised _____ *Practising*
Minister _____
Telephone number _____

Next of kin (name) _____ *Mrs Sylvia Fox*
Relationship to patient _____ *Wife*
Address _____ *Same address*
Telephone numbers _____ *10001*
Contact at night/in emergency   YES/~~NO~~

Occupation (or father) _____ *Inland Revenue Officer*
Marital status _____ *Married*
Children (or place in family) _____ *2 (1 married)*
Other dependants _____
Pets _____
School (children only) _____
Hobbies _____
Clubs _____ *School PTA*
Favourite pastime _____
Does patient smoke?   YES/NO

Table 3.6 (cont.)

Speech difficulty/language barrier

Dysphasia   Dysarthria

Accommodation

Lives alone   ~~YES~~/NO

Part III/EMI/Old People's Homes/Rented

Other _____ *Semi-detached house* _____

Consultant _____ *Mr Dorset* _____

House officer _____ *Dr Wood* _____

Presenting condition _____ *Severe chest pain* _____

History of present complaint and reason for admission

Slight dyspepsia during past week.
Suspected myocardial infarction
and cardiogenic shock

Past medical history
_____ *Fit and well* _____

Allergies   *None*

Current medication
_____ *N/a* _____

What patient says is the reason for admission and attitude to admission

Patient's expectations

Any problems at home while/because patient is in hospital?

Relevant home conditions (e.g. stairs)
_____ *Stairs* _____

Visiting problems

Care at home

Community nurse _____

No. _____

Name of GP _____ *Dr Grove* _____

Address *The Surgery, Culcott Rd, Manchester*

Other services involved

Home help _____   Day hospital _____

Laundry _____   Day centre/club _____

Inco supplies _____   Health visitor _____

Aids _____   Social worker _____

Meals on wheels _____   Voluntary worker _____

Daily living

Diet

Special _____

Food or drink dislikes _____

Appetite: ☑ GOOD   ☐ POOR

Remarks _____

Sleep

How many hours normally? _____ *7* _____

Sedation _____

What else helps? _____

Elimination

Bowels: Continent/Incontinent

How often opened? _____ *Daily* _____

Any medication? _____ *None* _____

Urinary: Continent/Incontinent

If incontinent; Day/Night/If not taken, how frequently? _____

Nocturia/Dysuria/Frequency/Urgency

Remarks _____

Female patients — Menstruation

Post-menopausal   Taking the pill

Regular   Irregular

Amenorrhoea   Dysmenorrhoea

Next period due: _____

Uses: STs Tampons

Hearing

Hearing aid: YES/<u>NO</u>

Remarks _____

Vision

Glasses/Contact lens: <u>YES</u>/NO

Remarks _____ *For reading* _____

Oral

Dentures or crowns: YES/<u>NO</u>

Any problems with mouth or teeth?

Mobility

Help needed with:

Walking/Standing/In/Out of bed/Bathing/Dressing

In/Out of chair/

Feeding/Other: _____

Remarks _____ *Normally active* _____

Prosthesis/appliance

Type of appliance _____

Help needed _____

General appearance

<u>Normal</u>   Dehydrated   Acutely ill

Obese   Thin   Emaciated

Remarks _____ *Slightly overweight* _____

Skin

Satisfactory	Broken areas	Dehydrated
Rash	Oedematous	Jaundiced
<u>Pallor</u>	Other *Cold and clammy*	
	(including bruising)	

Remarks _____

Level of consciousness

Orientated	<u>Semi-conscious</u>
Confused	Unconscious

Remarks _____

Mental assessment (if appropriate) *Unable to elicit*

Mood

Elated	Irritable	Agitated
Cheerful	Anxious	Aggressive
Miserable	Withdrawn	Suspicious
Apathetic		

Thought content

Hallucinations/Delusions/Paranoid Ideas

_____

Orientation

Time/Place/Person

Very confused   Slightly confused

Any particular time of day? _____

Confabulation _____

Remarks _____

Surveillance   Physical/Emotional

Information obtained from _____ *Mrs Fox*

Relationship to patient _____ *Wife*

By _____ *L.Smith*

Position/level of training _____

Date _____ *6·7·86*

Time _____

TREATMENT

The care plan (Table 3.7) shows the treatment Mr Fox requires.

Table 3.7   Care plan for Mr Fox

Problem	Objective	Plan of care	Rationale
1. Patient shocked due to reduced cardiac output	Improve cardiac output and support circulation until improvement is achieved	(a) Position lying flat	(a) Aids blood circulation to the brain
		(b) Promote rest, minimise patient activity, anticipate needs	(b) Reduces demand on the heart
		(c) Prepare for commencement of an intravenous infusion	(c) Provides intravenous route for administration of emergency drugs
		(d) Have available resuscitation equipment and drugs for use if fibrillation or cardiac arrest occurs	(d) Further myocardial infarction could occur
		(e) Give oxygen via mask at high concentration	(e) Ensure arterial blood contains high concentration of oxygen to maintain tissue perfusion
		(f) Give analgesia as prescribed, e.g., diamorphine	(f) Relieves pain which otherwise increases state of shock
	Detect changes in patient's condition	(a) Measure and record heart action by observation of pulse and heart conduction with a cardiac monitor	(a) Detects changes and permits prompt treatment for abnormalities
		(b) Measure and record respirations, blood pressure, temperature	(b) Respirations return to normal as acidosis is corrected. Blood pressure rises as cardiac output improves. Rise in temperature could indicate inflammatory response in damaged tissue
2. Potential problem of overloading the circulation of the blood	Prevent overloading of the circulation and detect early signs	(a) Record fluid intake and output	(a) While patient is shocked, oliguria will be present
		(b) Observe for sacral oedema, raised jugular venous pressure	(b) and (c) Shock permits the release of antidiuretic hormone and aldosterone, which causes retention of sodium and water
		(c) Weigh patient daily when condition permits	

Table 3.7 (cont.)

Problem	Objective	Plan of care	Rationale
3. Anxious patient and wife	Reduce anxiety	Give Mr Fox full explanation as his condition improves. Discuss further care and treatment with him and his wife. Arrange for wife to stay at hospital overnight and offer facilities for contacting daughter at home	Gives confidence in hospital staff and relieves fear of the unknown. Gains their cooperation. Provides opportunity for wife to be near husband during stressful time

MR FOX'S RECOVERY

Mr Fox's condition stabilises, no cardiac arrhythmias are detected, his pulse appears stronger though still rapid, the blood pressure rises to 100/80 mmHg and respirations are slower. He continues oxygen therapy which seems to have eased his distress and he says the chest pain is not so severe. He remains pale but his skin is no longer clammy or cyanosed. The doctor decides that Mr Fox should be transferred to the coronary care unit for further monitoring of progress.

The most likely outcome of Mr Fox's myocardial infarction is that he will make a steady recovery to normal activity during which time he will be taught to work, exercise, eat and drink, with moderation. He needs to avoid smoking entirely and avoid excessive emotional stress if possible. (For further reading see J. Macleod (Ed.), *Davidson's Principles and Practice of Medicine*, 14th edition, Churchill Livingstone, London, 1984.)

POSSIBLE COMPLICATIONS OF MYOCARDIAL INFARCTION

Consideration should be given to the possibility of complications of myocardial infarction occurring such as:
- Cardiac arrhythmias.
- Left ventricular failure.
- Emboli from a mural thrombus.
- Rupture of ventricle.
- Further coronary thrombosis.

All these complications could cause recurrence of cardiogenic shock.

2 Patient histories illustrating further problems related to cardiogenic shock

This part of the chapter comprises patient histories, self-testing questions and suggested answers.

An adult with left ventricular failure

Mr Hardwicke, aged 78 years, is a retired hospital porter who lives with his wife in a council flat near the hospital where he used to work. Just after he retired he visited his doctor for a routine medical check-up and was found to be moderately hypertensive with blood pressure 160/110 mmHg. Investigations were confined to examination of the fundus of his eyes, which were normal, and urinalysis, which revealed a trace of albumin. He was prescribed an antihypertensive drug, a diuretic, and was advised to reduce his weight by a calorie-controlled diet. His hypertension was controlled on this regime until six months ago, when he had to have his medication changed to methyldopa as he had become severely hypertensive. Since this visit to his doctor he has felt progressively unwell, with dyspnoea on effort; he also noticed that his sleep had been disturbed and he seemed to need three or four pillows to enable him to sleep. He seemed to lack energy and tended to feel the cold.

One night he wakes up with a feeling of suffocation, fighting for breath, wheezing and coughing frothy sputum. He disturbs his wife when trying to get to the window for more air. Mrs Hardwicke rings the doctor on call, who visits and examines Mr Hardwicke. The doctor makes the following findings:
- Frightened, distressed elderly gentleman.
- Respiration rapid, laboured and with a productive cough.
- Chest examination showed evidence of pulmonary oedema.
- Pulse rate rapid and weak.
- Blood pressure much lower than normal, 130/80 mmHg.
- Skin pale, cold and clammy.

The doctor makes a diagnosis of left ventricular failure due to long history of hypertension. He administers intravenous aminophylline to relax broncho-spasm and intravenous frusemide to relieve the pulmonary oedema. He stays with Mr Hardwicke to observe the effects of these medicines. As the diuretic starts to have effect, Mr Hardwicke produces a large quantity of urine and his breathing gradually improves. The doctor shows Mrs Hardwicke how to prop her husband well up in bed to allow as much tissue fluid as possible to drain away from the lungs. He explains to Mrs Hardwicke that he will call again in the morning and will arrange for the district nurse to visit.

The doctor informs the district nurse that Mr Hardwicke has developed left ventricular failure (cardiac asthma) the previous night. He informs her of the medication given and explains that Mr Hardwicke has poor cardiac output but that if he is kept at rest it will be sufficient to maintain adequate tissue perfusion.

SELF-TESTING QUESTIONS

BRIEF ANALYSIS AND GUIDELINES TO SUITABLE ANSWERS

Question 1

1. Devise a care plan for Mr Hardwicke to be nursed in his own home.

Your answer should include:
(a) Ensure rest in bed.
(b) Provide facilities for attention to hygiene and elimination.
(c) Advise regarding position for sleep and obtain back rest if possible from social services department or Red Cross.
(d) Assist wife to change Mr Hardwicke's position regularly and arrange for provision of sheepskin and bed cradle to help prevent pressure sores.
(e) Advise Mrs Hardwicke that her husband's diet should be light, easily digestible and salt-restricted (by omitting salt from her cooking).
(f) Ask her to check that Mr Hardwicke passes urine.
(g) After initial care the district nurse needs to do a full assessment of the home situation to see if there is a need for referral to the medical social worker and/or geriatric health visitor to provide financial aid, ongoing support and home care assistant while Mrs Hardwicke is engaged in caring for her husband.

Question 2

2. When he was first diagnosed as having hypertension, Mr Hardwicke had his eyes and urine examined. Explain the significance of these tests. What other investigations could have been carried out?

For eye changes in hypertension see suitable textbook. Renal disease can be cause *or* effect of hypertension.

For other investigations see suitable textbook. In a younger patient a 24 hour collection of urine may be done to estimate catecholamines, which are end products of adrenaline and noradrenaline, for the exclusion of phaeochromocytoma (tumour of the adrenal medulla).

Question 3

3. Mr Hardwicke developed left ventricular failure resulting from his hypertension. Discuss other possible complications of hypertension.

For summary see J. Macleod (Ed.), *Davidson's Principles and Practice of Medicine*, 14th edition, Churchill Livingstone, London, 1984.

Question 4

4. How would you explain to a junior nurse the method of estimating and recording a blood pressure?

Refer to Fact Sheet 1, page 110.

Question 5

5. During Mr Hardwicke's attack of left ventricular failure his blood pressure was 130/80 mmHg, which was much lower than his normal 160/110 mmHg. Explain why this happened.

Mr Hardwicke developed cardiogenic shock when the left ventricle failed to maintain cardiac output (see patient study at the beginning of the chapter, page 92). The reason why a blood pressure of 130/80 mmHg had such severe effects was because his body had adjusted to a state of hypertension.

Question 6

6. Describe the action of antihypertensive drugs and discuss their side-effects.

Refer to your teacher for guidance and a suitable pharmacology textbook.

7. Discuss the advantages and disadvantages of home or hospital care for Mr Hardwicke.

Question 7
Home care
(a) Advantages include:
- Familiar surroundings.
- Social contact with wife.
- Reduces disturbance and promotes rest.

(b) Disadvantages include:
- Absence of sophisticated monitoring equipment.
- Delay in obtaining medical aid.
- Extra burden on wife who is also elderly.

Hospital care
(a) Advantages include:
- 24-hour care and monitoring available.
- Prompt attention to complications if they arise.

(b) Disadvantages include:
- Unfamiliar surroundings.
- Disturbance in getting him there.
- Unfamiliar medical staff.
- Possibility of disorientation especially at night, with regressive behaviour.
- Social contact with wife reduced.

Fact Sheet 1   Estimating a blood pressure

1. Choose the correct size of cuff; too short a cuff will give a falsely high reading; too long a one, a falsely low.
   To get an accurate reading, the inflatable bag should encircle the arm completely and its centre should be over the brachial artery.
2. The patient should sit or lie as comfortably as possible. All clothing should be removed from the right arm and it should be supported so that the brachial artery at the antecubital fossa is at about the same level as the heart (Figure 3.18a). If the artery is much below the heart, a falsely high reading will be obtained; if above, a falsely low one.
3. The brachial artery should be felt for and identified in the antecubital fossa (front of elbow) and the cuff secured firmly round the arm (Figure 3.18b).
4. The radial pulse is then found with one hand and the cuff inflated to about 30 mm above the level at which the pulse disappears.
5. The cuff is then deflated and the reading on the sphygmomanometer at which the pulse reappears is recorded. This is the *systolic blood pressure by palpation*.
6. A stethoscope bell is placed over the artery, and the cuff inflated to about 30 mm above the systolic pressure recorded by palpation. (The bell should be clear of cuff and clothing or rubbing against them will make a distracting noise, Figure 3.18c.)
7. The valve is released slowly so that pressure falls at about 3 mm/second.
8. Interpretations of what is *heard* as the pressure is released are shown in Figure 3.18d.

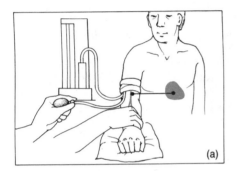

(a)

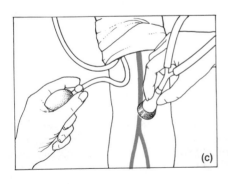

2.5 cm

(b)

(c)

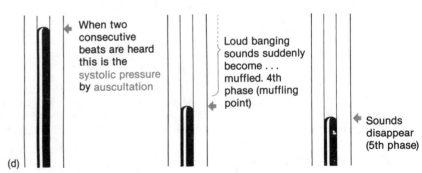

When two consecutive beats are heard this is the systolic pressure by auscultation

Loud banging sounds suddenly become . . . muffled. 4th phase (muffling point)

Sounds disappear (5th phase)

(d)

Figure 3.18   Estimating a patient's blood pressure

An adult with right ventricular failure

Mr Chandler is 66 years old and has had chronic bronchitis for the last 10 years. For the past 4 years he has had acute exacerbations which have necessitated antibiotic therapy and on one occasion hospital admission was required. At that time he developed symptoms of right-sided heart failure and digoxin and a diuretic were prescribed. Since then he has been suffering with severe dyspnoea and orthopnoea, and occasionally his ankles swell. His wife gets increasingly worried about his condition as she notices that he is becoming reluctant to eat, has increasing weakness and is unable to go out.

Mrs Chandler calls the doctor, who finds his condition has deteriorated, with cyanosis, engorged jugular veins, enlarged liver and gross ankle and sacral oedema. Mr Chandler says that his urine output is much less than normal. The doctor gives Mr Chandler an intramuscular injection of frusemide and arranges for his transfer to hospital.

SELF-TESTING QUESTIONS

1. Describe the effects of right ventricular failure and possible causes.

2. Discuss the assessment you would make of Mr Chandler in the accident and emergency department.

3. Describe the total management of Mr Chandler while in the accident and emergency department.

4. Following admission to the medical ward Mr Chandler fails to respond to treatment, his cardiac output continues to fall and he enters irreversible cardiogenic shock. Write a care plan for Mr Chandler for this period until he dies.

5. Explain the abnormal physiology of the presence of oedema in right-sided heart failure.

BRIEF ANALYSIS AND GUIDELINES TO SUITABLE ANSWERS

Question 1
For further reading refer to J. C. Houston, *Short Textbook of Medicine,* 7th edition, Hodder and Stoughton, London, 1982.

Question 2
Your answer should include the following assessments:
(a) State of shock by skin colour and temperature, pulse rate and volume, respiration rate, depth and difficulty, blood pressure, degree of cerebral hypoxia.
(b) Features of lung and heart disease such as cough and sputum, presence of secondary lung infection or pulmonary oedema, oedema of sacrum and ankles, when urine last passed.
(c) General physical and social features such as nutritional state, Norton Scale and wife's understanding of his critical condition.

Question 3
Your answer should include:
(a) Management of his cardiogenic shock (refer to Chapter 3, page 107, *but as Mr Chandler has chronic lung disease oxygen therapy must be in controlled low concentration only, as prescribed by the doctor.* See Table 2.1 (page 57) and Table 2.3 (page 60), for explanation.
(b) Management of digoxin and diuretic therapy in this emergency situation.
(c) Management of patient receiving intravenous aminophylline to relieve bronchospasm.
(d) Support of patient during electrocardiograph and chest x-ray.

Question 4
Care plan should include:
(a) Care and comfort of Mr Chandler, physically, psychologically, spiritually and socially.
(b) Prepare Mrs Chandler for her husband's death and arrange support as required.
Refer to G. Garrett, *Health Needs of the Elderly,* in the Essentials of Nursing Series, Macmillan Education, 1987.

Question 5
Refer to J. H. Green, *Basic Clinical Physiology*, 3rd edition, Oxford University Press, London, 1979.

Chapter 4

Nursing patients with disturbances of consciousness

Normal function of the nervous system

The nervous system provides the most rapid means of communication within the body. It is divided into the *central nervous system* (CNS), which is a concentrated mass of nerve tissue; and the *peripheral nerves*, which transmit information from the body's *receptors* to the CNS and appropriate messages from the CNS to the *effectors* in response to the sensory information.

1 Nerve structure

The functional unit of the nervous system is the *neuron*. The basic structure is similar for all neurons, but this pattern is considerably modified to serve the different functions of neurons in different parts of the nervous system. Figure 4.1 shows a motor neuron with *dendrites* (short processes for inter-communication), *cell body* with a nucleus, and *axon,* the long nerve process or *fibre*, which can transmit impulses over long distances, for example, from the CNS to the foot.

This pattern is slightly different in the *sensory* and *intermediate* nerves, as shown in Figure 4.2 a and b.

(a) The nerve cell and its impulse

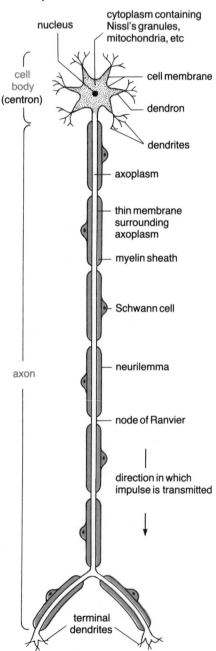

Figure 4.1   A motor neuron

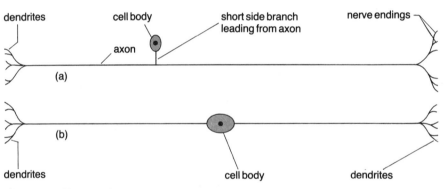

Figure 4.2   Neurons. (a) Sensory and (b) intermediate

The nucleus of the nerve cell lacks a *centromere,* a structure which is important in cell division, and so nerve cells cannot replicate themselves. The number of nerve cells in the body is therefore finite and is fixed in early childhood. From this time the number of neurons can only decrease, and from about the age of 30 there is a steady decline in their numbers.

The axon of the neuron is wrapped in one of two ways. The majority of nerves have a fatty *myelin sheath* which is composed of lipoprotein 'bandages' wrapped around the nerve. These are produced by the *Schwann cells* which lie alongside all nerves outside the CNS. The myelin sheath is interrupted at roughly one millimetre intervals by constrictions called *nodes of Ranvier.* Within the CNS, myelination is carried out by the *oligodendrocytes* (Figure 4.4).

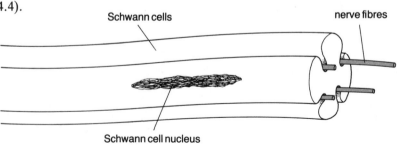

Figure 4.3   Unmyelinated nerve fibres

Some fibres, although they have Schwann cells, remain unmyelinated. They tend to form groups which sink into the substance of the Schwann cell, taking in folds of the cell membrane with them (Figure 4.3). Unmyelinated fibres are found in the autonomic nervous system and in sensory nerves carrying information about pain and smell. In the CNS the nerve cells are surrounded by *neuroglial cells* which wrap, support, insulate and protect them (Figure 4.4). They also supply them with nutrients and remove waste products. The neuroglial cells are well supplied with capillaries.

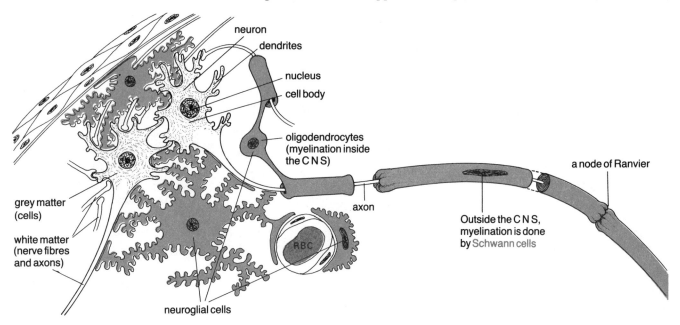

Figure 4.4   *A myelinated neuron within and outside the central nervous system*

Many intermediate nerve cells within the CNS have very short or non-existent axons.

2   Transmission of the nerve impulse

In its resting state, the axon maintains an electrical potential difference across the membrane of about -70 millivolts (the interior of the cell negative with respect to the environment of the cell). This charge (called the *resting potential*) is maintained by the cell membrane, which actively pumps out any sodium ions (Na^+) that may leak in. This *sodium pump mechanism* consumes energy.

When the axon receives a suitable stimulus the membrane becomes more permeable to Na^+ ions, which, being ten times more concentrated outside the cell, diffuse into the cell so rapidly that the fibre becomes positively charged at that point. This is the *action potential* and is about $+40$ millivolts. This depolarisation is a localised phenomenon, but the inflow of Na^+ ions sets up small local circuits across the neighbouring parts of the cell membrane. This excitation causes the cycle to be repeated in the neighbouring portion of the nerve and so the action potential is propagated along the axon, as shown in Figure 4.5.

As the axon becomes flooded with Na^+ ions, potassium ions (K^+) begin to leave. This marks the beginning of the recovery process which results in the restoration of the axon's negative resting potential. The axon membrane once again becomes impermeable to Na^+ ions, and the sodium pump starts up again. As Na^+ ions are rapidly extruded from the axon, the membrane becomes *repolarised,* i.e., restored to its resting potential. The K^+ ions passively diffuse back into the axon and the balance is restored. The whole process is complete in 2 milliseconds.

A nerve impulse can travel in either direction, but it normally travels one way as it is usually initiated at the end of the axon. After repolarisation, there is a short *refractory period* in which a second impulse cannot be transmitted, and this prevents the return spread of the impulse travelling along the axon (see Figure 4.6). Transmission of a nerve impulse is an 'all-or-nothing' phenomenon: it always has the same size and velocity for a given nerve, and is always transmitted if initiated (in the healthy neuron). The only variable is the

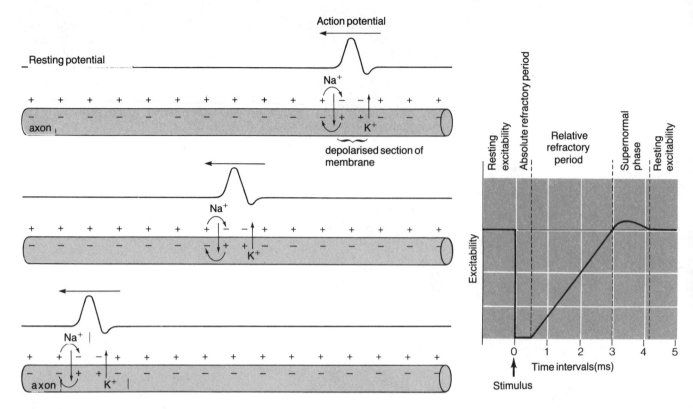

Figure 4.5   Stages in the propagation of the nerve impulse

Figure 4.6   Excitability of the nerve after impulse

frequency of impulses, and it is this which gives the patterning or coding of information carried by nerves. Generally, the greater the frequency of impulses along a given pathway, the more important and powerful a message is seen to be by the CNS. A limit to the frequency of impulses is imposed by the length of the refractory period. The refractory period has two parts: the *absolute refractory period* in which the axon is completely incapable of transmitting an impulse, and the following *relative refractory period* during which an impulse can be initiated, as long as the stimulus is strong enough, i.e., stronger than the normal *threshold stimulus* for that nerve.

The speed with which a nerve impulse is transmitted varies considerably, depending primarily on the diameter of the axon and the presence or absence of a myelin sheath. Generally, the greater the axon diameter, the greater the speed of transmission. If an axon is myelinated, the impulse is considerably faster than in a comparable unmyelinated axon, because the impulse seems to leap between the nodes of Ranvier. This process is known as *saltatory conduction,* and depolarisation occurs at these points of the axon only.

3   The synapse

The points at which nerves connect with each other and to muscles and glands are called *synapses* and transmission of the nerve impulse across these short gaps is effected by the release of chemical transmitters by the pre-synaptic neuron, and the detection of the transmitters by the post-synaptic neurons. An electrical impulse is not strong enough to jump across the synaptic gap. Synaptic transmission is illustrated in Figure 4.7.

There are several different chemical transmitters in the nervous system, but at the majority of synapses *acetylcholine* is released. This causes depolarisation of the neighbouring post-synaptic membrane, which, to prevent acetylcholine lingering, produces *cholinesterase,* an enzyme which inactivates acetylcholine.

The number of synapses in an effective communication circle can be as few as two, as in the simple knee-jerk *reflex arc*. Here only one *internuncial* neuron in the CNS connects the sensory neuron with the motor neuron, and consequently the variation of activity is limited.

Usually, the pattern of connections is much more complex with a range of diverse information input and the facility for continuously varied modification

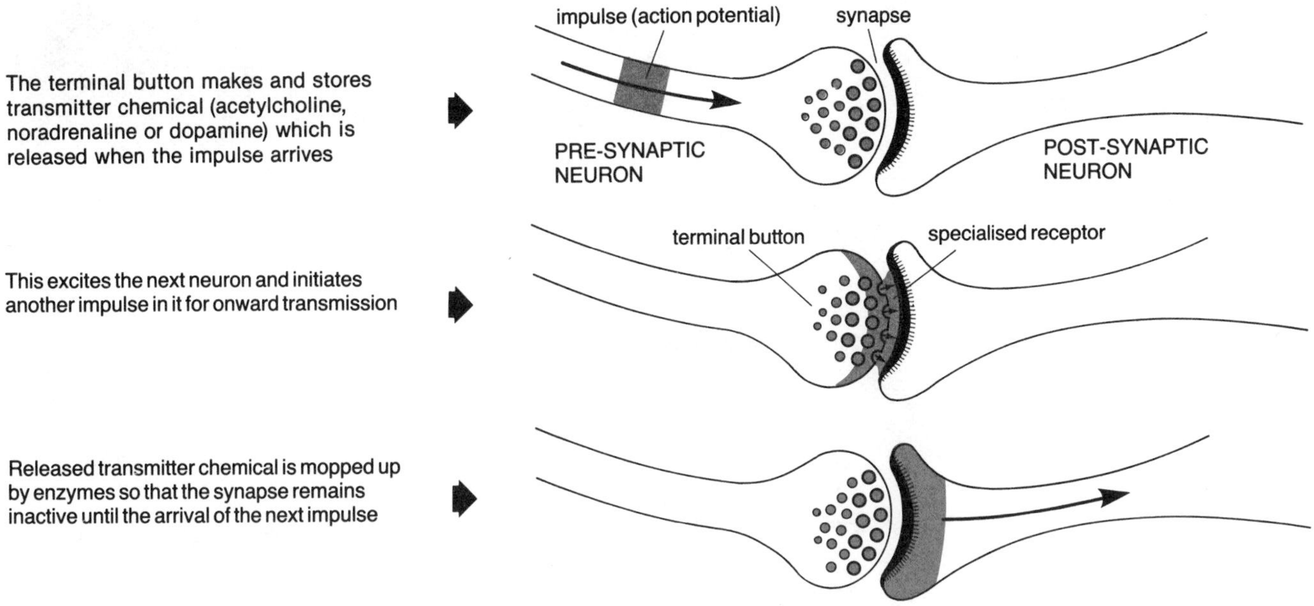

The terminal button makes and stores transmitter chemical (acetylcholine, noradrenaline or dopamine) which is released when the impulse arrives

This excites the next neuron and initiates another impulse in it for onward transmission

Released transmitter chemical is mopped up by enzymes so that the synapse remains inactive until the arrival of the next impulse

impulse (action potential) synapse

PRE-SYNAPTIC NEURON

POST-SYNAPTIC NEURON

terminal button specialised receptor

Figure 4.7 Synaptic transmission

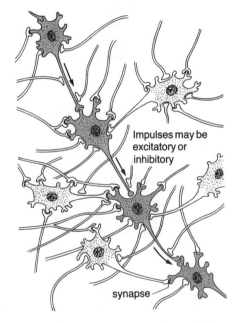

Impulses may be excitatory or inhibitory

synapse

Figure 4.8 Arrangement of synapses in the brain

of action. Chemical transmission between nerves at the synapse may be *inhibitory*, and information from one source may effectively overrule information coming from another source so that the CNS responds to a *selective* message and not to all the information available. The sensation of *pain* can sometimes be blocked or reduced by stimulation of inhibitory nerves which connect with the same nerve pathway. This is discussed, in detail, in D. Ottoson, *Physiology of the Nervous System*, Macmillan, London, 1982.

In the brain, the pattern of nerves and the arrangement of different transmitters is particularly complex (Figure 4.8). Release and detection of neurotransmitters occurs in localised regions and not only at synapses, and it seems that, in addition to the all-or-nothing type of nervous impulse, some brain cells generate 'waves' of depolarisation in localised areas which are not subject to the all-or-nothing rule. Some sensory and motor pathways have been clearly identified in the CNS (see pages 119 and 120) but, for many higher brain functions, no such clear nerve pathway can be established and such functions may actually continue unimpaired after excision of or lesions in parts of the brain. The exact physiological nature of memory, emotion and intellect is a field of considerable research and interest with, so far, few clear answers.

(b) Structure and function of the central nervous system

The nervous system is largely responsible for communication, both within the body and between the body and its surroundings. Information is transmitted via afferent nervous pathways regarding conditions outside and inside the body. This is compared with information stored from previous experience and then adjustments in body state and behaviour are made in response to instructions sent via the efferent nerves.

The collation and comparison of information, the storage of information from previous experience and the generation of responses to stimuli are functions carried out exclusively by the CNS (Figure 4.9), which consists of the *brain* and the *spinal cord*.

The brain

The brain is a soft mass of tissue weighing approximately 1.4 kg in the adult and it lies within the rigid bony structure of the cranium, protected also by the meninges (see page 120). For description, the brain may be divided into three anatomical parts: the cerebrum, the cerebellum and the brain stem.

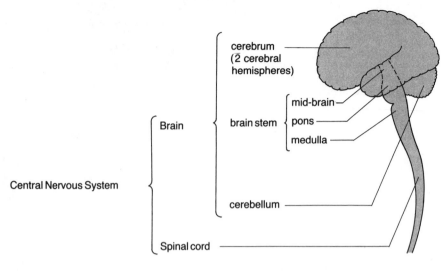

Figure 4.9 Central nervous system

The cerebrum

This is the largest part (Figure 4.10) and is formed by two hemispheres—the left and right. These are partially divided from each other by the longitudinal sinus, below which they are joined together by the corpus callosum, a broad band of nerve fibres. Each hemisphere is greatly folded, or convoluted, increasing the surface area. The grooves (depressions) are called *sulci*, and separate the ridges of the brain tissue, called *gyri*. The outer surface is called the *cerebral cortex* and is composed of nerve cells (grey matter); below this is

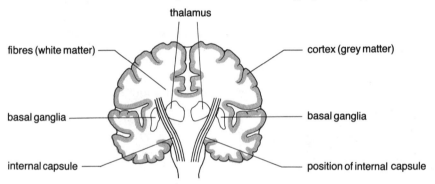

Figure 4.10 Section through the cerebrum

the white matter, which is composed of nerve fibres which connect areas of the cerebrum called *lobes*, and which make connections between each cerebral hemisphere and also between these and the cerebellum and the brain stem. Within this white matter is the internal capsule carrying both sensory impulses from the body to the cerebral cortex and motor-nerve impulses from the cortex to the body via the spinal cord.

The functions of the cerebrum are very complex and scientists continue to explore the links between human behaviour and neural physiology. It is known that in most adults, one cerebral hemisphere tends to be dominant, and that actions on one side of the body are controlled by the opposite cerebral hemisphere, e.g. right- or left-handedness. A right-handed person has a more highly developed cortex for motor functions of the hand in the left cerebral hemisphere, and for language abilities, including speech and reading.

Other areas of the cerebral cortex form lobes in each hemisphere, which are named after the bones of the skull which protect them, and they are identified with specific functions:

- the *temporal* lobes with taste, smell and hearing—and, in the dominant hemisphere, with understanding the spoken word.
- the *occipital* lobes with primary areas for vision.
- the *parietal* lobes, behind the central sulcus, with receiving sensory impulses from the opposite side of the body from muscles, tendons, joints and skin, and interpreted as sensations of size, shape and texture, and also with the sense of position in the environment.

- the *frontal* lobes, in front of the central sulcus, which are concerned with motor activity, i.e. voluntary movement on the opposite side of the body. Part of the cortex in this area is concerned with speech movements.

    The frontal lobes are also association areas, i.e. linking sensory and motor functions, and storing and interpreting information as a basis for memory, intellectual and creative activities.

Embedded within the cerebrum, but not part of it, are the basal ganglia: the *caudate* and *lentiform nuclei*. These are nerve cells concerned with the regulation of movement. The *thalamus* (grey matter) is important in sensory perception, e.g. pain and pressure; close to this are the pituitary gland controlling the endocrine system and the hypothalamus concerned with control of the autonomic nervous system (see Figure 4.11).

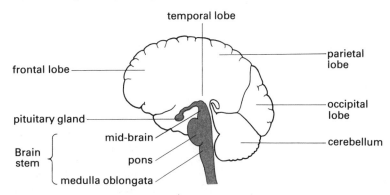

Figure 4.11   Section through brain showing approximate areas of lobes and the positions of certain structures

Within the underpart of the cerebral hemispheres, parts of the gyri of the cortex, parts of the thalamus, the olfactory nerves and the hypothalamus are all linked to form the *limbic* system. This plays a part in emotional and autonomic response and in subconscious motor and sensory activity.

The cerebellum

This forms one-tenth of the mass of the brain. It is formed by a thin cortex of grey matter (nerve cells) and the core is white matter (nerve fibres). Groups of these nerve fibres form the *cerebellar peduncles* connecting the cerebellum to the cerebrum and the brain stem. The cerebellum is partially divided into two hemispheres by a fold of dura mater—the *falx cerebelli*. The part joining the two hemispheres is called the *vermis*.

The function of the cerebellum is to control muscular co-ordination, maintaining posture, balance and equilibrium. It receives sensory impulses from muscles, tendons, joints and the semi-circular canals in the inner ear, and controls motor activity enabling fine movements, and smooth, precise actions. Unlike the cerebrum, each hemisphere of the cerebellum is concerned with the *same* side of the body.

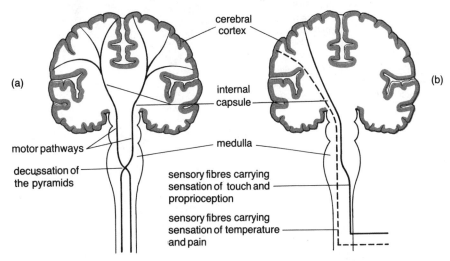

Figure 4.12   Motor and sensory pathways from and to the cerebral hemispheres. (a) Motor pathways from the cerebral cortex and (b) sensory pathways to the cerebral cortex

117

The brain stem

There are three parts of the brain stem: the *mid-brain*, the *pons varolii* and the *medulla oblongata*.

Within the roof of the mid-brain are reflex centres for sight and hearing. The base is formed by the cerebral peduncles which are large bundles of nerve fibres connecting the cerebrum with the rest of the brain and the spinal cord. Within the mid-brain lies the third, and part of the fourth, ventricle. The pons is mainly composed of nerve fibres some of which run transversely to connect the lobes of the cerebellum with each other and with the cerebral cortex. The medulla is continuous with the spinal cord, and links it with the rest of the brain. It consists mainly of nerve fibres, but within its core lie collections of grey matter (nuclei of some important cranial nerves) and the vital centres concerned with reflex activity. These are the *respiratory* centre (controlling the rate and depth of respiration), the *vasomotor* centre (controlling the size of blood vessels) and the *cardiac* centre (controlling the rate and strength of the heart beat). The fourth ventricle lies within the medulla.

In the medulla, some of the motor fibres and some sensory fibres cross from one side of the brain stem to the other at the *decussation of the pyramids* (Figure 4.12a). The sensory fibres crossing here are concerned with touch and position; those concerned with pain, pressure and temperature have crossed in the spinal cord (Figure 4.12b).

The *reticular formation* is an important network of nerve cells and their fibres which is continuous within the medulla, the remainder of the brain stem, the thalamus and the cerebral cortex. This network includes both the vital centres and the centres for reflex actions such as coughing, swallowing, vomiting and sneezing. It prevents all sensory impulses from reaching the cortex, and it screens and selects to prevent overload; it is also important in maintaining consciousness. Many cranial nerves originate within the medulla.

Tone is the resistance of a muscle to being stretched passively (e.g., by gravity), i.e., it prevents a live body from flopping like a dead one. It is a state of partial contraction. An important part of the mechanism producing tone is the spindle. When the muscle is stretched (increasing the distance between origin and insertion) the spindle is also lengthened and this information is sent to the ...

... spinal cord where the impulse is passed to a fast-conducting alpha-efferent motor nerve fibre which causes a group of muscle fibres to contract. This restores the muscle to its previous length and the spindle stops discharging.

If this mechanism operated without the adjustment, obviously no movement would be possible. The spindle is continuously reset by impulses arriving from centres in the brain. These are transmitted by the slower-conducting gamma-efferent fibres to the muscle fibres within the spindle (intrafusal) which govern the length of the spindle and thus its sensory discharge.

Adaption is relatively slow (though only taking fractions of a second) and is thus very suitable for the maintenance of balance and posture

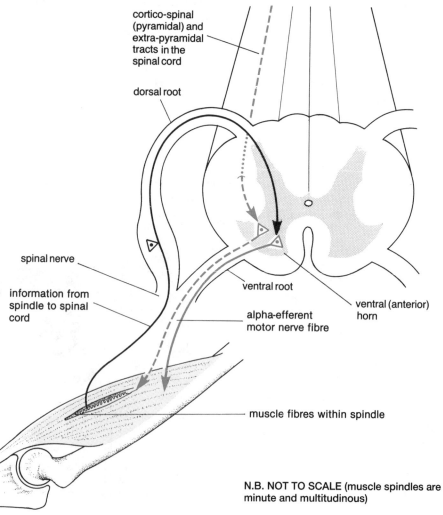

cortico-spinal (pyramidal) and extra-pyramidal tracts in the spinal cord

dorsal root

spinal nerve

information from spindle to spinal cord

ventral root

alpha-efferent motor nerve fibre

ventral (anterior) horn

muscle fibres within spindle

N.B. NOT TO SCALE (muscle spindles are minute and multitudinous)

PULL OF GRAVITY

Figure 4.13   Maintenance of muscle tone

2 The spinal cord

The spinal cord extends from the upper border of the first cervical vertebra to the lower border of the first lumbar vertebra. It is on average 1 centimetre in diameter, and has thirty-one pairs of *spinal nerves* branching from it. These carry both motor and sensory nerves.

Compared with the brain, the functions of the spinal cord seem relatively simple and limited. Sensory and motor information to and from the brain is carried by the spinal cord from and to parts of the body below the brain, but the spinal cord actually forms the link between a considerable amount of sensory information and motor output for several important reflex functions, mainly associated with posture and locomotion. As an example, Figure 4.13 shows the maintenance of muscle tone.

3 Sensory and motor pathways in the CNS

Sensory reception and the chief sensory pathways (see Figure 4.14)

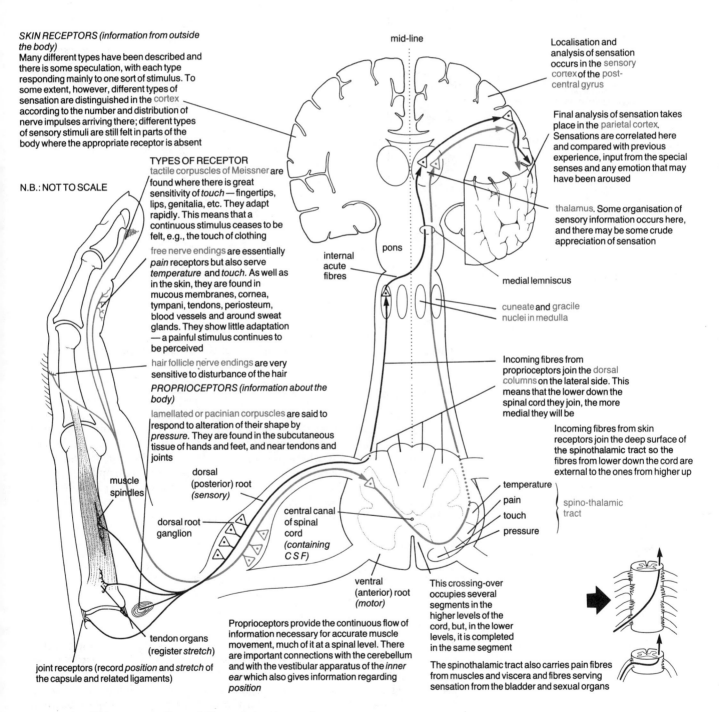

SKIN RECEPTORS (information from outside the body)
Many different types have been described and there is some speculation, with each type responding mainly to one sort of stimulus. To some extent, however, different types of sensation are distinguished in the cortex according to the number and distribution of nerve impulses arriving there; different types of sensory stimuli are still felt in parts of the body where the appropriate receptor is absent

N.B.: NOT TO SCALE

TYPES OF RECEPTOR
tactile corpuscles of Meissner are found where there is great sensitivity of *touch* — fingertips, lips, genitalia, etc. They adapt rapidly. This means that a continuous stimulus ceases to be felt, e.g., the touch of clothing

free nerve endings are essentially *pain* receptors but also serve *temperature* and *touch*. As well as in the skin, they are found in mucous membranes, cornea, tympani, tendons, periosteum, blood vessels and around sweat glands. They show little adaptation — a painful stimulus continues to be perceived

hair follicle nerve endings are very sensitive to disturbance of the hair

PROPRIOCEPTORS (information about the body)

lamellated or pacinian corpuscles are said to respond to alteration of their shape by *pressure*. They are found in the subcutaneous tissue of hands and feet, and near tendons and joints

muscle spindles

dorsal (posterior) root (sensory)

dorsal root ganglion

central canal of spinal cord (containing C S F)

ventral (anterior) root (motor)

tendon organs (register *stretch*)

joint receptors (record *position* and *stretch* of the capsule and related ligaments)

Proprioceptors provide the continuous flow of information necessary for accurate muscle movement, much of it at a spinal level. There are important connections with the cerebellum and with the vestibular apparatus of the *inner ear* which also gives information regarding *position*

mid-line

Localisation and analysis of sensation occurs in the sensory cortex of the post-central gyrus

Final analysis of sensation takes place in the parietal cortex. Sensations are correlated here and compared with previous experience, input from the special senses and any emotion that may have been aroused

thalamus. Some organisation of sensory information occurs here, and there may be some crude appreciation of sensation

pons

internal acute fibres

medial lemniscus

cuneate and gracile nuclei in medulla

Incoming fibres from proprioceptors join the dorsal columns on the lateral side. This means that the lower down the spinal cord they join, the more medial they will be

Incoming fibres from skin receptors join the deep surface of the spinothalamic tract so the fibres from lower down the cord are external to the ones from higher up

temperature
pain
touch
pressure

spino-thalamic tract

This crossing-over occupies several segments in the higher levels of the cord, but, in the lower levels, it is completed in the same segment

The spinothalamic tract also carries pain fibres from muscles and viscera and fibres serving sensation from the bladder and sexual organs

Figure 4.14 Main sensory pathways in the central nervous system

Motor pathways involved in voluntary movement

The motor cortex is responsible for conscious muscular action, e.g. unfamiliar hand movements (Figure 4.15). For these movements to be performed properly, the rest of the body must give maximum co-operation. These semi-conscious and postural patterns are controlled by the cerebellum and the basal ganglia. Two significant nerve groups are the *pyramidal tract* which exercises voluntary control over motor functions and the *extrapyramidal tracts* which mainly inhibit action and are concerned with involuntary control of motor activities contributing to movement. Parkinson's disease, and the 'extrapyramidal side effects' of certain drugs, cause reduction in this inhibition resulting in muscular rigidity and tremors at rest.

For these movements to be performed properly, the rest of the body must give maximum cooperation. These *semi-conscious* and *postural* patterns are under the control of the basal ganglia and the cerebellum

There are very complex interconnections between the different parts of the control system, and efficient operation requires continuous input of sensory information from the eyes, from the vestibular balancing system of the inner ear and from muscle and joint receptors

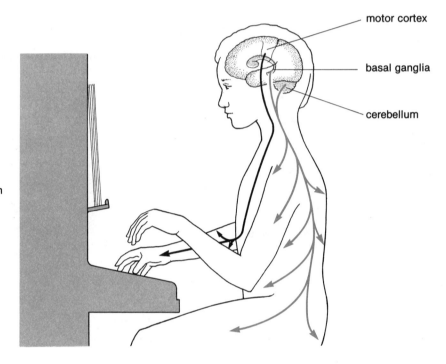

Figure 4.15   Control of voluntary movement

4   The meninges

These are three membranes which protect the brain and spinal cord (Figures 4.16 and 4.17).

The dura mater

This is a tough, fibrous membrane forming two layers within the skull. The outer (or periosteal) layer forms the periosteum lining the cranium. The inner (or meningeal) layer is adherent to this except where the venous sinuses run between the layers, and where the innermost layer dips down in the *sulci* (e.g. the *falx cerebri*) to separate parts of the cerebral hemispheres, and to separate the cerebrum from the cerebellum. The entire venous drainage of the brain occurs within the venous sinuses. There is a potential space between the dura and the arachnoid called the *subdural space*.

The arachnoid mater

The *arachnoid* (spidery) layer forms a loose, net-like covering for the brain, and parts of it are attached to the pia. Between the arachnoid and the pia mater is the *subarachnoid space* containing cerebrospinal fluid.

The pia mater

This 'tender' membrane is very delicate and is firmly attached to the brain. It consists of a plexus of blood vessels in loose linking tissue. It dips into the sulci and, by protruding into the ventricles of the brain, it forms the *choroid plexuses*. These secrete the cerebrospinal fluid (CSF) which fills the ventricles and the central canal of the spinal cord, and the *subarachnoid* space between the arachnoid and pia, thus completely surrounding the CNS.

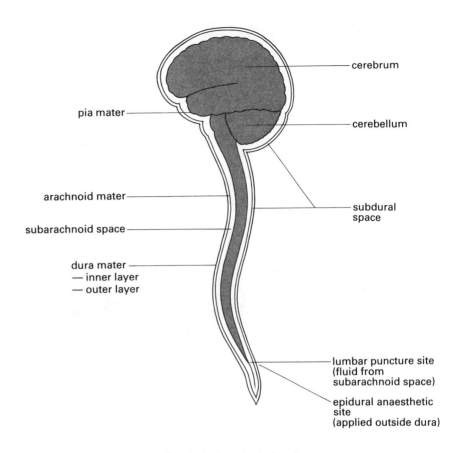

Figure 4.16 Meninges surrounding the brain and spinal cord

Labels for Figure 4.16:
- cerebrum
- cerebellum
- pia mater
- arachnoid mater
- subdural space
- subarachnoid space
- dura mater
  — inner layer
  — outer layer
- lumbar puncture site (fluid from subarachnoid space)
- epidural anaesthetic site (applied outside dura)

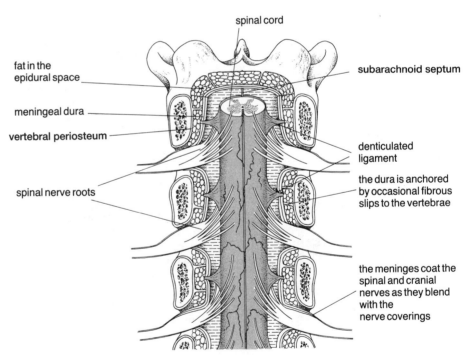

Figure 4.17 Meninges surrounding the spinal cord

Labels for Figure 4.17:
- spinal cord
- fat in the epidural space
- subarachnoid septum
- meningeal dura
- vertebral periosteum
- denticulated ligament
- the dura is anchored by occasional fibrous slips to the vertebrae
- spinal nerve roots
- the meninges coat the spinal and cranial nerves as they blend with the nerve coverings

The spinal cord is not allowed to hang loosely in the vertebral column, but is stabilised by fibrous projections of the pia. The *subarachnoid septum* connects it incompletely to the arachnoid mater, and the *denticulate ligament* attaches it to the dura, which is anchored by occasional fibrous slips to the vertebrae.

The fat of the *epidural space* between the meningeal dura and the vertebral periosteum packs the spinal cord within the mobile vertebral column and contains many veins. An anaesthetic injected into this space will block the spinal nerve roots that traverse it.

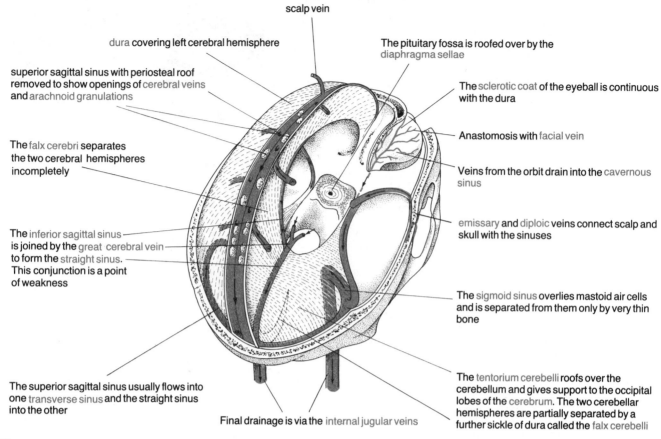

scalp vein

dura covering left cerebral hemisphere

The pituitary fossa is roofed over by the diaphragma sellae

superior sagittal sinus with periosteal roof removed to show openings of cerebral veins and arachnoid granulations

The sclerotic coat of the eyeball is continuous with the dura

The falx cerebri separates the two cerebral hemispheres incompletely

Anastomosis with facial vein

Veins from the orbit drain into the cavernous sinus

The inferior sagittal sinus is joined by the great cerebral vein to form the straight sinus. This conjunction is a point of weakness

emissary and diploic veins connect scalp and skull with the sinuses

The sigmoid sinus overlies mastoid air cells and is separated from them only by very thin bone

The superior sagittal sinus usually flows into one transverse sinus and the straight sinus into the other

Final drainage is via the internal jugular veins

The tentorium cerebelli roofs over the cerebellum and gives support to the occipital lobes of the cerebrum. The two cerebellar hemispheres are partially separated by a further sickle of dura called the falx cerebelli

Figure 4.18   Venous sinuses

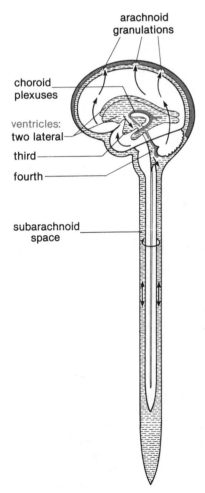

arachnoid granulations

choroid plexuses

ventricles:
two lateral

third

fourth

subarachnoid space

Figure 4.19   Cerebrospinal fluid

The venous sinuses (Figure 4.18) are channels between the two layers of the dura. They are lined with endothelium, but have no valves, and the walls, being dura, have no muscles. Flow in the sinuses is partly due to gravity, and partly to the 'force from behind' of the arterial blood pressure in the brain. In the *cavernous sinus* flow is also assisted by the pulsations of the carotid artery.

The *arachnoid granulations,* located in the longitudinal fissure, transmit the cerebrospinal fluid from the subarachnoid space to the blood in the superior sagittal sinus.

5   The cerebrospinal fluid (CSF)

CSF is a clear liquid similar in composition to plasma, since it contains water, minerals, lymphocytes, glucose and protein. It is formed from blood by the action of the *choroid plexuses* of the lateral, third and fourth *ventricles*. Approximately 550 ml of CSF is produced in 24 hours, and at any one time its total volume is 200 ml. It flows around the subarachnoid space surrounding both the brain and the spinal cord (Figure 4.19) and is reabsorbed into the blood via the arachnoid granulations. In the spinal cord, CSF probably drains back into the veins of the epidural space.

Functions of the CSF

The functions of the CSF are outlined below.

- It acts as a shock absorber for the CNS, forming a fluid cushion.
- It forms an exchange medium between blood and brain, keeping the brain's biochemical environment relatively constant despite changes in the blood.
- It helps to support the brain, which is thirty times lighter in CSF than in air.
- Pressure changes in the brain can be buffered by changing rates of CSF production and adsorption.

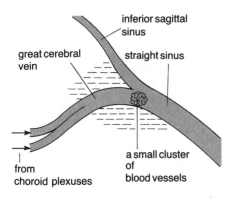

Figure 4.20 Control of CSF production and absorption

Regulation of CSF production is carried out by modifying the blood pressure in the choroid plexuses. A small cluster of blood vessels protrudes into the lumen of the straight sinus. Congestion of this cluster causes it to act like a ball-valve, causing back-pressure to the plexuses and hence increased production of CSF (Figure 4.20). There are others at other sites close to the choroid plexuses.

6   Blood supply to the brain

The brain needs a large blood supply, and receives 750 ml/minute. If the flow of blood to the brain stops, unconsciousness occurs within ten seconds. At normal temperatures, irreversible brain damage occurs after about three minutes of anoxia (lack of oxygen). At lower temperatures the brain can survive anoxia for longer periods, as has been observed in people nearly drowned in icy water. The body is sometimes cooled deliberately, thus reducing its metabolic requirements to prolong the permitted period of anoxia when brain or heart surgery is being done.

Figure 4.21 illustrates the layout of the brain's arterial supply.

The communicating arteries of the circle of Willis (colourless in Figure 4.21) vary in size, and are potential alternative channels rather than actual ones. This is why a radio-opaque substance, injected into one internal carotid artery, will show up on an arteriogram in its own 'territory' without overlap. Alterations in pressure as a result of pathological change will open them up.

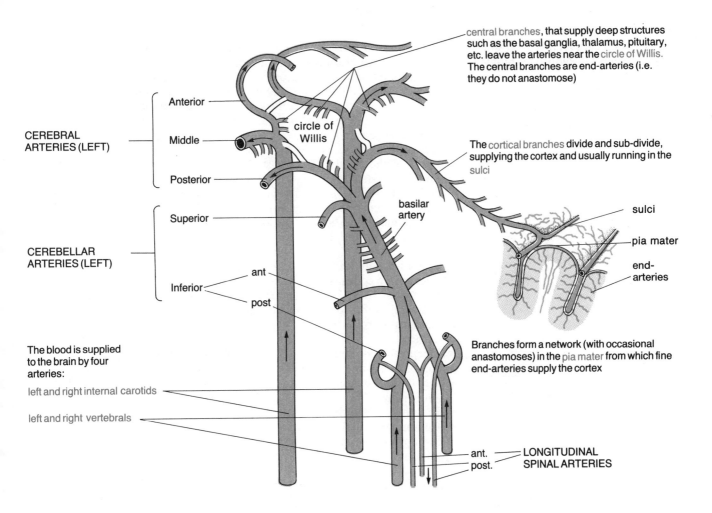

Figure 4.21   Blood supply to the brain

The patients with disturbances of consciousness

(a) Disturbances of consciousness in patients with
conditions caused by
accident, infection or drug
overdose

1   Patient study and care plan for an adult with cerebrovascular accident

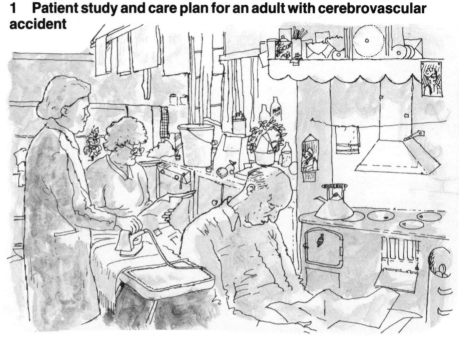

Figure 4.22   Mrs Robinson

History of social, psychological and physical events leading to the present condition

The patient chosen for this section to illustrate disturbance of consciousness is an adult with cerebrovascular accident.

Mrs Robinson (Figure 4.22), aged 72 years, lives with her 80-year-old husband and his sister, Mrs Edwards, a widow aged 78 years, in a large Victorian house in a neglected area of a major city. The upper part of the house is let as bedsitters, occupied by two students. The house has a flight of six steps up to the front door and the only bathroom and toilet is on the first floor. There is a small garden at the rear but as the house is built on a hill there are several steps up to it. The nearest shops are at the bottom of a steep hill but on a bus route. The hospital is at the far side of the city centre. Mrs Robinson, the most active member of the family, does most of the shopping, cooking and housework although her sister-in-law has taken responsibility for the family's washing and ironing. Mr Robinson enjoys propagating seeds and cuttings in his small greenhouse but is no longer able to look after the heavy work in the garden.

After a morning's housework Mrs Robinson was found by her sister-in-law on the floor in the kitchen. Mrs Edwards was unable to rouse her and was frightened by Mrs Robinson's noisy breathing and odd colour. She called her brother and went next door to ask the neighbour to get help. They tried to make Mrs Robinson comfortable on the floor but were both very anxious by the time the doctor arrived. The doctor examined Mrs Robinson and, suspecting that she had had a cerebrovascular accident, arranged for her immediate transfer to the medical ward of the local hospital.

On arrival the following observations are made:

- Deeply unconscious.
- Limbs flaccid and reflexes absent.
- Pupils equal but reacting
  sluggishly.
- Breathing stertorous.
- Colour pale and slightly cyanosed.
- Swallowing and coughing reflexes
  absent.
- Incontinent of urine.
- Pulse 90 beats per minute.
- Blood pressure 130/90 mmHg.
- Temperature 36.8°C.

Explanation of abnormal physiology and pathology

You should revise the normal structure and function of the central nervous system and its blood supply, and see Table 4.1.

Any interruption of the blood supply to the brain *or* any injury to the nerve cells and/or nerve pathways within the brain *or* any increase of pressure within the cranium will result in loss of, or reduction in, the function of that part of the brain affected and the organs and tissues supplied by the affected nerves.

Table 4.1

Normal physiology	Abnormal physiology
(a) Conscious state, aware of surroundings and responsive to stimuli, depends on healthy brain tissue and good blood supply	Sudden loss of consciousness due to haemorrhage from a cerebral artery which results in lack of blood to the area of brain tissue distal to the site of rupture of the vessel
(b) Central nervous system, motor nerves maintain muscle tone and activity	Pressure of leaking blood on motor pathways interrupts nerve impulses to the muscles on the opposite side of the body, causing loss of muscle tone and flaccid paralysis
(c) Sensory nerve pathways bring information of pain, touch, temperature and pressure from the body to the brain	Pressure of leaking blood on the sensory pathways interrupts the impulses bringing information to the brain from the opposite side of the body
(d) Protective reflexes situated in the medulla oblongata operate below the level of consciousness to protect against, for example, inhalation of saliva or vomit	Pressure within the cranium rises due to the haemorrhage which compresses the medulla oblongata. This inhibits the swallowing and coughing reflexes
(e) Vital centres such as respiratory, vasomotor and temperature-regulating function in conjunction with the autonomic nervous system	Damage to brain tissue or raised intracranial pressure compresses the nerve centres and inhibits activity, causing difficulty in breathing, poor temperature control and changes in the blood pressure
(f) Oculomotor nerve (3rd cranial nerve) controls the size of the pupils to regulate the amount of light to the retina	Damage or pressure on the oculomotor nerve can cause sluggish reaction of the pupil to light or unequal pupil response to light
(g) Centres in the dominant hemisphere of the brain permit articulation of speech	Damage or pressure on the dominant hemisphere may result in dysphasia

Care plan

PREPARATION FOR PATIENT WITH CEREBROVASCULAR ACCIDENT

Nursing history and assessment
This is shown in Table 4.2.

Table 4.2   *Nursing history and assessment sheet for Mrs Elsie Robinson*

NURSING HISTORY AND ASSESSMENT SHEET
Record No. _____ 33333 _____

PATIENT LABEL
Mr/Mrs/Miss _____ Elsie Robinson _____
Address _____ 16 Bellevue Terrace, Churchtown _____
Male/Female   Age _____ 72 _____
Date of Birth _____ 6·6·14 _____

Date of admission/~~first visit~~
_____ 3·10·86 _____
Time _____
Type: ☐ Routine ☑ Emergency
  Transfer from: _____

Religion _____ C/E _____
Practising/baptised _____ Practising _____
Minister _____
Telephone number _____

Next of kin (name) _____ Mr Arthur Robinson _____
Relationship to patient _____ Husband _____
Address _____ Same address _____

Telephone numbers _____ 4567 (Neighbour- _____
Contact at night/in emergency YES/NO   Mrs Orr)

Occupation (or father) _____ Housewife _____
Marital status _____ Married _____
Children (or place in family) _____
Other dependants _____
Pets _____
School (children only) _____
Hobbies _____
Clubs _____
Favourite pastime _____
Does patient smoke?   YES/NO

Speech difficulty/language barrier

Dysphasia   Dysarthria

Accommodation

Lives alone   YES/NO

Part III/EMI/Old People's Homes/Rented
Other _____ Large Victorian terraced house _____

Table 4.2 (cont.)

Consultant ___ *Mr Cornwall* ___

House officer ___ *Dr Robins* ___

Presenting condition ___ *Unconscious* ___
Cerebrovascular accident

History of present complaint and reason for admission
___ *N/a* ___

Past medical history
___ *N/a* ___

Allergies *None*

Current medication
___ *None* ___

What patient says is the reason for admission and attitude to admission

Patient's expectations *N/a*

Any problems at home while/because patient is in hospital?

Relevant home conditions (e.g. stairs)
Steps to front door, steps to garden.
House on steep hill

Visiting problems
___ *No transport* ___

Care at home

Community nurse ___

No. ___

Name of GP ___ *Dr Bloggs* ___

Address ___ *The Health Centre, Churchtown* ___

Other services involved *To be assessed*

Home help ___ Day hospital ___

Laundry ___ Day centre/club ___

Inco supplies ___ Health visitor ___

Aids ___ Social worker ___

Meals on wheels ___ Voluntary worker ___

Daily living

Diet

Special ___

Food or drink dislikes ___

Appetite: ☐ GOOD ☐ POOR
Remarks ___ *Previously normal* ___

Sleep

How many hours normally? ___ *6* ___

Sedation ___

What else helps? ___

Elimination

Bowels: Continent/~~Incontinent~~

How often opened? ___ *Daily normally* ___

Any medication? ___ *No* ___

Urinary: Continent/~~Incontinent~~

If incontinent; Day/Night/If not taken, how frequently? ___

Nocturia/Dysuria/Frequency/Urgency

Remarks ___

Female patients — Menstruation

Post-menopausal   Taking the pill

Regular   Irregular

Amenorrhoea   Dysmenorrhoea

Next period due: ___

Uses: STs Tampons

Hearing

Hearing aid: YES/NO

Remarks ___

Vision

Glasses/Contact lens: YES/NO

Remarks ___

Oral

Dentures or crowns: YES/NO

Any problems with mouth or teeth?

___

Mobility

Help needed with:

Walking/Standing/In/Out of bed/Bathing/Dressing

In/Out of chair/

Feeding/Other: ___

Remarks ___ *Unconscious (normally active)*

Prosthesis/appliance

Type of appliance ___

Help needed ___

General appearance

Normal   Dehydrated   Acutely ill

Obese   Thin   Emaciated

Remarks ___

Skin

Satisfactory   Broken areas   Dehydrated

Rash   Oedematous   Jaundiced

Pallor   Other *Cold, slightly cyanosed*
(including bruising)

Remarks ___

<table>
<tr><td colspan="3">Level of consciousness</td><td colspan="2">Orientation</td></tr>
</table>

Level of consciousness

Orientated   Semi-conscious

Confused   <u>Unconscious</u>

Remarks _____

Mental assessment (if appropriate) *Unconscious*

Mood

Elated   Irritable   Agitated

Cheerful   Anxious   Aggressive

Miserable   Withdrawn   Suspicious

Apathetic

Thought content

Hallucinations/Delusions/Paranoid Ideas

_____

Orientation

Time/Place/Person   Very confused   Slightly confused

Any particular time of day? _____

Confabulation _____

Remarks _____

Surveillance   Physical/Emotional

Information obtained from *Mr Robinson and Mrs Edwards*

Relationship to patient *Husband, Sister-in-law*

By _____ *J.A. Jones* _____

Position/level of training _____

Date _____ *3·10·86* _____

Time _____

TREATMENT

The care plan for Mrs Robinson is shown in Table 4.3. It is most important that before and during every procedure Mrs Robinson is spoken to by the nurse responsible for her care to provide a stimulating environment to aid rehabilitation.

Table 4.3   Care plan for Mrs Robinson

Problem	Objective	Plan of care	Rationale
1. Unconscious patient unable to maintain own airway and has lost swallowing and coughing reflex	Maintain clear airway	(a) Position Mrs Robinson semi-prone without pillow	(a) Saliva and possible vomit less likely to be inhaled—prevents tongue from falling backward and blocking pharynx
		(b) Remove dentures	(b) Prevents inhalation of dentures
		(c) Prepare apparatus for pharyngeal suction	(c) To remove saliva and/or vomit
		(d) Administer oxygen therapy as prescribed	(d) Provides oxygen-enriched air
		(e) Have oropharyngeal airway available	(e) May be difficult to stop tongue dropping backward if jaw lax
2. Unconscious patient unable to move or feel	Prevent pressure sores, contractures of joints, muscle wasting, venous stasis, hypostatic pneumonia and urinary stasis. Prevent trauma to insensitive skin	(a) Turn and reposition Mrs Robinson at least 2-hourly	(a) Relieves pressure over bony prominences, aids ventilation and drainage of lungs, encourages venous return, permits inspection of skin
		(b) Provide aids such as ripple mattress, sheepskin, bed cradle, extra pillows	(b) Reduces pressure, helps to protect insensitive skin
		(c) Support all limbs and joints including fingers in a natural position	(c) Prevents contractures, foot drop, wrist drop
		(d) With physiotherapist put all joints through full range of movement twice a day	(d) Prevents adhesions and stiffness of joints and muscle atrophy
		(e) Avoid over-extension of joints when turning or moving patient	(e) Flaccid paralysis around joints may allow joint to dislocate or damage supporting ligaments and tendons, making rehabilitation a slower process
3. Unconscious patient unable to control bladder function	Prevent complications of incontinence and ensure bladder emptying	(a) Insert urinary catheter and connect to closed drainage	(a) Prevents urine contact with skin and ensures bladder emptying
		(b) Record on fluid balance chart the amount of urine drained	(b) Provides record for estimating fluid balance
		(c) Carry out catheter toilet and vulval hygiene three times a day	(c) Helps to prevent ascending infection into bladder

Table 4.3 (cont.)

Problem	Objective	Plan of care	Rationale
4. Unconscious patient unable to eat and drink	Maintain adequate hydration and nutrition	(a) Pass nasogastric tube and give 3-hourly intragastric feeds to cover daily requirements for protein, carbohydrate, fat, vitamins and minerals. For Mrs Robinson this could be per 24 hours: 1000 calories which should contain not more than 35-40 grams of protein in 2000 millilitres of fluid. If diarrhoea occurs reduce glucose content and if necessary reduce lactase also	(a) Provides artificial route for administration of nutrients and water which patient can then digest and absorb
		(b) Check that tube is patent and in the stomach prior to each feed and put 25 millilitres of water down the tube before and after each feed	(b) Prevents introduction of feed into trachea. Water ensures patency of tube by clearing debris
		(c) Give not more than 250 millilitres of warmed liquid at each feed	(c) Prevents over-distension of stomach and possible regurgitation
		(d) Do not turn patient immediately after feeding	(d) Prevents regurgitation
		(e) Record balance of feed and water on fluid balance chart	(e) Provides record of fluid intake
5. Unconscious patient unable to control bowel function	Prevent constipation and faecal impaction	(a) Give adequate fluid intake	(a) Minimises water reabsorption from the large intestine and so keeps stool soft
		(b) Give suppositories every third day if no bowel action	(b) Keeps lower bowel empty
6. Patient at risk of extension of cerebral lesion	Monitor patient's condition to detect changes	Measure and record the following, frequency of observations as appropriate:	
		(a) Pulse	(a) Falling pulse rate indicates increasing intracranial pressure
		(b) Blood pressure	(b) Rising blood pressure indicates increasing intracranial pressure
		(c) Respirations	(c) Slowing in Cheyne–Stokes indicates increasing intracranial pressure
		(d) Temperature	(d) Pyrexia could indicate infection in chest or urinary tract, or interference with temperature-regulating centre in brain
		(e) Level of consciousness	(e) Changes in response to stimuli indicate improvement or deterioration
		(f) Pupil size and reaction to light	(f) Refer to section on abnormal physiology
		(g) Type and extent of paralysis	(g) Flaccid paralysis changes to spastic paralysis as time passes. Danger of severe contractures occurring. Lesion usually affects one side of brain, therefore gives hemiparesis or hemiplegia on opposite side
7. Patient unable to care for personal hygiene	Provide care of skin, mouth, eyes and hair	(a) Bed bath daily and repeat if sweating	(a) Prevents accumulation of sweat, dead skin cells and haven for pathogenic microorganisms. Allows inspection of the skin for pressure or abrasions

Problem	Objective	Plan of care	Rationale
		(b) Mouth care at least 4-hourly with attention to procedure and suction available	(b) Ensures clean mucous membrane, prevents stomatitis, parotitis and allows inspection. Attention to procedure minimises risk of inhalation
		(c) Give nasal toilet 3-hourly and check that naso-gastric tube is not dragging on nostril and skin of face	(c) Tube irritates mucous membrane in nostril and can cause pressure sore
		(d) Swab eyes with sterile normal saline or water 4-hourly and keep lids closed	(d) Removes debris, prevents infection and corneal abrasions
		(e) Brush and arrange hair as necessary. Wash or use dry shampoo if period of unconsciousness is prolonged	(e) Stops hair knotting and causing pressure, improves appearance
8. Anxious, elderly and frail relatives who have no transport	Reassurance of relatives and advice regarding visiting and communication	(a) Arrange for Mr Robinson and Mrs Edwards to meet the doctor and senior nurse for discussion and explanation of Mrs Robinson's condition	(a) Reassures, relieves initial anxiety and establishes relationship with hospital staff
		(b) Provide ongoing information to both relatives	(b) Keeps relatives up to date with changes in condition
		(c) Make sure relatives have ward telephone number and advise to ring for information each day at least	(c) As above, both are elderly and unable to visit daily
		(d) Offer referral to medical social worker regarding travelling difficulties and home arrangements	(d) May be able to arrange volunteer driver to bring them to hospital. May need home support services
		(e) Make arrangements for communication in emergency, day or night, if relatives require. Make sure all staff are aware of arrangements	(e) Mrs Robinson's husband cannot be contacted by telephone, and as he is elderly he may not want to be called at night. Also, communication with him involves a neighbour with a telephone

Mrs Robinson's recovery and rehabilitation

Mrs Robinson remains deeply unconscious for five days and then starts to open her eyes. Some spontaneous movement of the left side of her body returns. The right hemiplegia becomes more obvious. She starts to suck anything put in her mouth and seems to be swallowing her saliva. Her eyes appear to focus but she makes no attempt to speak. She has a worried expression on her face and becomes agitated when approached. Having become aware of the nasogastric tube and urinary catheter, she attempts to remove both. Oral fluids are gradually reintroduced and when sufficient fluid is taken for daily requirements the nasogastric tube is removed. She experiences difficulty with dribbling due to paralysis of facial muscles. A rehabilitation programme is started, involving the nursing staff, physiotherapist, speech therapist and occupational therapist for preparation for return to daily living, that is: regaining balance in bed, in chair and standing; teaching to walk and manage stairs; visiting the toilet; eating and drinking at table; washing and dressing; developing ability to talk and communicate. The urinary catheter was removed when Mrs Robinson was able to use the sani-chair.

During this time the medical social worker and occupational therapist carry out a home assessment to determine the feasibility of Mrs Robinson's returning home if left with residual hemiplegia or dysphagia. Joint discussion between nursing staff, medical staff, paramedical staff and relatives decides the support services which will be required for transfer to the community.

It is advisable to revise the Bobath technique for the care of patients following cerebrovascular accident.

2 Patient histories illustrating further problems related to disturbances of consciousness

This part of the chapter comprises patient histories, self-testing questions and suggested answers.

A young person with meningococcal meningitis

Sally Spencer, aged 18 years, was on a camping holiday with two friends when she began to feel unwell with a headache, vomiting, a stiff neck and backache. As she felt feverish, she thought she was suffering from influenza but she rapidly became so unwell, irritable and drowsy that her friends were worried and took her to the local hospital.

On arrival, examination and history reveal the following signs and symptoms of meningeal irritation.

1. Signs of meningeal irritation:
   - Neck rigidity: passive flexion of the neck is impossible due to stretching the inflamed routes of the cervical nerves.
   - Kernig's sign positive: if the patient's thigh is flexed to 90° from the abdomen, it is then impossible to straighten the knee passively due to spasm of the hamstring muscles; this manoeuvre stretches the roots of the sciatic nerve, which are inflamed at their exits from the spinal meninges.
   - Irritability and resentment of interference.
   - Drowsiness and confusion.
2. Symptoms of meningeal irritation:
   - Headache.
   - Photophobia.
   - Vomiting.
   - Pyrexia — 39°C.
   - Pain in back and limbs.

Sally is admitted for further investigations and care and her relatives are informed.

Further investigations include:

1. Lumbar puncture.
2. Nose and throat swabs for bacteriology.
3. Blood sample for culture and sensitivity.
4. Urine sample for analysis, culture and sensitivity, and microscopy.
5. Sputum specimen for culture and sensitivity if obtainable.

The doctor diagnoses Sally as having meningitis, probably due to meningococci, and starts treatments pending the bacteriology results. He prescribes sulphonamides, a high loading dose initially and then four-hourly intramuscularly. As Sally's condition is obviously deteriorating into coma, intrathecal penicillin is also prescribed.

SELF-TESTING QUESTIONS

BRIEF ANALYSIS AND GUIDELINES TO SUITABLE ANSWERS

1. Devise a care plan for:
   (a) Sally's unconscious state
   (b) Sally's febrile state
   (c) Sally's possibly infectious condition.

Question 1
(a) Refer to previous care plan for Mrs Robinson (pages 127–129).
(b) Your answer should include:
   - Light bedclothes and use of bed cradle.
   - Frequent sponging of face and hands.
   - Well-ventilated room.
   - Use of fan and/or tepid sponging if prescribed.
(c) Include the following procedures:
   - Protection of staff, visitors and other patients by isolation and use of protective clothing.
   - Teaching of careful handwashing.
   - Use of disposable equipment with attention to agreed hospital procedure.

2. Laboratory results reveal the following in the cerebrospinal fluid: a turbid fluid under pressure containing increased number of white blood cells, with isolation of the meningococcus, protein content raised and glucose lower than normal. Other investigations revealed nothing abnormal.

Describe later specific complications of meningococcal meningitis.

3. Describe the likely outcome of Sally's condition.

Question 2

Later complications of meningococcal meningitis are those of septicaemia as follows:

(a) The appearance of a petechial rash before the third day of illness, which can spread to form large haemorrhagic patches on limbs and trunk. Infection of one or more joints may occur.

(b) Conjunctivitis.

(c) A severe complication is adrenal failure due to haemorrhage into the adrenal gland cortex.

Question 3

(a) If treatment is prompt, and supportive nursing is given, Sally will regain consciousness over a period of days and will require several weeks' convalescence and rehabilitation.

(b) Residual effects of meningitis are rare. Septicaemia can result in aplastic anaemia and/or adrenal failure and death. It can also lead to encephalitis, deafness or pericarditis, and, in infants, it may result in hydrocephalus.

An adult patient with a head injury due to a road traffic accident

Mr Stephen Sikorski, aged 60 years, of Polish descent, has lived in Britain since 1950. He is married and lives with his wife and his father who is now 85 years old. Mr Sikorski was brought into the accident and emergency department deeply unconscious, having been knocked down by a car while he was crossing the road.

Assessment reveals the following:
- Lacerations to face and scalp.
- Unconscious and not responding to voice or painful stimuli.
- Pupils equal but reacting sluggishly to light.
- Breathing quickly (no dentures or loose teeth).
- Pulse and blood pressure within normal limits.
- No other obvious injuries.

An x-ray of the skull is performed but no bony injury is revealed. Mr Sikorski is transferred to the trauma ward and his relatives are informed of his admission.

SELF-TESTING QUESTIONS

1. Describe the significance of the observations you would make of Mr Sikorski following admission to the ward.

BRIEF ANALYSIS AND GUIDELINES TO SUITABLE ANSWERS

Question 1

Your answer should include:

(a) Reference to abnormal physiology and rationale for observations in patient study for Mrs Robinson: see pages 120 and 123.

(b) Observe for leakage of blood and/or cerebrospinal fluid via the nose or ears. Test fluid for glucose to identify cerebrospinal fluid.

(c) Prompt action *must* be taken in event of the following:
- Pupils fail to respond to light.
- Blood pressure rises with concurrent fall in pulse rate.
- Leakage of cerebrospinal fluid occurs.

This could indicate extradural haematoma and tear in the meninges which would need urgent surgical intervention (see Fact Sheet 2, page 132).

Question 2

See Fact Sheet 2 on page 132.

2. Distinguish between:
- Extradural haematoma.
- Subdural haematoma.
- Concussion.

3. Discuss the possible difficulties that could be encountered as Mr Sikorski regains consciousness.

Question 3

Mr Sikorski may be disorientated, aggressive, forgetful, liable to fall out of bed. He could inflict injury on himself or others due to confusion. He could have amnesia and possibly difficulty in recognising family and friends. Initially he may revert to his first language. He may have residual disfigurement from facial lacerations.

Fact Sheet 2   Cerebral haematomas and concussion

EXTRA-DURAL HAEMOTOMA – a typical history

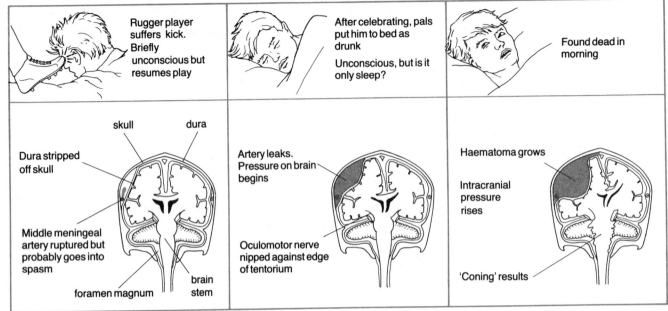

Figure 4.23   Extra-dural haematoma: a typical history

EXTRA-DURAL HAEMATOMA (Figure 4.23)

Brain injury can be fatal either when there is gross tissue disruption or when, although structural damage is less severe, the intracranial pressure rises. This can be due either to cerebral oedema or to the accumulation of blood—extra-durally, sub-durally or within the brain. The largest exit from the rigid skull is the foramen magnum so movement of the brain is towards it. As the temporal lobes are pushed down, the oculomotor nerve of one side gets caught against the sharp edge of the tentorium cerebelli. This leads first to interference with the autonomic component of the nerve, the pupil becoming constricted, then dilated and fixed to light. If intracranial pressure continues to rise, this will happen to the other IIIrd nerve and the pupil it supplies. Then the medulla and pons get jammed into the foramen magnum, the vital centres become ischaemic, the pulse slows, blood pressure rises, and death ensues. Because of the typical shape of a brain which has been squashed like this, this is called 'coning'.

Deterioration in a patient with head injury requires urgent action. A difficult surgical differential diagnosis has to be made: if the cause of the pressure is haemorrhage, the skull can be opened and clots evacuated; if it is oedema, a dehydrating agent is used—usually the osmotic diuretic mannitol; and of course the wrong decision makes this worse—opening the skull causes an oedematous brain to mushroom out of the burr-hole, and dehydrating a brain with vascular damage just gives more room to the blood and worsens the situation that way.

SUB-DURAL HAEMATOMA: A TYPICAL HISTORY

An elderly lady has a fainting attack and hits her head on the radiator. She recovers fully but 10 days later her relatives notice that she is drowsy, forgetful and not her usual bright self. She is seen by her doctor who decides to keep her under observation as he suspects that her previous head injury has caused a small sub-dural haematoma (i.e., blood clot situated between the dura and pia maters). During the next four weeks she gradually recovers but remembers little of her illness. The haematoma is reabsorbed with no residual effects.

CONCUSSION

Colloquially, this term is used for any type of unconsciousness following a bang on the head. Strictly speaking, however, it refers to a brief state of unconsciousness lasting only a few hours and with no permanent damage to the brain. After the patient recovers consciousness, he may be confused for up to 24 hours and will have no memory of this period (post-traumatic amnesia). He also loses his memory of events just before the injury (retrograde amnesia). The extent of the amnesia depends on the severity of the injury.

A young person, unconscious following an overdose of aspirin

Jennifer Ladbrook, a 17-year-old schoolgirl, is studying for the General Certificate of Education at 'A' level standard. She is finding the course difficult and wishes to leave school now and start work with her friends as a clerk in the local printing works. Her parents are anxious for her to complete the 'A' level course and are not prepared to support her if she leaves school early. Jennifer has a boyfriend whom she has known for 2 years; he has just left school and gone 200 miles away to college.

Jennifer normally studies in her bedroom each evening and her mother takes her a warm drink last thing at night. Yesterday evening Mrs Ladbrook found Jennifer's bedroom door locked and could not get her to answer when she knocked. Mr Ladbrook was able to force the door. They found Jennifer on her bed unconscious with an empty aspirin bottle in the wastebin. They rang for an ambulance and she was taken to the hospital accompanied by her distraught parents.

On examination, her skin is found to be flushed and sweating, pulse full and bounding; and she is hyperventilating.

SELF-TESTING QUESTIONS

BRIEF ANALYSIS AND GUIDELINES TO SUITABLE ANSWERS

1. Describe the immediate management of Jennifer on arrival in the accident and emergency department.

Question 1
Your answer should include:
(a) Care and monitoring of an unconscious patient.
(b) Removal of gastric contents by stomach washout after insertion of cuffed endotracheal tube to prevent inhalation of gastric contents into the lungs. All washings should be saved for inspection and analysis.
(c) Commencement of artificial ventilation by intermittent positive pressure respirator if required.
(d) Commencement of intravenous infusion to correct dehydration from sweating and promote a diuresis of alkaline urine to rid the body of salicylates. The infusion should be of sodium lactate, normal saline and 5% dextrose in rotation at an initial rate of two litres per hour.
(e) Measurement of urine output following catheterisation. If no diuresis occurs it may indicate impaired renal function due to salicylate poisoning and haemodialysis may be required.

Question 2

2. (a) Describe the possible difficulties that could be encountered as Jennifer regains consciousness and (b) discuss what psychological and psychiatric care could be given.

(a) Jennifer's reaction on regaining consciousness could include:
  ● Severe withdrawal and regressive behaviour.
  ● Depression.
  ● Aggression.
  ● Apprehension regarding seeing parents.
  ● Guilt and regret.
  ● Rejection of parents or other support.
(b) Psychological and psychiatric help should be given by empathetic staff.
  ● Staff should show tolerance and understanding of Jennifer's behaviour and attempted suicide.
  ● Staff should be willing to let her talk and should monitor discreet observation of Jennifer's emotional state.
  ● She should be referred to school counsellor and for psychiatric opinion.
  ● Parents should have opportunity to discuss Jennifer's future with Jennifer and medical and school staff.

3. Describe common reasons for taking an overdose of drugs.

Question 3

Your answer should include discussion of accidental and deliberate overdose.

(a) Accidental overdose:
- In children.
- In the elderly.
- In the forgetful.

(b) Deliberate overdose:
- To end life.
- As a call for help.
- To manipulate a situation.

4. Describe the effects and immediate treatment of other common poisons that can be taken as an overdose.

Question 4

Common medicines which may be taken as an overdose include:
- Tricyclic antidepressants, e.g. amitriptyline.
- Ferrous compounds, especially by children.
- Diazepam.
- Paracetamol.

See pharmacology textbook for effects of overdose and possible antidotes. For specific supportive therapy consult J. Macleod (Ed.), *Davidson's Principles and Practice of Medicine*, 14th edition, Churchill Livingstone, London, 1984, and/or Regional Drug Information Centre.

Chapter 5

Nursing patients with general effects from local injury or disease

Normal body defences against injury and disease

(a) The skin

The skin is one of the most versatile organs of the body. It covers the whole body surface, including the cornea, and lines the body orifices. The average adult has two square metres of skin. It varies in thickness between half a centimetre (soles of the feet) and half a millimetre (eyelids).

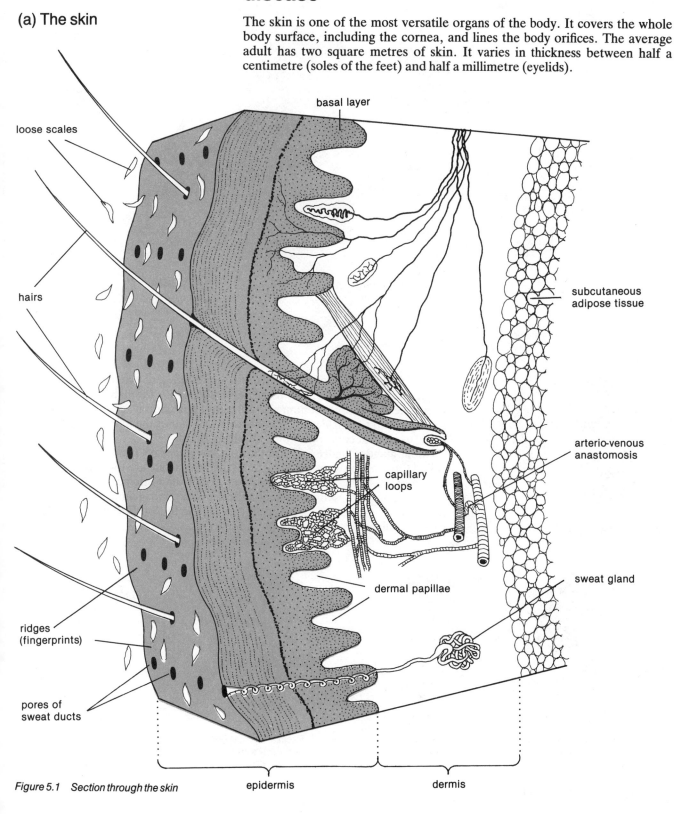

Figure 5.1 Section through the skin

1 Structure and modifications

The skin is composed of two layers: the outer *epidermis* and the inner *dermis* (Figure 5.1).

The cells of the *basal layer* of the epidermis are constantly dividing and moving towards the surface. Here they become *keratinised* (hardened by protein change) and are being constantly lost by the normal abrasion which the skin receives. About one gram of dead cells is shed per day.

The basal layer also contains *melanocytes* which produce the pigment *melanin*, giving the skin its coloration. Melanin production is stimulated by the ultraviolet light in sunlight. The action of ultraviolet light also stimulates the production of vitamin D by sterols in the skin.

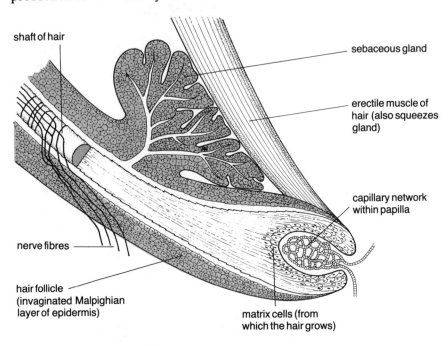
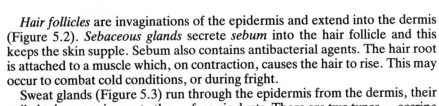

shaft of hair

sebaceous gland

erectile muscle of hair (also squeezes gland)

capillary network within papilla

nerve fibres

hair follicle (invaginated Malpighian layer of epidermis)

matrix cells (from which the hair grows)

Figure 5.2   Root of a hair

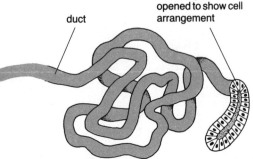

duct

terminal portion opened to show cell arrangement

Figure 5.3   Sweat gland

Hair follicles are invaginations of the epidermis and extend into the dermis (Figure 5.2). *Sebaceous glands* secrete *sebum* into the hair follicle and this keeps the skin supple. Sebum also contains antibacterial agents. The hair root is attached to a muscle which, on contraction, causes the hair to rise. This may occur to combat cold conditions, or during fright.

Sweat glands (Figure 5.3) run through the epidermis from the dermis, their coiled tubes opening on to the surface via ducts. There are two types — eccrine and apocrine. These secrete a solution of salts and uric acid with a pH of 6. Secretion of sweat is under sympathetic nervous control, and enables the body to lose excess water and keep itself cool. Some foodstuff aromatics including garlic are also released in sweat.

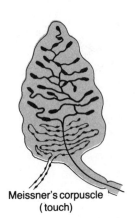

Meissner's corpuscle (touch)

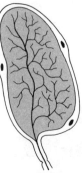

Ruffini end organ (heat and cold)

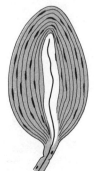

Pacinian corpuscle in deep layers of derma (pressure)

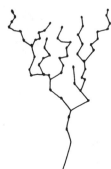

Free nerve endings in Malpighian layer (touch and pain)

Figure 5.4   Sensory nerve endings

In the dermis there are numerous nerve endings (Figure 5.4), some of which are modified to form sensory receptors which are variously stimulated by change in temperature, touch and pressure.

The capillaries of the dermis are involved with heat loss or conservation; they dilate to facilitate heat loss and constrict to conserve heat. These capillaries also dilate when there is alcohol present in the blood — causing redness of the skin and increasing heat loss. For this reason the St Bernard dogs' traditional brandy would have been a very real danger to a person suffering from exposure!

The skin has various modifications and specialised structures. The *cornea* of the eye, for example, is composed of clear cells which are some distance from the nearest capillaries. The nail is a hardening of the horny zone of the epidermis and grows from its root at the nail matrix at 2–4 mm per month (Figure 5.5). The *mammary gland* (breast) is a modified apocrine gland.

2 Functions of the skin

The functions of the skin are outlined below.
- *Protection* against invasion by microorganisms, and damage due to injury or ultraviolet light.
- *Waterproofing:* keeping body fluids in and water out.
- *Sensory organ:* detecting pain, touch, temperature change and pressure.
- *Excretion* and *secretion* via the sweat and sebaceous glands.
- *Temperature control* by the movement of hairs, production of sweat and control of dermal capillaries.
- *Production of vitamin D.*

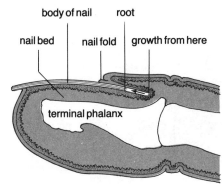

Figure 5.5   Growth of a nail

(b) The lymphatic system

As blood is pumped around the circulatory system, fluid is forced out of the capillaries and forms the extracellular fluid. The *lymphatic system* serves as the

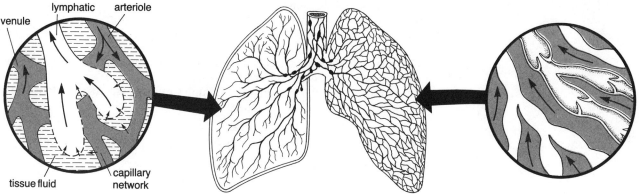

Figure 5.6   Lymph vessels

drain by which this fluid can be returned to the blood. It takes the form of a series of thin-walled and blind-ending collecting vessels, the *lymphatics,* which join to form larger vessels, and which tend to accompany blood vessels, bringing extracellular fluid back from all parts of the body. The lymph vessels (Figure 5.6) have valves at regular intervals and this gives them a beaded appearance when full.

The flow of lymph through the vessels is maintained chiefly by muscular activity. At rest, there is almost no lymph flow. Lymph vessels are not present in tissue which does not move, and are also lacking in striated muscle (Figure 5.7).

Lymph is a clear fluid except in the *lacteals*, which are the lymph vessels which drain the digestive system. The lymph fluid here is called *chyle;* it contains absorbed fat and looks milky.

Large protein molecules, foreign particles (such as dust in the lungs or bacteria) and cancer cells can pass into the lymphatic system. These substances accumulate in the *lymph nodes* (Figure 5.8) into which lymph is poured from the larger lymph vessels. Lymph nodes possess large numbers of lymphocytes and phagocytic endothelial cells and are important in the defence of the body against disease. They may become inflamed during infection. Lymph nodes also appear to produce *antibodies*, which will be discussed further on page 215.

Figure 5.7   Distribution of lymph vessels. These are present in all parts of the body except those parts shown

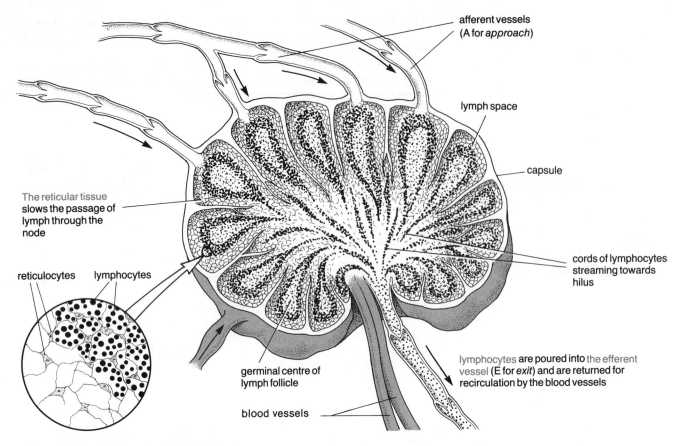

afferent vessels
(A for *approach*)

lymph space

capsule

cords of lymphocytes
streaming towards
hilus

The reticular tissue
slows the passage of
lymph through the
node

reticulocytes   lymphocytes

lymphocytes are poured into the efferent
vessel (E for *exit*) and are returned for
recirculation by the blood vessels

germinal centre of
lymph follicle

blood vessels

Figure 5.8   Section through a lymph node

Eventually, all the lymph collects into two large channels which return it to the circulatory system via the right and left subclavian veins.

Various organs are associated with the lymphatic system: the *tonsils* and *adenoids,* and the *thymus gland.*

Tonsils and adenoids are specialised masses of lymph tissue. Lymph vessels travel from them towards the cervical nodes.

The thymus is similar in structure to lymph tissue and has an important role in the control of the immune response.

The patients with general effects from local injury or disease

(a) Effects from pathogenic organisms, carcinoma, enlarged prostate gland and varicose veins

1   Patient study and care plan for a young adult with acute pyelonephritis

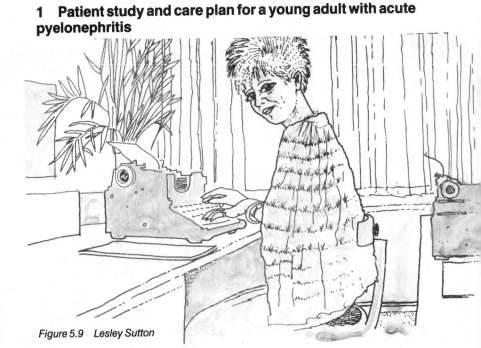

Figure 5.9   Lesley Sutton

History of social, psychological and physical events leading to the present condition

The patient chosen in this section to illustrate general effects from local injury or disease is an adult with acute pyelonephritis.

Lesley Sutton (Figure 5.9), aged 20 years, shares a flat with two girlfriends and works as a typist in a typing pool for an accountancy firm. She recently began a course of antibiotics for a urinary tract infection but failed to complete the course as her symptoms subsided after three days. On waking one morning of the following week, Lesley had aching pains in both loins and lower abdomen. She felt hot but shivery and developed frequency of micturition and experienced pain on passing urine. Lesley asked her friends to contact her boss and she attended the morning surgery of her GP.

The GP examined Lesley and discussed her history. While she was with her doctor Lesley experienced a severe rigor, following which he arranged transfer to the local hospital as there would be no one to care for her in her flat, and she required further investigations and treatment.

On arrival at hospital Lesley is admitted to a medical ward where the following investigations are immediately carried out.

Investigation	Results
Laboratory examination of urine for cultural sensitivity and microscopy	Identification of *E.coli* in urine, sensitive to ampicillin. Microscopy showed presence of pus cells
Blood for: full blood count haemoglobin urea and electrolytes	Red cells and platelets normal but increased white cell count. Haemoglobin, urea and electrolytes normal

Explanation of abnormal physiology and pathology

It is advisable to revise the normal tissue response to injury and the body defences against injury and infection, and see Table 5.1.

Table 5.1

Normal physiology	Abnormal physiology
(a) Intact skin and mucous membranes	Invasion of pathogenic microorganisms through mucous lining of urinary tract
(b) Any injury or entry of a foreign protein causes the capillaries in the area to constrict initially and then, within a few seconds, dilate. Then the circulation slows, causing local redness and increase in heat. The walls of the capillaries become permeable, allowing fluid exudate to bathe the tissue spaces which dilute any toxins present. This increase of fluid at the site causes swelling. The swelling causes pressure on any nerve endings in the area, resulting in pain. The white cells migrate to the area and pass through the permeable walls of the capillaries by a process called diapedesis to phagocytose the invading pathogenic organism	Successful invasion of microorganisms stimulates normal physiological response but due to insufficient white blood cells and/or virulence of invading organism, and incomplete course of antibiotics, the organism was able to survive sufficiently to damage local tissues and multiply. Dead white cells, tissue cells and bacteria liquefy to form pus which passes into the urine
(c) Resolution usually follows with constriction of capillaries and reabsorption of remaining exudate so redness, heat, swelling and pain disappear	The inflammatory response does not resolve; therefore heat, redness, swelling and pain affecting the mucous lining persist and spread throughout the lining of the urinary tract
(d) Normally organisms in the bloodstream are phagocytosed by monocytes and the cells of the reticulo-endothelial system present in the liver, spleen and bone marrow. Lymph nodes normally filter microorganisms and destroy them	(i) Successful breaching of the local defences allows the bacteria and/or the toxins from the bacteria to enter the blood stream, lympatic system and the cavity of the urinary tract (ii) Once the organisms or toxins have successfully invaded the bloodstream, general effects occur: ● rise in body temperature ● headache ● general malaise ● sweating ● nausea ● rapid pulse ● anorexia (iii) Inflamed mucous membranes result in pain in loins and bladder, frequency of micturition, pain on micturition

Care plan

PREPARATION FOR PATIENT WITH ACUTE PYELONEPHRITIS

Following the immediate investigations, the care plan shown in Table 5.3 is brought into action.

Nursing history and assessment
Table 5.2 shows Lesley's completed sheet.

Table 5.2 Nursing history and assessment sheet for Miss Lesley Sutton

NURSING HISTORY AND ASSESSMENT SHEET

Record No. _77777_

PATIENT LABEL

Mr/Mrs/Miss _Lesley SUTTON_

Address _Top flat, 263 Vauxhall Rd, London_

Male/Female   Age _20 years_

Date of Birth _12.7.66_

Date of admission/~~first visit~~

_3.11.86_

Time _____

Type: ☐ Routine ☑ Emergency

Transfer from: _____

Religion _R/C_

Practising/baptised _Practising_

Minister _____

Telephone number _____

Next of kin (name) _Mrs and Mrs Sutton_

Relationship to patient _Parents_

Address _11 Kings Crescent, Leigh, Bathshire_

Telephone numbers _45678_

Contact at night/in emergency   YES/~~NO~~

Occupation (or father) _Typist (full time)_

Marital status _Single_

Children (or place in family) _____

Other dependants _____

Pets _____

School (children only) _____

Hobbies _____

Clubs _____

Favourite pastime _____

Does patient smoke?   YES/<u>NO</u>

Speech difficulty/language barrier

Dysphasia   Dysarthria

Accommodation

Lives alone   YES/<u>NO</u>

Part III/EMI/Old People's Homes/<u>Rented</u>

Consultant _Mr Hampshire_

House officer _Dr Stead_

Presenting condition _Urinary tract infection_

History of present complaint and reason for admission

Urinary tract infection 1 week ago. Failed to complete course of ampicillin.
Hot, shivery, frequency of micturition and pain, severe rigor

Past medical history

Healthy

Allergies _None_

Current medication

None

What patient says is the reason for admission and attitude to admission

Urinary tract infection

Patient's expectations _Expects to recover quickly and return to work a.s.a.p._

Any problems at home while/because patient is in hospital? _N/a_

Relevant home conditions (e.g. stairs)

_____

_____

Visiting problems

_____

Care at home

Community nurse _____

No. _____

Name of GP _Dr Jones_

Address _The Health Centre, Vauxhall Rd, London_

Other services involved

Home help _____	Day hospital _____
Laundry _____	Day centre/club _____
Inco supplies _____	Health visitor _____
Aids _____	Social worker _____
Meals on wheels _____	Voluntary worker _____

Daily living

Diet

Special _____

Food or drink dislikes _____

Appetite: ☑GOOD ☐POOR

Remarks _____

Sleep

How many hours normally? ___9___

Sedation _____

What else helps? _____

Elimination

Bowels: Continent/Incontinent

How often opened? ___Daily___

Any medication? _____

Urinary: Continent/Incontinent *Normally*

If incontinent; Day/Night/If not taken, how frequently? _____

Nocturia/Dysuria/Frequency/Urgency

Remarks _____

Female patients — Menstruation

Post-menopausal   Taking the pill

Regular   Irregular

Amenorrhoea   Dysmenorrhoea

Next period due: ___12·11·86___

Uses: STs Tampons

Hearing

Hearing aid: YES/NO

Remarks _____

Vision

Glasses/Contact lens: YES/NO

Remarks _____

Oral

Dentures or crowns: YES/NO

Any problems with mouth or teeth?

_____

Mobility

Help needed with:

Walking/Standing/In/Out of bed/Bathing/Dressing

In/Out of chair/

Feeding/Other: _____

Remarks ___Normally active___

Prosthesis/appliance

Type of appliance _____

Help needed _____

General appearance

Normal   Dehydrated   Acutely ill

Obese   Thin   Emaciated

Remarks _____

Skin

Satisfactory   Broken areas   Dehydrated

Rash   Oedematous   Jaundiced

Pallor   Other ___Flushed___
                    (including bruising)

Remarks _____

Level of consciousness

Orientated   Semi-conscious

Confused   Unconscious

Remarks _____

Mental assessment (if appropriate)

Mood

Elated   Irritable   Agitated

Cheerful   Anxious   Aggressive

Miserable   Withdrawn   Suspicious

Apathetic

Thought content

Hallucinations/Delusions/Paranoid Ideas

_____

Orientation

Time/Place/Person *Yes*

Very confused   Slightly confused

Any particular time of day? _____

Confabulation _____

Remarks _____

Surveillance   Physical/Emotional

Information obtained from ___Patient___

Relationship to patient _____

By ___M. White___

Position/level of training _____

Date ___3·11·86___

Time _____

141

Table 5.3 Care plan for Lesley on admission to the ward

Problem	Objective	Plan of care	Rationale
1. Arrival of a patient with a local urinary tract infection	To cure the infection	(a) Administer antibiotics as prescribed. Observe wanted and unwanted effects	(a) *Escherichia coli* is sensitive to Ampicillin.
		(b) Give at least three litres of fluids daily. Record balance chart	(b) Increased fluid intake has the effect of increasing urine output which flushes debris from the urinary tract. Provides a record of amount of fluid taken
		(c) Test urine daily for albumin, blood and specific gravity	(c) Provides a record of progress of infection which could spread to kidney tissue
		(d) Obtain urine specimen for repeat microscopy as requested	(d) Monitors effect of treatment
2. Patient in a febrile state	Minimise discomfort and reduce temperature if possible	(a) Light bed clothes	(a) Encourages loss of body heat by radiation
		(b) Well-ventilated room	(b) Encourages loss of heat by convection
		(c) Cool by tepid sponging and use of fan as prescribed	(c) Encourages loss of heat by evaporation and convection
		(d) Provide clean bed linen and clothes as appropriate	(d) Encourages loss of heat by conduction and provides comfort by removing sweaty clothes
		(e) Give cool fluids hourly. Record amount drunk on fluid balance chart	(e) Replaces fluid loss by sweating. Increases urine output which flushes debris from urinary tract. Assists in reducing body temperature
		(f) Give prescribed anti-pyretic and analgesic, e.g., paracetamol	(f) Assists in lowering body temperature and relieves pain and possible headache
3. Reluctant to eat	Ensure adequate dietary intake	Give light cool foods, e.g., ice cream, yoghurt, jelly, milk shakes	Provides easily digested adequate nutrition, minimises overheating, and promotes healing
4. Acutely ill young person	Provide rest and comfort	Rest in bed. Encourage Lesley to change position frequently	Resting the body promotes tissue repair. Changing position in bed prevents complications of bed rest, e.g., pressure sores
5. Unable to attend to own hygiene	To assist her to attend to personal hygiene	(a) Assist with blanket bath in bed daily	(a) Removes sweat and dead skin cells which can harbour microorganisms
		(b) Provide frequent mouthwashes and facilities to clean teeth	(b) Mouth liable to be dry and become infected due to febrile state
6. Patient anxious regarding outcome of illness and when she will be able to return to work	Relieve anxiety	(a) Explanation of present illness and reason for treatment	(a) Assists patient's understanding of her illness and promotes her cooperation in treatment
		(b) Provide a medical certificate for her employer	(b) Gives information to her place of work and enables her to claim for sickness benefit
		(c) Provide ongoing information as to effects of treatment	(c) Reassures patient and enables planning for return to home and work

RECOVERY AND ADVICE ON DISCHARGE

Within a few days Lesley's temperature returns to normal; loin and bladder pain, frequency and dysuria have all disappeared. Her appetite starts to return to normal and she starts to be up and about. Plans are made for her discharge within a few days so long as she continues taking the antibiotics as prescribed for a further week (two weeks in all). Lesley is advised to visit her GP at the health centre in one month's time for a check-up and repeat urine specimen for laboratory investigation. She is informed that if her symptoms recur she should promptly seek medical advice, as persistent urinary tract infections require a complete urological investigation.

2 Patient histories illustrating further problems related to general effect from local injury or disease.

This part of the chapter comprises patient histories, self-testing questions and guidelines for suggested answers.

A child with osteomyelitis

Gerry Rowland, aged 14 years, lives with his parents and four sisters in a traveller's van. They live as itinerants, settling on established sites for a few weeks only at a time before moving on to find other work. One day Gerry hurt the lower part of his left leg on an old piece of metal. The injury required suturing at the local hospital. He was given an injection of tetanus toxoid and advised to return to the hospital the following week for removal of sutures. He didn't return to the hospital because the family had moved on and his sutures were removed by his grandmother while on the road. Three weeks after the accident Gerry complained of increasing bone pain in the lower part of his left leg. He is reluctant to bear weight on it and is distressed when it is moved. Gerry's mother noticed that his leg felt hot to touch and the old wound was discharging pus. That evening Gerry became feverish and nauseated; he felt weak and refused to let anyone touch his leg. His parents became worried and brought him in to the local hospital.

On arrival at hospital investigations reveal the following:

Investigation	Results
X-ray of lower leg	Periosteal reaction and bone destruction in lower tibia, suggestive of osteomyelitis
Full blood count	Slight reduction in number of red blood cells, increased white cell count, platelets normal
Blood culture	Positive, growth of *Staphylococcus aureus*

The doctor examines Gerry and makes a diagnosis of osteomyelitis. He explains to Gerry and his parents that the condition needs treatment in the form of antibiotic therapy, immobilisation of affected limb and possible surgical decompression and drainage of the infected bony area.

SELF-TESTING QUESTIONS

1. (a) Describe the normal physiological response to infection in a bone.
(b) How does the infection spread to the rest of the body?

2. Devise a care plan for Gerry for the first 48 hours after his admission to hospital.

BRIEF ANALYSIS AND GUIDELINES TO SUITABLE ANSWERS

Question 1

(a) Your answer should state that the normal physiological response is the same as in any tissue except that bone cannot swell under the pressure of increased fluid exudate. This causes pressure on the essential blood supply in the bone within the Haversian system and canals, followed by occlusion of the blood supply, and death of the bone as a result.

If the condition is untreated, pockets of infection are walled off by the laying down of new bone (involucrum), and chronic sinuses may form which may drain onto the surface. Complete healing does not occur until all dead bone has been destroyed, discharged or excised.

(b) Infection spreads to rest of the bone via the bloodstream, and lymphatics, as seen in patient study on pages 138–139.

Question 2

Your answer should include:

(a) Care of the febrile patient, hygiene, rest and nutrition as in major care plan.

(b) Specific care of the affected limb:
- Immobilisation and relief of any pressure on any aspect of the limb by use of a plaster of Paris back slab.
- Relief of pain by appropriate analgesia, intravenous or intramuscular route.
- Wound swab for confirmation of causative organism; regular wound toilet with strict attention to aseptic technique, giving analgesic coverage, for example, use of Entonox.

- Local observations of limb for alteration of redness and swelling.
- Appropriate antibiotics intravenously.
- Practice anti-cross-infection measures.
- If surgical intervention is necessary to drain the wound, ideally Gerry should be nursed in a cubicle to reduce risk of cross-infection to other patients.
- Encourage parents to participate in Gerry's care. Provide ongoing explanation and reassurance to all of them.

Question 3

3. What support should be given to Gerry's parents prior to and after his discharge from hospital?

Your answer should include:

(a) Instruction of parents in all procedures which may be required at home. These may be changes of dressings, application of splint and use of crutches, supervision of leg exercises.

(b) The giving of detailed written information of Gerry's treatment and past condition to enable appropriate follow-up management if family move to another area.

(c) Instruction of parents in details of possible complications, return of previous symptoms, stiffness of joints and deformity.

(d) Alert local district nurse to the need to follow up the after-care of Gerry at home, particularly as he is likely to be a temporary resident only.

(e) Offer follow-up appointment at physiotherapy department and discuss with parents the need for Gerry to practise leg exercises after discharge.

An adult with carcinoma of the breast

Mrs Elizabeth Harvey, aged 45 years, who is a member of the local District Health Authority, lives with her husband, who is a businessman and a city councillor. Mrs Harvey has an active and busy life and avoids going immediately to her doctor when she finds a painless lump in her left breast. However, several weeks later she finds a small nodule in her left axilla and the lump in her breast has become slightly larger. She goes to her doctor, who confirms her fear that she is likely to have a carcinoma of her left breast with spread to her axilla. Her doctor arranges for her to be admitted to hospital within the next few days and discusses with her the possible treatment she will receive. Mrs Harvey returns home distressed and discusses her fear with her husband, who cancels her arrangements for the next few weeks.

The following investigations are arranged for Mrs Harvey prior to her admission to hospital:

Investigation	Results
Mammogram	Confirms mass detected in left breast
Chest x-ray	Normal
Skeletal survey	Normal

Mrs Harvey arrives as planned into hospital to the surgical ward. Having discussed the results of the recent investigations with her doctor, she is to have a left simple mastectomy and removal of node in the left axilla.

BRIEF ANALYSIS AND GUIDELINES TO SUITABLE ANSWERS

Question 1

1. Describe what you understand by the term *carcinoma*.

Explanation of the term carcinoma.

Normal	Abnormal (carcinoma)
Cellular division is a normal process for growth and repair of tissues. It is ordered and controlled, maintaining a constant balance between cells being worn out and destroyed and new cells being made	Cellular division goes out of control and becomes invasive, disorderly and the normal balance is disturbed. Repeated division of abnormal cells leads to development of a tumour or growth. Carcinoma is a tumour of epithelial tissue.

2. Explain the possible local effects of a carcinoma in the breast.

Question 2

Local effects:

(a) Uncontrolled cellular division, microscopic at first but becomes palpable as tumour enlarges.

(b) Tumour invades surrounding structures and can become fixed to overlying skin, or underlying muscle, or nipple.

(c) Nipple may invert and/or bleed.

(d) Dimpling of the skin occurs — peau d'orange — due to tension on ligaments of Cooper.

(e) May eventually spread to ribs or may fungate on to surface of skin.

(f) There is little local tissue response to the invading tumour cells.

3. Explain the possible systemic effects of a carcinoma of the breast and describe how they may come about.

Question 3

Possible systemic effects may be summarised in the following way. A tumour from the primary carcinoma can be carried in the lymphatic vessels to the nearest lymph nodes, where it can lodge and start dividing, forming a secondary deposit (metastasis). Alternatively, a tumour cell can be carried in the blood stream to any point of the body, for example, the spinal column, brain, lungs, liver, where a secondary tumour can develop. Eventually the patient may become cachectic and develop carcinomatosis.

4. Describe the nurse's role in (a) the specific pre-operative and (b) the specific post-operative care that would be required for Mrs Harvey.

Question 4

(a) In pre-operative care your answer should include:
- Discussion of possible outcomes with both Mr and Mrs Harvey.
- Arrange for Mrs Harvey to see the appliance officer to discuss suitable and acceptable prosthesis.
- Ensure that area for surgery is clearly marked by doctor.

(b) In post-operative care your answer should include:
- Management of drainage tubes and wound.
- Suitable arm exercises.
- Attention to privacy and adjustment to altered body image.
- Check that appliance is suitable and ready for patient's discharge.
- Give useful addresses, e.g., Mastectomy Association.

An adult with carcinoma of the rectum

Mr Arthur Lewis, aged 70 years, is a retired gas fitter. He lives alone in a small terraced cottage in an outlying village. He has been a widower for 10 years and has no children. The cottage is in need of modernisation and has an outside toilet only but a sitz bath has been installed in the smallest bedroom. Over the past year Mr Lewis noticed a change in bowel activity with episodes of diarrhoea and constipation. Increasingly, he feels that there is incomplete emptying of the bowel after a bowel action and he tries to correct this with aperients. He becomes more concerned when he starts to notice a trace of blood and slime with the stool. He becomes listless, pale and loses some weight, and reluctantly takes the advice of his younger sister who makes an appointment for him to see the GP. On examination the doctor discovers a mass in the wall of the rectum and general examination of Mr Lewis reveals an elderly, anaemic man who has recently lost weight.

The GP arranges for his admission to the local hospital for further investigations and treatment. Sigmoidoscopy and biopsy confirm a carcinoma of the lower rectum which has ulcerated through the mucous lining, causing bleeding and excessive mucus secretion. The surrounding mucous lining is red and slightly oedematous. The doctor discusses the findings with Mr Lewis and explains that total removal of the rectum is necessary, leaving Mr Lewis with a permanent colostomy.

SELF-TESTING QUESTIONS

1. Describe the possible outcomes if Mr Lewis continued to be untreated.

BRIEF ANALYSIS AND GUIDELINES TO SUITABLE ANSWERS

Question 1

The possible outcomes may be described under local effects and general effects.

Local effects:

(a) Gradual extension of the tumour through the wall of the rectum and into the lumen which may eventually cause obstruction and severe constipation.

(b) Outward spread of the tumour can involve the prostate gland, bladder, seminal vesicles and ureters and also the sacral plexus, causing intractable pain.

General effects:

(a) Via the bloodstream to any part of the body but more usually to the liver, lungs or adrenal glands.

(b) Via the lymphatic system to the local lymph nodes initially but if spread is not halted these will spread to more distant nodes and again into the bloodstream.

(c) Bleeding from the tumour will cause increasing anaemia, reducing the oxygen-carrying capacity of the blood. Widespread malignancy causes cachexia, a condition in which the patient develops anorexia, debility and failure of the immune mechanisms, which contribute to his rapid decline.

Question 2

2. Devise a care plan for Mr Lewis to prepare him for surgery.

Your answer should include the following:

(a) Care of an anxious, elderly, malnourished, anaemic gentleman who has difficulties with elimination.

(b) Preparation of the bowel for surgery by rectal washouts, possible low residue diet and antibiotics.

(c) There is a possible need for pre-operative blood transfusion.

(d) Opportunity should be given to meet the stoma-therapist for discussion regarding the site of the stoma and future management.

(e) Mr Lewis should be referred to the medical social worker for urgent assessment of his home situation.

Question 3

3. Devise a care plan for Mr Lewis following abdominoperineal excision of rectum.

Your answer should give details of immediate care and later care.

(a) Immediate care should include:
  - Comfort and hygiene.
  - Observation for shock and bleeding.
  - Pain relief.
  - Management of intravenous therapy, nasogastric tube, urinary catheter, wounds and wound drainage.
  - Management and observation of the stoma for oedema, retraction, bleeding, colour and function.
  - General care to prevent complications of bed rest.

(b) Later care should include:
  - Mobilisation.
  - Re-introduction of diet.
  - Removal of intravenous infusion, nasogastric tube, urinary catheter and wound drainage tubes.
  - Removal of sutures.
  - Teaching Mr Lewis how to care for his colostomy and give contact with Colostomy Association and stoma-therapist.
  - Liaison with medical social worker for transfer to the community — consideration to be given to facilities at home and possibility of obtaining local authority grant for home improvement.
  - Arranging for district nurse to establish a hygiene regime.

Further reading

Capra, L. G., *The Care of the Cancer Patient*, Macmillan Education, London, 2nd edn (1986).

Tiffany, R. (Ed.), *Oncology for Nurses and Health Care Professionals*, volume 2, *Care and Support*, Allen and Unwin, London, 1978.

An adult with uterine fibroids

Miss Mary Clark, aged 45 years, is a geography teacher in a large comprehensive school. She lives in a maisonette near the school and her interests include hill-walking and membership of the local amateur dramatic society. She has always enjoyed good health until recently when she developed menorrhagia and a shorter menstrual cycle. The heavy blood loss was making her anaemic and tired. She was seen by the gynaecologist, who diagnosed uterine fibroids and advised that she should have a total hysterectomy. While waiting for admission the doctor prescribed her iron tablets to help correct her anaemia.

Three months later she is admitted from the waiting list for surgery. Routine pre-operative investigations include:

1. Full blood count and haemoglobin.
2. Blood grouping and cross-matching.
3. Urine test for culture, sensitivity and microscopy.
4. High vaginal swab for culture and sensitivity.
5. Cervical smear for cytology.

Results were within normal limits.

The operation is discussed with her and she is assured that her ovaries will not need to be removed and therefore she will eventually experience the menopause as normal.

SELF-TESTING QUESTIONS

1. Explain what you understand by the term fibroid, and describe how it is different from a carcinoma.

2. Describe the specific post-operative management of Miss Clark following a hysterectomy.

BRIEF ANALYSIS AND GUIDELINES TO SUITABLE ANSWERS

Question 1

Fibroids are benign tumours formed from local cellular divisions within the fibrous tissue of the uterus. Fibroids grow slowly and often stop growing altogether. Size can vary from small to very large; they may be single or multiple; and they may be embedded within the organ or pedunculated. They do not infiltrate through local tissue but may push tissue aside and form a capsule around themselves. Invasion of lymphatic channels or blood vessels does not occur and therefore there is no spread to other parts of the body. They cause problems due to their position and size. Multiple fibroids within the uterus cause enlargement of the uterus with increased surface area of the lining endometrium and therefore heavy bleeding during menstruation.

Question 2

Your answer should include attention to the physical, psychological and social aspects.

(a) Physical aspects:
   • Care of a surgical wound.
   • Care of bladder and bowels after pelvic surgery.
   • Vulval hygiene and monitoring of vaginal blood loss.
(b) Psychological aspects:
   • Reactions to loss of female reproduction organ.
(c) Social aspects:
   • Miss Clark lives alone and will probably need convalescent care and may need to be away from school for most of a term.
   • She should be advised to avoid heavy lifting such as that involved in shopping.

An adult with benign hypertrophy of the prostate gland

Mr John Gibbard, aged 65 years, has recently retired from his job as a pharmacist. He has been looking forward to his retirement and forthcoming visit to America with his wife to visit their son and family. Six months before they were due to go to America he started to develop urinary symptoms: frequency of micturition during day and night, poor stream and difficulty in emptying his bladder completely. After a social evening with friends in the local pub he awoke during the night with a full bladder but was unable to pass urine. He became distressed and agitated and woke his wife. The doctor was contacted and he arranged for Mr Gibbard to be admitted to hospital.

On admission Mr Gibbard is found to be in severe pain with acute retention of urine, the bladder is distended and palpable above the symphysis pubis. Rectal examination reveals an enlarged prostate gland; and Mr Gibbard is prepared for the insertion of a supra-pubic catheter and controlled decompression of the bladder. He is transferred to the surgical ward feeling much more comfortable and allowed to rest. The next morning the need for the following investigations are discussed:

1. Cystoscopy, biopsy of prostate gland and retrograde pyelogram.
2. Blood urea and electrolytes.
3. Haemoglobin and full blood count.
4. Specimen of urine for culture, sensitivity and microscopy.

Closed bladder drainage is continued and Mr Gibbard is encouraged to drink a minimum of three litres of fluid daily.

1. Mr Gibbard has an enlarged prostate gland surrounding the neck of the bladder. What are the possible effects on the urinary tract and kidneys?

Question 1

Your answer should include:

(a) Difficulty in emptying the bladder which can lead to sudden acute retention of urine or retention with overflow.

(b) Development of frequency, poor stream and emptying of the bladder leading to a continual residue of urine in the bladder.

(c) Stasis of residual urine can lead to infection.

(d) Back pressure from the bladder causes eventual development of hydro ureters or hydronephrosis and kidney damage.

(e) Kidney damage will result in a raised blood urea, due to its failure to excrete protein waste products.

2. Mr Gibbard's enlarged prostate was diagnosed by rectal examination. Explain the anatomical relationships of the prostate gland and the rectum.

Question 2

Refer to your teacher for guidance to a suitable textbook.

3. Discuss the advantages and disadvantages of urethral versus supra-pubic catheterisation.

Question 3

(a) Urethral catheterisation can cause trauma to the urethra and prostate. The procedure may be impossible due to urethral stricture or compression. Urethral mucosa is sensitive to interference and reacts to constant irritation of an indwelling catheter. This may lead to the development of a urinary tract infection.

(b) Supra-pubic catheterisation is used when urethral catheterisation is either difficult or impossible. It avoids trauma to the urethra but involves a surgical procedure through the abdominal wall. The risk of urinary tract infection appears to be lessened.

4. Describe the major differences between a benign and a malignant tumour of the prostate gland.

Question 4

For your answer refer to S. Collins and E. Parker, *An Introduction to Nursing*, this series, p 55.

5. Mr Gibbard has a benign tumour of the prostate gland removed surgically. Devise a care plan for his management in the post-operative period.

Question 5

The care plan should include the following aspects:

(a) Monitoring and management of shock.

(b) Management of the bladder drainage apparatus including:
   - Prevention of sepsis.
   - Monitoring of blood loss and action if haemorrhage or formation of blood clot occurs.
   - Measuring and recording urine output.

(c) Prevention of complications of an elderly person being confined to bed.

(d) Discussion of possible after-effects such as:
   - Dribbling of urine for a period of approximately 6 weeks.
   - Sterility but usually no impotence.

(e) Convalescence prior to Mr Gibbard's visit to America.

N.B. Renal stones can cause similar effects to those resulting from an enlarged prostate (see Question 1) if they obstruct the urethra or *both* ureters.

An adult with varicose veins

Mrs Edith Duke, aged 30 years, is a housewife and mother of four young children. There have been marital problems over the past year and Mrs Duke has now been left to cope with the children. She is receiving Social Security benefits and the health visitor is visiting her regularly. She had varicose veins during each of her pregnancies, but they recovered after each child was born until two years ago, when the youngest was born. The distension of the veins, pain and dragging sensation in her legs has got steadily worse and she now has a patch of discoloration on the medial aspect of the right lower leg. She has been wearing support tights but her doctor now advises treatment by injection of a sclerosing agent.

An outpatient appointment is arranged and a neighbour agrees to look after the two youngest children for the afternoon of the appointment and to collect the others from school.

SELF-TESTING QUESTIONS

1. (a) What are varicose veins?
   (b) Explain how they can occur.
   (c) What are the possible complications?

BRIEF ANALYSIS AND GUIDELINES TO SUITABLE ANSWERS

Question 1

(a) Varicose veins are distended, tortuous superficial veins due to stasis in the long and short saphenous veins of the leg.
(b) Stasis can be due to:
   - Congenital laxity of the walls of the veins.
   - Incompetence of the valves.
   - Pressure on the pelvic veins inhibiting venous return due to: obesity, pregnancy, pelvic tumours, chronic constipation.
   - Standing for long periods.
(c) Possible complications are as follows:
   - Rupture and haemorrhage.
   - Varicose eczema and ulceration due to increased venous pressure, especially in the capillary beds, causing leakage of blood cells into the tissue spaces. The blood cells break down, releasing pigments which stain the skin. Secondary bacterial infection can occur in the poorly drained tissues leading to ulceration. The infection causes tissue response of redness, heat, swelling and loss of function.

2. Describe the nurse's responsibilities while caring for Mrs Duke in the outpatient department.

Question 2

The nurse's responsibilities include:
(a) Explanation of the procedure to Mrs Duke.
(b) Preparation of the equipment needed.
(c) Positioning Mrs Duke and her lower limbs to empty the veins of blood.
(d) Comfort and support during the procedure.
(e) Ensuring that the leg is well supported by pressure bandage and that circulation to toes is adequate.
(f) Advice should include:
   - Keeping the support bandage in place and dry.
   - Elevating the leg when sitting.
   - Walking at regular intervals throughout the day.
   - Avoiding standing still for long periods.
   - Reminding Mrs Duke to let the health visitor know that she has now received treatment.
   - Avoiding sitting with legs crossed.

Chapter 6

Nursing patients with disturbance of metabolism

Normal functions of the liver, pancreas and thyroid gland

'Metabolism' refers to all of the body's normal processes which result in:

1. The provision of oxygen, nutrients and water to all cells of the body.
2. The utilisation of these by all cells to produce and use energy, body proteins (both structural and non-structural), storage products and waste products.
3. The elimination of the waste products.

These processes are controlled and regulated to suit the body's precise requirements at any one time, and the primary result of normal metabolism is the maintenance of the body in health and good repair to enable the person to undertake the activities of daily living.

The processes of metabolism enable the body's internal physical and chemical environment to be kept close to the necessary norm at all times, even if there is a change in the external environment. This control is called *homeostasis*.

(a) The liver

The liver weighs about 1.5 kg (3–4% of body weight) and is the largest organ in the body (Figure 6.1). It is essential to life, and carries out numerous different important metabolic processes. Because of its great activity, it has a very large blood supply, receiving 1.5 litres of blood per minute. Because of its

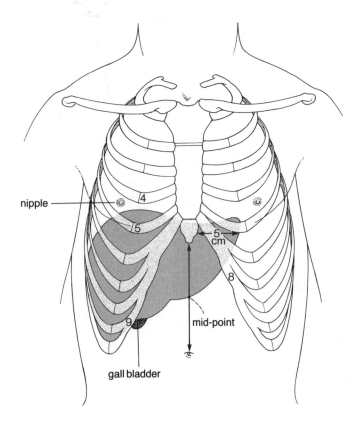

Figure 6.1   Position of the liver

vascularity, it is extremely pliable, easily torn by trauma and difficult to operate upon, as it will not hold stitches. The liver has a great capacity for regeneration: a loss of more than 80% can be made good and two weeks after hemihepatectomy its size is restored to normal, requiring the production of 50–100 grams of liver tissue per day.

1 Functions

It has been estimated that the liver has over 500 functions. The most significant are described below.

Regulation of glucose, lipids and amino acids

GLUCOSE

If the hormone *insulin,* which is produced by the pancreas, is present, the liver cells take up and convert excess glucose to *glycogen* for storage. If carbohydrates are present together with an excess of glucose, the liver will produce glycerol, for fat production.

LIPIDS

The liver cells can take up lipids and either break them down or modify them and send them to adipose tissue to be stored.

AMINO ACIDS

Amino acids and proteins (which are built up from amino acids) cannot be stored, and any amino acids surplus to the body's immediate requirements are broken down by the liver to form urea which is carried in the blood to the kidneys, where it is eliminated from the body.

Production of bile

Bile is produced by liver cells and stored in the gall bladder. It consists of bile salts produced from cholesterol, which emulsify fats in the small intestine to enable the water soluble enzyme *lipase* to act upon them. Bile also contains several important excretory products which are eliminated from the body in the faeces. Secretion of the bile (Figure 6.2a, b) into the small intestine via the bile duct is controlled by the vagus nerve and by hormones produced by the small intestine when fatty acids are present. These act both to relax the *sphincter of Oddi* at the junction between the bile duct and the small intestine, and to contract the gall bladder.

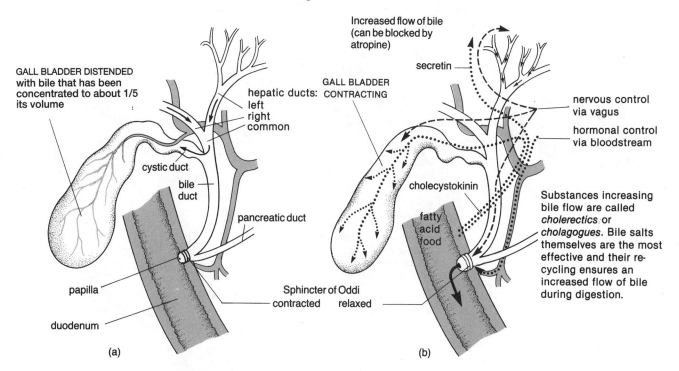

Figure 6.2   Flow of bile. (a) During tasting and (b) 20 minutes after a fatty meal

Formation of cholesterol

Cholesterol is an important constituent of cell membranes and is produced from fat by the liver cells. Excess cholesterol is excreted in the bile, but if there is a considerable excess it may be deposited in the gall bladder and bile duct and in the walls of arteries, causing obstructions. If the bile duct becomes obstructed, jaundice results. If arteries have depositions, the smooth flow of blood is impaired and blood clots or *thromboses* may form.

Heat production

The liver has a continuously high metabolic rate and consequently has a slightly higher temperature than the rest of the body. The large quantity of blood which flows through the liver is therefore warmed.

Role in red blood cell formation

In the foetus, red blood cells are produced by the liver. In the adult they are produced in red bone marrow but the liver continues to produce a chemical substance called the *haematinic* principle which is essential in red blood cell formation. Vitamin B12 must be present in the liver for the production of the haematinic principle.

Elimination of sex hormones

Some sex hormones are modified by the liver; others are excreted in the bile or via the kidneys.

Bilirubin metabolism

Old red blood cells are broken down by phagocytic cells in the spleen, liver and bone marrow. Haemoglobin is broken down in the liver cells, which store the globin and iron molecules and convert the remainder of the 'haem' groups to *biliverdin,* a green pigment which is then converted to *bilirubin*. This is passed into the bile and gives it its characteristic golden colour.

Blood storage

The veins of the liver can expand to serve as a *blood reservoir*. The total volume of the liver can vary between 300 cm^3 and 1500 cm^3.

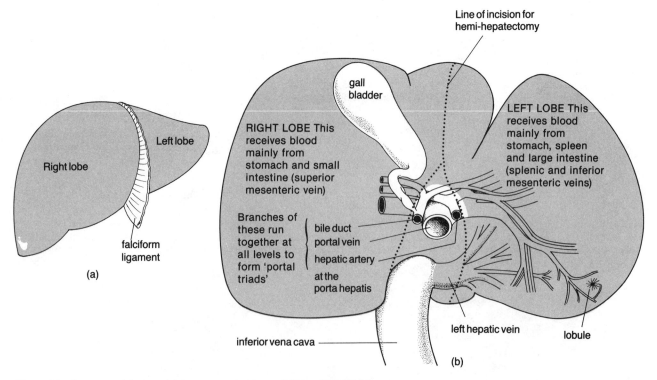

Figure 6.3   Structure of the liver. (a) Anatomical division and (b) functional division

Production of some plasma proteins

These include *fibrinogen*, required for blood clotting, albumin and globulin.

Vitamin and mineral storage

Vitamins A, D and B12 can be stored by the liver, which also stores some minerals including potassium, iron and copper.

2 Structure

The structure of the liver (Figure 6.3a, b) is directly related to the functions described. It receives blood from both the hepatic artery (oxygenated) and the *hepatic portal vein* (rich in food materials from the gut). Blood from the liver leaves via the *hepatic vein*.

Liver cells are highly specialised, and are arranged into liver *lobules* (Figure 6.4a, b) which are roughly cylindrical in shape and approximately 1 mm in diameter. Their structure enables each liver cell to have close contact with blood (in the *sinusoids*) and with the *canaliculi* (fine channels) into which bile products are passed.

Attached to the walls of the sinusoids are the specialised *Kupffer cells*, which are phagocytic cells and part of the *reticulo-endothelial* system, whose task it is to destroy old red blood cells. All other liver functions are carried out by the liver cells.

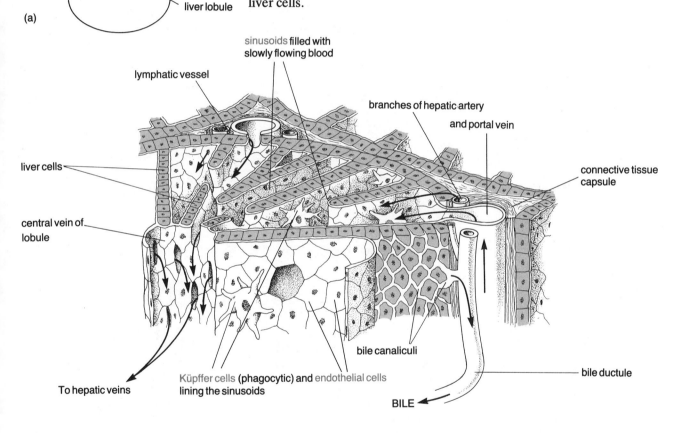

(a) liver lobule

Figure 6.4 A liver lobule. (a) Complete lobule and (b) part of a lobule showing blood flow

(b) A note on hormones

The hormones are the 'chemical messengers' of the body. They are produced by *endocrine glands* (which are ductless), passed into the bloodstream, and exert an effect on a target organ. The rate of secretion of hormones varies widely over the 24-hour period: for example, adrenocorticoids are produced at a high rate in the morning. Some disorders may result from a change in the rhythm and rate of hormone secretion throughout the day, with little or no change in the *total* daily hormone production. Blood hormone levels should therefore be monitored regularly throughout the day, and hormone-containing drugs are best administered in frequent small doses.

Hormones are usually carried in the blood bound to a carrier protein to inactivate them. These form a reservoir from which free hormone can be released. They are broken down in the liver and excreted in bile or urine.

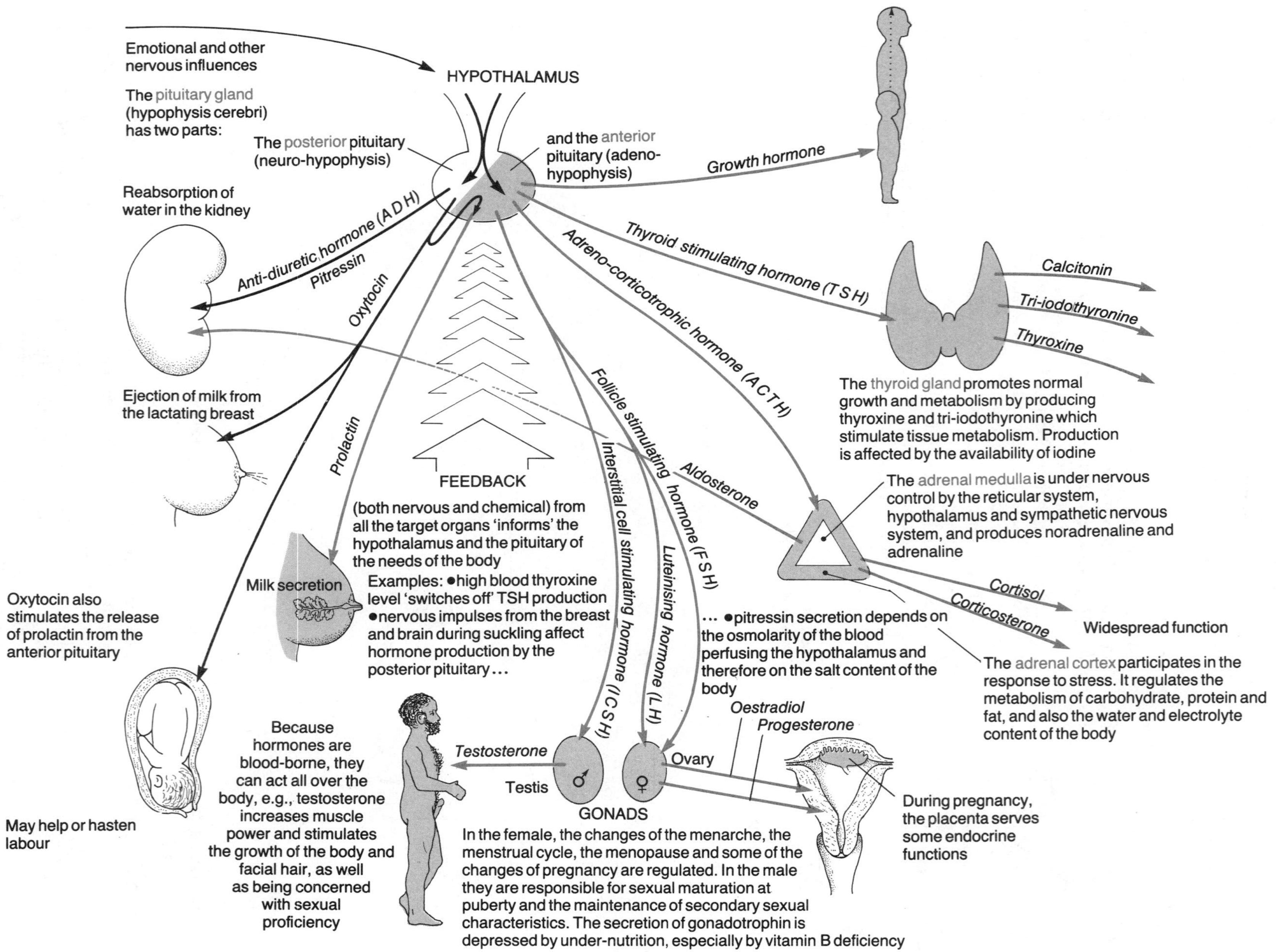

Figure 6.5   Important hormone functions controlled by the pituitary gland and hypothalamus

Emotional and other nervous influences

The pituitary gland (hypophysis cerebri) has two parts:

The posterior pituitary (neuro-hypophysis)

and the anterior pituitary (adeno-hypophysis)

HYPOTHALAMUS

Growth hormone

Thyroid stimulating hormone (TSH)

Adreno-corticotrophic hormone (ACTH)

Calcitonin

Tri-iodothyronine

Thyroxine

The thyroid gland promotes normal growth and metabolism by producing thyroxine and tri-iodothyronine which stimulate tissue metabolism. Production is affected by the availability of iodine

The adrenal medulla is under nervous control by the reticular system, hypothalamus and sympathetic nervous system, and produces noradrenaline and adrenaline

Cortisol

Corticosterone   Widespread function

Aldosterone

The adrenal cortex participates in the response to stress. It regulates the metabolism of carbohydrate, protein and fat, and also the water and electrolyte content of the body

• pitressin secretion depends on the osmolarity of the blood perfusing the hypothalamus and therefore on the salt content of the body

During pregnancy, the placenta serves some endocrine functions

Oestradiol

Progesterone

Ovary

Follicle stimulating hormone (FSH)

Luteinising hormone (LH)

Interstitial cell stimulating hormone (ICSH)

GONADS

Testis

Testosterone

♀

♂

In the female, the changes of the menarche, the menstrual cycle, the menopause and some of the changes of pregnancy are regulated. In the male they are responsible for sexual maturation at puberty and the maintenance of secondary sexual characteristics. The secretion of gonadotrophin is depressed by under-nutrition, especially by vitamin B deficiency

FEEDBACK

(both nervous and chemical) from all the target organs 'informs' the hypothalamus and the pituitary of the needs of the body

Examples: • high blood thyroxine level 'switches off' TSH production • nervous impulses from the breast and brain during suckling affect hormone production by the posterior pituitary . . .

Anti-diuretic hormone (ADH)

Pitressin

Oxytocin

Prolactin

Reabsorption of water in the kidney

Ejection of milk from the lactating breast

Milk secretion

Because hormones are blood-borne, they can act all over the body, e.g., testosterone increases muscle power and stimulates the growth of the body and facial hair, as well as being concerned with sexual proficiency

Oxytocin also stimulates the release of prolactin from the anterior pituitary

May help or hasten labour

154

The mode of action of hormones on their target cells is not completely understood, and may vary between different hormones. The membranes of the cells of the target organ are certainly involved in the chain of events, and it is possible that hormones combine with special sites on the membrane, to cause change in cell membrane function. For example: insulin makes liver cells more permeable to glucose; oxytocin causes the release of calcium ions (Ca^{2+}) in uterine muscle, causing excitation of the muscle and hence contraction.

Figure 6.5 summarises some of the important hormone functions, and also illustrates the role of the *pituitary gland* as the main coordinator of the endocrine system. Some endocrine glands are also under nervous control, adding considerable versatility to the system.

(c) The pancreas

The pancreas is a soft pink gland situated at the back of the upper abdomen (Figure 6.6). It has two secretory parts, the *islets of Langerhans* which make up an endocrine (ductless) gland secreting *hormones (insulin* and *glucagon)* into the bloodstream, and the acini cells which form an exocrine gland with a duct to the duodenum along which the *pancreatic enzymes* pass (see Figure 6.7). The enzymes produced by the pancreas are *trypsin, chymotrypsin* (involved with protein breakdown), *carboxypeptidase* (peptide breakdown), *lipase* (fat breakdown) and *amylase* (hydrolysis of starch).

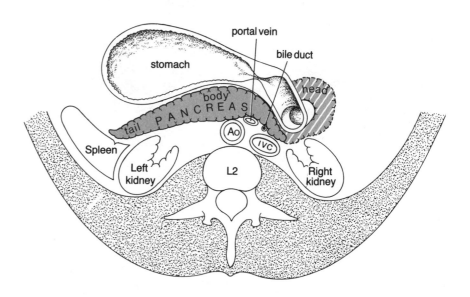

Figure 6.6   Position of the pancreas

The hormones produced by the islets of Langerhans are both involved with glucose metabolism. Insulin facilitates the uptake of glucose by liver and muscle cells, and the production from glucose of glycogen. This results in a reduction in blood sugar. Glucagon facilitates the breakdown of glycogen, and thus increases blood sugar. A normal person secretes about 50 units of insulin per day. The rate of insulin production is controlled primarily in respect of the level of glucose in the blood (Figure 6.8). An increase in blood sugar stimulates insulin production; a drop in blood sugar results in a drop in insulin production. Parasympathetic nervous stimulation (via the vagus nerve) also stimulates insulin production, and this may itself be stimulated by a drop in blood sugar. Sympathetic nerve stimulation (via the splanchnic nerves) releases adrenaline and inhibits insulin production; as does adrenaline production by the adrenal medulla.

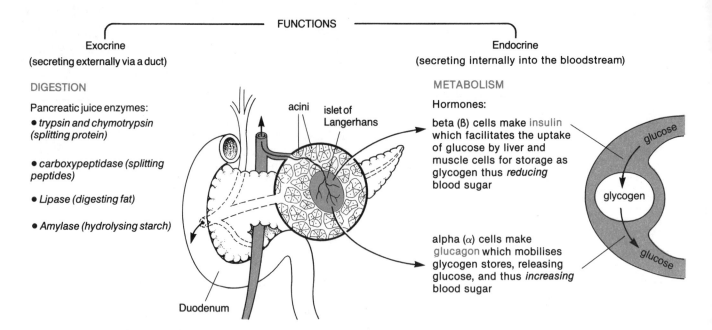

FUNCTIONS

Exocrine
(secreting externally via a duct)

Endocrine
(secreting internally into the bloodstream)

DIGESTION

Pancreatic juice enzymes:
- *trypsin and chymotrypsin (splitting protein)*
- *carboxypeptidase (splitting peptides)*
- *Lipase (digesting fat)*
- *Amylase (hydrolysing starch)*

acini   islet of Langerhans

Duodenum

METABOLISM

Hormones:

beta (ß) cells make insulin which facilitates the uptake of glucose by liver and muscle cells for storage as glycogen thus *reducing* blood sugar

alpha (α) cells make glucagon which mobilises glycogen stores, releasing glucose, and thus *increasing* blood sugar

glucose

glycogen

glucose

Figure 6.7   Functions of the pancreas

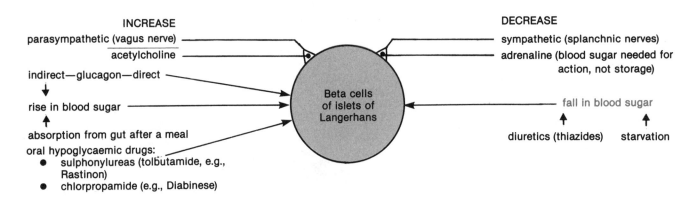

INCREASE

parasympathetic (vagus nerve)

acetylcholine

indirect—glucagon—direct
↓
rise in blood sugar
↑
absorption from gut after a meal

oral hypoglycaemic drugs:
- sulphonylureas (tolbutamide, e.g., Rastinon)
- chlorpropamide (e.g., Diabinese)

Beta cells of islets of Langerhans

DECREASE

sympathetic (splanchnic nerves)

adrenaline (blood sugar needed for action, not storage)

fall in blood sugar
↑   ↑
diuretics (thiazides)   starvation

Figure 6.8   Control of insulin secretion

(d) The thyroid gland

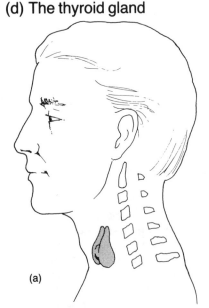

(a)

*Figure 6.9   Position of the thyroid gland.
(a) In the neck and (b) relative to other structures*

The thyroid is an endocrine (i.e. ductless) gland (Figure 6.9a, b) which is under the control of the pituitary gland. The thyroid produces two similar hormones, *tri-iodothyronine* (T_3) and *thyroxine* (T_4), and also calcitonin which has a role in calcium balance.

T_3 and T_4 are involved with energy metabolism and both contain iodine, which is needed by the thyroid gland for their production. Four times more T_4 is produced than T_3, and both are stored when not required in the colloid of the follicles in the gland.

The pituitary gland produces *thyroid stimulating hormone* (TSH) which stimulates breakdown of the colloid by enzymes, and hence release of T_3 and T_4. TSH also stimulates uptake of iodine by the thyroid gland, and production is stimulated by *thyroid releasing factor* (TRF) which is produced by the hypothalamus when T_3 and T_4 levels in the blood are low.

T_3 and T_4 influence the metabolism of all tissues, ensuring normal mental development, bone growth and maintenance, and sexual maturity at puberty. They also heighten the effect of adrenaline and noradrenaline which both cause an increase in the rate of heart beat. The conversion of glycogen to glucose in the liver is increased, as is peripheral use of glucose by all tissues and protein breakdown.

Iodides must be present in the diet and are found in sea-fish, milk, vegetables grown in iodine-rich soil, eggs, and iodised table-salt. Lack of iodine results in the formation of a goitre, poor growth and slow metabolism. The thyroid enlarges and can be felt, and the neck appears thick.

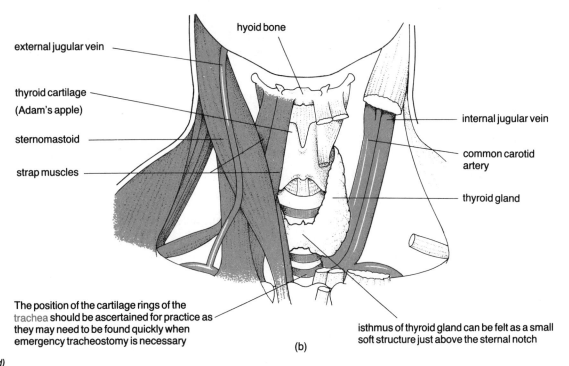

external jugular vein

thyroid cartilage
(Adam's apple)

sternomastoid

strap muscles

hyoid bone

internal jugular vein

common carotid
artery

thyroid gland

The position of the cartilage rings of the trachea should be ascertained for practice as they may need to be found quickly when emergency tracheostomy is necessary

isthmus of thyroid gland can be felt as a small soft structure just above the sternal notch

(b)

Figure 6.9 (continued)

The patients with disturbances of metabolism

(a) Disturbance of functions of the liver

1 Patient study and care plan for an adult with liver failure

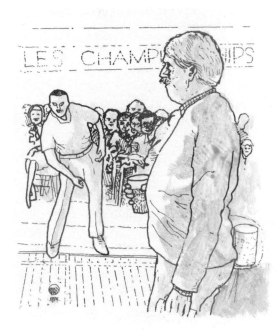

Figure 6.10 Mr Geoffrey Collins

History of social, psychological and physical events leading to the present condition

The patient chosen for this section to illustrate disturbance of the functions of the liver is an adult with liver failure.

Mr Geoffrey Collins (Figure 6.10), aged 50 years, lives with his wife in a council house on the outskirts of a city. Their two children are married and live in the city. He is a member of the local skittle club and he has drunk alcohol moderately all his life. His past history includes episodes of alcoholic gastritis, which occur after a bout of drinking; he suffers from epigastric pain, loss of appetite at breakfast, and mucus vomiting in the mornings. During the last few months he has noticed a loss of weight but his abdomen seemed to be getting bigger. One morning he vomited blood and felt weak and dizzy; he made an appointment to see his doctor that morning.

The doctor examined Mr Collins and found the following:
- Slight jaundice.
- Enlarged liver and spleen.
- Mild ascites.
- Evidence of loss of weight and anaemia.
- Some spider naevi on upper arms and chest.
- Erythema of palms of hands.
- Dilated umbilical veins.

The doctor discussed the diagnosis of liver disease with Mr Collins and advised admission to hospital for investigation of his liver and gastric bleeding.

Explanation of abnormal physiology and pathology

It is advisable to revise the normal functions and structure of the liver, and see Table 6.1.

Table 6.1

Normal physiology	Abnormal physiology of liver failure
(a) *The liver manufactures:* (i) *Bile* which contains: • *pigments*—the waste products of destroyed red blood cells, excreted in the bile • *salts*—necessary for the emulsification of fats	Bile continues to be made but oedema of liver sinusoids can obstruct the flow of bile. Bilirubin therefore accumulates in the bloodstream resulting in jaundice. The body fails to emulsify fats, salts accumulate in the blood, causing skin irritation, and fatty bulky stools are excreted
(ii) *Plasma proteins* from assimilated amino acids: • *albumin*—maintains osmotic pressure of the blood and protein pool in the body	Liver unable to utilise amino acids to manufacture plasma proteins, resulting in reduction of production of albumin and a lowering of the osmotic pressure in the blood. This results in oedema and ascites and loss of protein pool for replacement of tissue cells
• *globulin*—necessary for the carriage of antibodies and nutrients	No alteration in blood levels of globulin
• *prothrombin* and *fibrinogen*—factors necessary for blood clotting	Reduced production of these factors leads to tendency to bleeding, within the gastrointestinal tract, skin and mucous membranes
(b) *The liver stores:* (i) *Iron and Vitamin B12* required for manufacture of haemoglobin and red blood cells	Stores not replaced, leads to failure of manufacture of red blood cells and progressive anaemia
(ii) *Glucose* as glycogen and forms glycogen from surplus protein and fat. It also converts stored glycogen back into glucose when blood glucose level drops	Liver failure leads to fall in blood glucose level as liver is unable to store glycogen and therefore there are no reserves to reconvert to glucose when blood levels fall
(iii) *Fat-soluble vitamins:* A, D, E, K	Failure of storage of these vitamins has effects on night vision, bones and clotting
(c) *The liver destroys:* (i) Red blood cells by the Kupffer cells in the liver sinusoids	No effect, other reticulo-endothelial tissue will carry out this function
(ii) *Some drugs,* e.g., barbiturates, Largactil, paracetamol	Prolonged action of ingested or injected drugs
(d) *The liver converts:* Blood ammonia from protein metabolism to urea for excretion via the kidney	Failure to convert ammonia to urea causes blood ammonia to accumulate and rise. High blood ammonia causes unconsciousness and coma (encephalopathy)
Hormones and enzymes (inactivates)	Continued circulation of androgens gives rise to spider naevi, palmar erythema and possibly gynaecomastia

Portal hypertension occurs as blood cannot pass through cirrhotic liver easily, increases ascites and causes oesophageal varices and/or haemorrhoids.

Care plan

PREPARATION FOR PATIENT WITH LIVER FAILURE

Mr Collins is admitted to hospital later that day, where the following investigations are made and results revealed.

Investigation	Result
Endoscopy	Some evidence of oesophageal varices, with no signs of recent bleeding. Severe gastritis with mucous lining still bleeding
Blood test for grouping and cross-matching Haemoglobin Serum bilirubin Liver function tests	Haemoglobin low Bilirubin slightly increased Serum alkaline phosphatase increased Plasma proteins: albumin decreased, globulin increased
Prothrombin time Urea Electrolytes	Prothrombin time increased Low blood urea Electrolytes within normal limits
Liver biopsy	Confirms cirrhotic changes

NURSING HISTORY AND ASSESSMENT

Table 6.2 shows the completed form for Mr Collins.

TREATMENT

Following the investigations the care plan described in Table 6.3 is implemented for Mr Collins's gastritis and liver failure.

Table 6.2 Nursing history and assessment sheet for Mr Collins

NURSING HISTORY AND ASSESSMENT SHEET
Record No. _293949_

PATIENT LABEL
Mr/~~Mrs/Miss~~ _Geoffrey Collins_
Address _10 Tulip Close, Edithmead_

Male/Female   Age _50_
Date of Birth _6·6·36_

Date of admission/~~first visit~~
_10·6·86_

Time _____
Type: ☐ Routine ☑ Emergency
Transfer from: _____

Religion _C/E_
Practising/baptised _Non-practising_
Minister _____
Telephone number _____

Next of kin (name) _Mrs Collins_
Relationship to patient _Wife_
Address _Same address_

Telephone numbers _87654_
Contact at night/in emergency   YES/~~NO~~

Occupation (or father) _Dock worker_
Marital status _Married_
Children (or place in family) _2 (both married)_
Other dependants _____
Pets _____
School (children only) _____
Hobbies _____
Clubs _Skittle club_
Favourite pastime _____
Does patient smoke?   YES/<u>NO</u>

Speech difficulty/language barrier

Dysphasia   Dysarthria

Accommodation

Lives alone   YES/<u>NO</u>
Part III/EMI/Old People's Homes/Rented
Other _____

Consultant _Mr York_
House officer _Dr Young_
Presenting condition _Gastric bleeding_

159

Table 6.2 (cont.)

History of present complaint and reason for admission

Recent weight loss but abdomen increasing in size. Vomited blood, weak and dizzy. Liver disease and gastric bleeding

Past medical history

Moderate drinker. Episodes of alcoholic gastritis

Allergies   *None*

Current medication

None

What patient says is the reason for admission and attitude to admission

Liver failure and bleeding. Slightly resentful

Patient's expectations

Any problems at home while/because patient is in hospital?

In short-time work at present.

Relevant home conditions (e.g. stairs)   *?Financial*

Visiting problems

Care at home

Community nurse _____

No. _____

Name of GP   *Dr Grant*

Address   *The Medical Centre, Edithmead*

Other services involved

Home help _____	Day hospital _____
Laundry _____	Day centre/club _____
Inco supplies _____	Health visitor _____
Aids _____	Social worker _____
Meals on wheels _____	Voluntary worker _____

Daily living

Diet

Special _____

Food or drink dislikes _____

Appetite: ☐ GOOD ☑ POOR

Remarks   *Poor appetite in early part of day*

Sleep

How many hours normally?   *6*

Sedation _____

What else helps? _____

Elimination

Bowels: Continent/Incontinent

How often opened?   *Daily*

Any medication? _____

Urinary: Continent/Incontinent

If incontinent; Day/Night/If not taken, how frequently? _____

Nocturia/Dysuria/Frequency/Urgency

Remarks _____

Female patients — Menstruation

Post-menopausal	Taking the pill
Regular	Irregular
Amenorrhoea	Dysmenorrhoea

Next period due: _____

Uses: STs Tampons

Hearing

Hearing aid: YES/NO

Remarks _____

Vision

Glasses/Contact lens: YES/NO

Remarks _____

Oral

Dentures or crowns: YES/NO

Any problems with mouth or teeth?

Mobility

Help needed with:

Walking/Standing/In/Out of bed/Bathing/Dressing

In/Out of chair/

Feeding/Other: _____

Remarks   *Usually active*

Prosthesis/appliance

Type of appliance _____

Help needed _____

General appearance

Normal	Dehydrated	Acutely ill
Obese	Thin	Emaciated

Remarks   *Weight loss during last few months*

Skin

Satisfactory	Broken areas	Dehydrated
Rash	Oedematous	Jaundiced *(slightly)*
Pallor	Other *Some itching*	
	(including bruising)	

Remarks _____

Level of consciousness

Orientated   Semi-conscious

Confused   Unconscious

Remarks ⎯⎯⎯⎯⎯⎯⎯⎯⎯⎯

Mental assessment (if appropriate)

Mood

Elated   Irritable   Agitated

Cheerful   Anxious   Aggressive

Miserable   Withdrawn   Suspicious

Apathetic

Thought content

Hallucinations/Delusions/Paranoid Ideas

⎯⎯⎯⎯⎯⎯⎯⎯⎯⎯⎯⎯⎯⎯⎯⎯

Orientation

Time/Place/Person

Very confused   Slightly confused

Any particular time of day? ⎯⎯⎯⎯⎯⎯

Confabulation ⎯⎯⎯⎯⎯⎯⎯⎯⎯

Remarks ⎯⎯⎯⎯⎯⎯⎯⎯⎯⎯⎯

Surveillance   Physical/Emotional

Information obtained from ⎯⎯ *Mrs Collins*

Relationship to patient ⎯⎯ *Wife*

By ⎯⎯ *MAR*

Position/level of training ⎯⎯⎯⎯⎯⎯

Date ⎯⎯ *10·6·86*

Time ⎯⎯⎯⎯⎯⎯⎯⎯⎯⎯⎯⎯

Table 6.3   *Care plan for Mr Collins while a patient in the medical ward*

Problem	Objective	Plan of care	Rationale
1. Patient slightly resentful about admission	Gain patient's confidence	(a) Discuss with Mr and Mrs Collins the need for admission and the details of future management	(a) Gives opportunity for patient and wife to express their fears
		(b) Reassure Mr Collins that his permission will be asked before any tests are carried out	(b) Encourages Mr Collins to relax and gain confidence
		(c) Introduce Mr Collins to other patients in the ward	(c) Encourages him to be sociable
		(d) Check his hearing aid is functioning	(d) To ensure he is able to socialise
2. Acute gastritis	Minimise the effects of gastritis	Give fluids of high calorie content, progressing to light, easily digested meals	Reduces irritation to gastric mucosa and maintains nutritional state
3. Tendency to bleed	Detect bleeding	(a) Observe vomit for blood, stools for melaena	(a) For early detection and prompt replacement therapy
		(b) Measure and record pulse and blood pressure	(b) Indicates internal haemorrhage by rise in pulse and drop in blood pressure
		(c) Daily urine test for blood	(c) and (d) For early detection for prompt treatment
		(d) Inspect skin and mucous membranes for bruising and bleeding	
		(e) Have available vitamin K and Pitressin	(e) Insufficient vitamin K available for clotting. Pitressin to vasoconstrict bleeding vessels in oesophagus
4. Acutely ill man with papery skin with slight ascites	Minimise discomfort and detect development of complications of bed rest	(a) Position sitting up supported with pillows	(a) Ascites can impair breathing
		(b) Turning and repositioning at regular intervals	(b) Reduces pressure on skin over bony prominences
		(c) Use of aids: ripple mattress, sheepskin, bed cradle	(c) Weight of ascites makes turning difficult
		(d) Detect early signs of pressure sores, skin abrasions, bruising, hypostatic pneumonia, urinary stasis	(d) Allows prompt change of care plan and treatment

Table 6.3 (cont.)

Problem	Objective	Plan of care	Rationale
5. Liver failure	Minimise effects of liver failure while maintaining adequate nutrition	Give high-protein, high-carbohydrate, possibly low-salt and with added iron and vitamins and low-fat in the form of frequent glucose drinks and light, easily digested food	High-protein diet improves protein synthesis and therefore plasma proteins; therefore improves clotting and reduces oedema. High-carbohydrate maintains blood glucose level. Glucose aids recovery of damaged liver cells. Low-salt assists in reduction of oedema. Iron and vitamin supplement because body at present unable to absorb and assimilate. If jaundiced probably insufficient bile salts to emulsify fats
6. Mild ascites	Detect increase in ascites	(a) Weigh daily	(a) Measures fluid retention
		(b) Measure girth daily	(b) Gives record of increase or decrease in ascites
		(c) Record fluid balance: if worsens give spironolactone as prescribed	(c) Provides record; patient has a tendency to develop oedema. Other diuretics can be used with care but there is a risk of hyperkalaemia which may precipitate encephalopathy (abdominal paracentesis is contraindicated as it inevitably removes protein and electrolytes)
7. Inability to detoxicate drugs	Avoid overdosing	Be constantly aware this is a hazard; use hypnotic and analgesic drugs with care	Action of all drugs will be prolonged and will accumulate in the blood
8. Potential hepatic encephalopathy	Detect early signs of encephalopathy	(a) Observe for lethargy, confusion, irrational behaviour, flapping tremor of outstretched hands, inability to draw geometrical figure	(a) Liver's inability to convert ammonia to urea. High levels of blood ammonia cause cerebral irritation and eventual coma
		(b) Observe for precipitating factors: gastrointestinal bleeding, intercurrent infection	(b) Blood in the alimentary tract contains protein which cannot be metabolised
		(c) If (b) occurs: (i) Stop all protein intake (or possibly reduce to 20 grams protein daily) (ii) Give colonic washout (iii) Have ready oral neomycin as prescribed	(c) If (b) occurs: (i) Protein is unable to be metabolised (ii) Removes protein waste from bowel (iii) Prevents production of ammonia from bacterial activity in the bowel

RECOVERY AND ADVICE

While Mr Collins is on the regime of this diet and rest, his gastritis improves, ascites disappears, his general nutritional state improves and energy returns. The doctor advises that in the long term Mr Collins should abstain from alcohol completely and suggests that he should contact Alcoholics Anonymous. The dietician advises Mr and Mrs Collins on a high-protein diet.

Long-term problems could result in portal hypertension from back pressure from severely fibrosed liver. This could initiate bleeding from oesophageal varices, return of ascites and gross enlargement of spleen. For further information refer to J. Macleod (Ed.), *Davidson's Principles and Practice of Medicine*, 14th edition, Churchill Livingstone, London, 1984.

2 Patient histories illustrating further problems related to disturbance of functions of the liver

This part of the chapter comprises patient histories, self-testing questions and guidelines for suggested answers.

A child with hepatitis due to virus type A (infective hepatitis)

Timothy White, aged 15 years, lives with his parents and two brothers on a new housing estate. He returns from a fortnight's summer camp and starts back to school. Three weeks later his mother notices that he is listless and anorexic. Over the next twenty-four hours Timothy develops a fever, complains of aching in back and limbs and feels sick. His mother thinks he has the 'flu, puts him to bed and keeps him away from school. Timothy's mother rings the doctor the next morning, who visits the house that day. Following examination he advises Timothy's mother to keep him warm in bed and to contact him again if she is worried. During the next few days Timothy continues to feel very unwell with a high fever, requiring frequent changes of bedclothes and cool washes, and is only able to tolerate clear fluids. Mrs White again becomes concerned and rings the doctor, who visits and examines Timothy. He discovers early signs of jaundice, enlarged liver, and a urine sample reveals a positive test for bilirubin.

The doctor informs Mrs White that Timothy has infective hepatitis, possibly contracted at summer camp.

He asks her to ensure that all members of the family take care with handwashing after visiting the toilet and warns that other members of the family may have already been infected. Over the next two days Timothy becomes increasingly jaundiced; his urine is dark brown in colour and stools are pale and bulky. However, during this time his temperature returns to normal and he begins to feel better. After a week the jaundice disappears, stools and urine return to normal and he begins to feel more his usual self. The doctor advises that Timothy should not return to school that term as a period of convalescence is required.

SELF-TESTING QUESTIONS

1. Virus type A causes inflammation of the liver cells and is spread by the faecal – oral route. How would you advise a family to minimise the risk of spread if one member was affected?

2. Describe the abnormal physiology of hepatitis due to virus type A (infective hepatitis).

BRIEF ANALYSIS AND GUIDELINES TO SUITABLE ANSWERS

Question 1
Your answer should include:
(a) Careful disposal of excreta from the infected person.
(b) Handwashing after bowel action and before each meal.
(c) Patient to keep own flannel and towels.
(d) Wash and dry patient's crockery and cutlery separately.
(e) Reduce number of visitors.

Question 2
Virus A enters the body via the gastrointestinal tract and settles in the liver cells. The liver becomes inflamed and oedematous, which blocks the sinusoids and bile canaliculi so preventing excretion of bile into the biliary tract and duodenum. The absence of bile results in pale, fatty, bulky stools. Bilirubin accumulates in the bloodstream and stains the skin yellow; conjugated bilirubin is excreted in the urine making it dark brown. Circulating bilirubin causes drowsiness and lethargy. The inflammation causes liver enlargement, pyrexia and anorexia.

A young adult with hepatitis due to virus type B (serum hepatitis)

Elaine Little, 19-year-old student nurse, lives in the nurses' residence attached to a large general hospital. She develops all the signs and symptoms of hepatitis (as described in previous patient history) but she gives no history of contact with hepatitis and she has been abroad on holiday recently. On close questioning she recalls pricking her finger on a blood-contaminated needle (approximately three months ago) that had been used for taking blood from a patient who was a medical laboratory technician. At the time of this incident Elaine failed to report to the staff health department and did not complete an incident form.

The doctor advises Elaine that hospital admission is required and arranges for a bed to be made available. She is admitted and nursed with all supportive therapy. Care is taken of blood samples taken from Elaine with attention to local hospital procedure.

SELF-TESTING QUESTIONS

1. Serum hepatitis is due to virus type B and is spread by contact with blood, saliva and sweat. (a) Describe how Elaine became infected with this virus and (b) give other possible examples of how infection may occur.

BRIEF ANALYSIS AND GUIDELINES TO SUITABLE ANSWERS

Question 1
(a) Elaine was infected by virus type B by inoculation from a needle contaminated with the blood of a laboratory technician who must have carried the Australian antigen (hepatitis associated with antigen, HAA). This antigen is thought to be the coat of the virus particle which can be present in apparently healthy individuals but transmission of the antigen to another person causes serum hepatitis.

(b) Other examples of transmission include:
- Between drug addicts sharing needles.
- Between patients and staff in haemodialysis units.
- Between laboratory staff.
- Between medical and nursing staff.

2. Why should Elaine have reported such a minor injury as a needle puncture?

Question 2
Any puncture wound from blood-contaminated needle, stillette, scalpel, and any blood contamination entering cuts or abrasions on a nurse's skin could put the nurse at risk from serum hepatitis.

At the time of the incident the patient from whom the contaminate has come should be identified and notes checked for presence of Australian antigen. If no history, blood sample may be taken for checking. Even in the absence of firm confirmation the nurse should receive hyperimmune gammaglobulin as protection.

An adult with acute cholecystitis associated with gallstones

Mrs Green, aged 45 years, lives with her husband and two teenage children in a farming community. During the last two years Mrs Green has suffered minor bouts of dyspepsia and difficulty in tolerating fat in her meals. For the last three days Mrs Green complained to her husband that she was feeling off-colour, slightly nauseated and shivery. During one night she woke up feeling hot and sick with severe pain in the upper right side of her abdomen. Her husband contacted their GP, who examined Mrs Green and recommended admission to hospital.

On arrival at the hospital Mrs Green appears very distressed, having been vomiting in the ambulance. On examination the doctor finds the following:
- A tender right hypochrondrium.
- Slightly yellow sclera of eyes.
- Temperature 39°C.
- Pulse 100 beats per minute.
- Respirations 24 per minute.
- Blood pressure normal.
- Tongue dry and coated.

The doctor orders the following investigations:

1. Blood examination for:
   - Urea and electrolytes.
   - Serum bilirubin.
   - Full blood count.
2. Intravenous infusion of dextrose saline.
3. Nasogastric tube.
4. Intravenous cholangiogram which showed the presence of stones in the gall bladder.

Diagnosis of acute cholecystitis is made, analgesics are given and antibiotic therapy commenced with explanation to Mr and Mrs Green.

SELF-TESTING QUESTIONS

BRIEF ANALYSIS AND GUIDELINES TO SUITABLE ANSWERS

1. Describe and illustrate the structure and function of the gall bladder and biliary tract.

Question 1
Refer to page 151.

2. Describe the metabolic function of bile.

Question 2
Refer to page 151, bile.

3. Explain the abnormal physiology of Mrs Green's present condition.

Question 3
Your answer should include an explanation of Mrs Green's pyrexia, abdominal pain, vomiting and yellow tinge to sclera.

4. Discover the various radiological investigations that can be carried out on the biliary tract and explain the reason for the choice of an intravenous cholangiogram for Mrs Green.

Question 4

Possible radiological investigations are as follows:

(a) Radiography of the abdomen: a plain x-ray of the abdomen which may show radio-opaque stones (30% approximately).

(b) Cholecystography: oral organic iodine-containing compound is used which is absorbed and secreted by the liver in the bile and concentrated in the normal gall bladder. If the gall bladder is functioning sufficiently to produce a shadow any non-opaque stones will probably be demonstrated.

(c) Cholangiography by one of three methods:
- Intravenous cholangiogram: the intravenous administration of a dye which is concentrated and excreted by the liver permits visualisation of the main biliary ducts and gall bladder. Often used in acute cholecystitis when the patient is vomiting and unable to tolerate oral preparations (as used for our patient, Mrs Green); following oral cholecystography when the gall bladder has been found to be non-functioning; or following cholecystectomy.
- Operative and post-operative cholangiogram for testing the patency of the biliary ducts by cannulating the ducts during surgery and via the T-tube post-operatively prior to its removal.
- Choledochopancreatography: retrograde cannulation of the common bile duct and pancreatic duct via the ampulla of Vater using a flexible fibre-optic endoscope.

5. Describe the possible composition of gall stones.

Question 5

There are three main groups:

(a) Cholesterol stones — normal constituent of bile which precipitates out of solution.

(b) Pigment stones — over-concentration, when there is excessive excretion of bilirubin by the liver (very rare).

(c) Mixed stones — most common, containing cholesterol, calcium and biluribin.

6. If a stone formed in the gall bladder passes into the common bile duct, describe the possible complications of this occurrence.

Question 6

Your answer should include:

(a) Description of biliary colic due to peristalsis in the ducts under the influence of the autonomic nervous system.

(b) Distension of the gall bladder due to accumulating bile which could lead to inflammation, perforation, peritonitis.

(c) Obstruction to the flow of bile from the liver causing back pressure on the bile canaliculi in the liver leading to raised serum bilirubin levels and eventually jaundice. The obstruction of the flow of bile into the duodenum causing pale stools and steatorrhoea, and failure of absorption of fat and fat-soluble vitamins (A, D, E and K).

7. Describe the effects to Mrs Green if she were to develop obstructive jaundice due to a gall stone obstructing her common bile duct.

Question 7

See answer to question 6 but extend this to include long-term effects of fat intolerance, deficiency of vitamins especially vitamin K, accumulation of bilirubin and bile salts in the blood.

(b) Disturbance of the metabolic function of the pancreas

History of social, psychological and physical events leading to the present condition.

The patient chosen for this section to illustrate disturbance of the metabolic function of the pancreas is a young adult with diabetes mellitus of juvenile onset.

1 Patient study and care plan for a young adult with diabetes mellitus of juvenile onset

Simon Gallagher (Figure 6.11), aged 16 years, is a healthy active schoolboy studying for his General Certificate of Education 'O' levels. He lives with his parents and younger sister in a council flat in a city suburb. He is a member of the local boy's football club and does a daily morning and evening newspaper round. Mrs Gallagher has become concerned with Simon's increasing tiredness and loss of weight and wonders if he is overtaxing himself with his examinations approaching. Simon reveals to her that he is having to visit the toilet at night on one or two occasions to pass large quantities of urine and is finding he is wanting

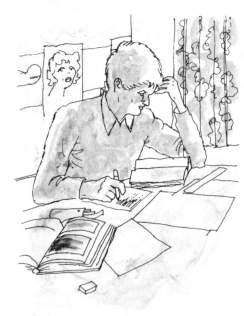

Figure 6.11   Simon Gallagher

to drink more than usual. She advises Simon to give up his paper round until his examinations are over. In the meantime he develops a large boil on the back of his neck which he tries to ignore while he is taking his examinations.

One afternoon he returns from school feeling ill, sick and feverish and goes to bed. His mother notices that Simon becomes increasingly dry and thirsty. He becomes drowsy during the evening and when she finds difficulty in rousing him she calls her GP.

The doctor examines Simon and finds the following:

- Semi-conscious state.
- Dry skin, tongue and lips.
- Distended abdomen.
- Deep sighing respirations.
- Rapid pulse.
- Low blood pressure.
- Breath fetid and sweet, smelling of acetone.
- Urinanalysis revealed presence of glucose and ketones.
- Blood from finger prick revealed raised glucose levels.

The doctor makes a diagnosis of hyperglycaemia due to diabetes mellitus and arranges for an ambulance to take Simon to hospital immediately. He explains Simon's condition to his parents who make arrangements to go to the hospital with him.

Explanation of abnormal physiology and pathology

It is advisable to revise the endocrine function of the pancreas (pages 155–156), and see Table 6.4.

Table 6.4

Normal physiology	Abnormal physiology and pathology
(a) Insulin stimulates the liver to manufacture glycogen from the glucose which reaches the liver by the blood from the alimentary tract. This action rapidly reduces the blood glucose level after each meal	Lack of insulin results in failure of stimulation of the liver to manufacture glycogen from the blood glucose; therefore the blood glucose level remains high
(b) Insulin makes the tissue cell walls permeable to glucose, allowing passage of glucose into the cell for metabolic activity for the production of energy	Lack of insulin results in impermeability of the cell walls to glucose, therefore depriving cells of their energy source and causing accumulation of glucose in the blood
(c) Carbohydrate is taken in the diet, is digested and absorbed into the blood in the form of glucose, maltose and sucrose. Once in the bloodstream under the action of insulin, glucose is stored in the liver as glycogen or is passed into the tissue cells for energy	Carbohydrate continues to be taken in the diet and is digested and absorbed into the bloodstream. Once in the bloodstream glucose fails to be converted to glycogen in the liver or pass into the tissue cells, therefore accumulates in the blood
(d) Under increased exercise or stress the body can mobilise glycogen from the liver back into the bloodstream due to the action of adrenaline	The patient who is stressed, e.g., due to the presence of infection, depletes his liver stores of glycogen so blood glucose level rises until stores are used up
(e) Normally blood glucose level: 2.5–4.7 mmol/l or 45–85 mg/100 ml	Blood glucose rises above normal limits
(f) Normally no glucose is excreted in the urine	(i) When blood glucose rises above 9.2 mmol/l excess glucose is excreted in the urine (this level is commonly referred to as the renal threshold) (ii) Glycosuria causes osmotic diuresis resulting in polyuria, nocturia, polydipsia and dehydration. Uncontrolled glycosuria causes hypovolaemic shock and excessive excretion of sodium and potassium and electrolyte imbalance (iii) Increased glucose concentration in tissue fluids provides an ideal culture medium for the growth of bacteria (iv) Glycosuria can cause inflammation of vulva, vagina, glans penis
(g) Output of insulin is controlled by the level of blood glucose. When the blood glucose levels rise after a meal the insulin output also rises to bring the blood glucose level back to normal	When the blood glucose level rises there is no rise in the output of insulin so the blood glucose level continues to rise
(h) Insulin stimulates the production of body protein from amino acids for the growth and repair of body tissue. It also stimulates the formation of adipose tissue from fatty acids	Lack of insulin causes failure of formation of new body protein and adipose tissue resulting in loss of weight and delayed healing

Normal physiology	Abnormal physiology and pathology
(i) For the metabolism of fat for heat and energy, carbohydrate has to be metabolised	Failure of metabolism of carbohydrate due to lack of insulin results in incomplete metabolism of fat. Partially oxidised fats combine to produce substances called *ketone bodies*, e.g., acetone, acetoacetic acid, which accumulate in the blood: (i) Ketone bodies are toxic to the brain and if they reach a high enough level will cause coma (ii) They are excreted in the urine and expired air (causing sweet-smelling breath) (iii) Accumulation of ketones causes acidosis and fall in plasma bicarbonate level (iv) Acidosis causes deep sighing respirations as the body attempts to correct the pH imbalance by excreting acid in the form of carbon dioxide

Care plan

PREPARATION AND TREATMENT FOR PATIENT WITH DIABETES MELLITUS

On arrival at the accident and emergency department treatment by intravenous therapy is commenced, to include the following:

1. Sodium lactate to correct acidosis.
2. Normal saline to correct dehydration.
3. Potassium to replace depleted potassium.
4. Insulin according to blood glucose level.
5. Antibiotics for infection.

Nursing history and assessment
The nursing history and assessment form is completed for Simon, as shown in Table 6.5.

Table 6.5 Nursing history and assessment sheet for Simon Gallagher

NURSING HISTORY AND ASSESSMENT SHEET
Record No. ___636363___

PATIENT LABEL
Mr/Mrs/Miss ___Simon GALLAGHER___
Address ___Flat 2A, The Towers, Oldchester___
Male/Female   Age ___16___
Date of Birth ___10.2.69___

Date of admission/first visit
___12.10.86___
Time _____
Type: ☐ Routine   ☑ Emergency
  Transfer from: _____
Religion ___Methodist___
Practising/baptised ___Practising___
Minister _____
Telephone number _____
Next of kin (name) ___Mr and Mrs T. Gallagher___
Relationship to patient ___Parents___
Address ___Same address___

Telephone numbers ___2266___
Contact at night/in emergency   YES/NO
Occupation (or father) ___Father - Building worker___
Marital status ___Single___
Children (or place in family) ___Eldest child___
Other dependants _____
Pets _____
School (children only) _____
Hobbies _____
Clubs ___Local boys' football club___
Favourite pastime _____
Does patient smoke?   YES/NO

Speech difficulty/language barrier

Dysphasia   Dysarthria

Accommodation

Lives alone   YES/NO
Part III/EMI/Old People's Homes/Rented
Other ___Flat___

Table 6.5 (cont.)

Consultant _Mr Hart_

House officer _Dr James_

Presenting condition _Semi - conscious_
Hyperglycaemic coma

History of present complaint and reason for admission
Polyuria for 3 weeks. Became sick, feverish, increasingly dry and thirsty, semi-conscious. Hyperglycaemia

Past medical history
Boil on neck

Allergies _None_

Current medication
None

What patient says is the reason for admission and attitude to admission
N/a semi - conscious

Patient's expectations

Any problems at home while/because patient is in hospital?

Relevant home conditions (e.g. stairs)

Visiting problems

Care at home

Community nurse

No.

Name of GP _Dr John_

Address _The Health Centre, Oldchester_

Other services involved

Home help _____ Day hospital _____

Laundry _____ Day centre/club _____

Inco supplies _____ Health visitor _____

Aids _____ Social worker _____

Meals on wheels _____ Voluntary worker _____

Daily living

Diet

Special _____

Food or drink dislikes _____

Appetite: ☐ GOOD ☐ POOR
Remarks _Previously normal_

Sleep

How many hours normally? _9_

Sedation _____

What else helps? _____

Elimination

Bowels: Continent/Incontinent

How often opened? _____

Any medication? _____

Urinary: Continent/Incontinent

If incontinent; Day/Night/If not taken, how frequently? _____

Nocturia/Dysuria/Frequency/Urgency

Remarks _Polyuria_

Female patients — Menstruation

Post-menopausal   Taking the pill

Regular   Irregular

Amenorrhoea   Dysmenorrhoea

Next period due: _____

Uses: STs Tampons

Hearing

Hearing aid: YES/NO

Remarks _____

Vision

Glasses/Contact lens: YES/NO

Remarks _____

Oral

Dentures or crowns: YES/NO

Any problems with mouth or teeth?
_No_

Mobility

Help needed with:

Walking/Standing/In/Out of bed/Bathing/Dressing

In/Out of chair/

Feeding/Other: _____

Remarks _Usually active_

Prosthesis/appliance

Type of appliance _____

Help needed _____

General appearance

Normal   Dehydrated   Acutely ill

Obese   Thin   Emaciated

Remarks _Recent weight loss_

Skin

Satisfactory   Broken areas   Dehydrated

Rash   Oedematous   Jaundiced

Pallor   Other _Dry tongue and lips_
                          (including bruising)

Remarks _____

Level of consciousness

Orientated	<u>Semi-conscious</u>
Confused	Unconscious

Remarks _____

Mental assessment (if appropriate) *N/a semi-conscious*

Mood

Elated	Irritable	Agitated
Cheerful	Anxious	Aggressive
Miserable	Withdrawn	Suspicious
Apathetic		

Thought content

Hallucinations/Delusions/Paranoid Ideas

_____

Orientation

Time/Place/Person

Very confused   Slightly confused

Any particular time of day? _____

Confabulation _____

Remarks _____

Surveillance   Physical/Emotional

Information obtained from ____ *Mr and Mrs Gallagher*

Relationship to patient ____ *Parents*

By ____ *M. GREEN*

Position/level of training _____

Date ____ *12·10·86*

Time _____

Treatment for semi-conscious patient

Following initiation of the treatment described above Simon is transferred to a medical ward for monitoring and stabilisation of his condition (see Table 6.6).

Table 6.6   Care plan for Simon Gallagher while a patient in a medical ward

Problem	Objective	Plan of care	Rationale
1. Patient in a semi-conscious state	Maintain his safety	(a) Place patient in semi-prone position	(a) Prevent inhalation of vomit or saliva
		(b) Have available oxygen and suction equipment	(b) Suction to remove secretions and prevent their inhalation. Oxygen for emergency use in case of asphyxiation or after use of suction
		(c) Fix cot sides in position	(c) Prevent patient falling out of bed
	To reduce fear and assist in re-establishing his orientation	(a) Talk to him when attending to his needs	(a) and (b) Stimulates Simon to respond either verbally or by gesture
		(b) Address him by name	
		(c) Ask parents to bring in his own personal effects	(c) and (d) Encourages parents to participate in Simon's recovery and re-establishes familiar motor patterns
		(d) Encourage parents to talk to Simon	
2. Dehydration	Relieve dehydration and monitor effects of replacement therapy	(a) Monitor rate of intravenous fluid regime	(a) Ensures sufficient intravenous fluids are given in the early stages of treatment (usually 1 litre of normal saline hourly)
		(b) Measure and record fluid intake and output	(b) Records amount for basis for further treatment
		(c) Check site of cannulation for signs of tissuing and inflammation	(c) Early detection of complications
	Prevent oral sepsis or discomfort	Give oral hygiene 2-hourly and apply lanolin to lips	Dry mouth and cracked lips can lead to the development of infection. Treatment is soothing and makes the mouth more comfortable
	Prevent damage to dry skin and detect any complications	(a) Wash and dry skin with care	(a) Removes dead skin cells and prevents the multiplication of pathogenic bacteria
		(b) Turn and reposition 2-hourly while Simon is too ill to do so	(b) and (c) Relieves pressure on bony prominences
		(c) Use aids, e.g., sheepskin, bed cradle	
		(d) Report skin abrasion or eruptions	(d) Enables prompt treatment to be carried out

Table 6.6 (cont.)

Problem	Objective	Plan of care	Rationale
3. Acidosis	Re-establish the normal acid–base balance	(a) Monitor rate of intravenous infusion	(a) Ensures prescribed fluids are given
		(b) Ensure blood samples have been taken for plasma bicarbonate levels	(b) Measures the effect of treatment (normal plasma bicarbonate 24–32 mmol/l)
		(c) Monitor rate and depth of respirations	(c) Indicates the return to normal
4. Electrolyte imbalance	Re-establish the normal electrolyte balance and monitor the effects by replacement therapy	(a) Give intravenous normal saline with added potassium as prescribed	(a) Replaces sodium and potassium lost in vomiting, sweating and in movement of fluids and electrolytes between the extracellular and intracellular fluid compartments which occur in dehydration
		(b) Monitor the possible effects to the heart from intravenous potassium by using a cardiac monitor and recording pulse rate and rhythm	(b) If too rapid an infusion of potassium is given, it can cause cardiac arrhythmias and arrest
		(c) Ensure blood samples are taken for serum electrolytes	(c) Measures the effect of treatment (normal sodium 136–148 mmol/l, potassium 3.8–5 mmol/l)
5. Patient not producing sufficient insulin for normal metabolic requirements	To initiate and then maintain replacement therapy of insulin	(a) Give soluble insulin intravenously as prescribed in controlled amounts to gradually reduce blood glucose levels	(a) Soluble insulin has rapid action and giving of controlled amounts of insulin prevents sudden hypoglycaemia
		(b) Monitor effects of treatment by: (i) Testing urine for glucose and ketone bodies (ii) Ensuring the taking of regular blood samples for estimation of glucose levels	(b) Measures the effect of treatment. Enables the change of intravenous fluids from normal saline to dextrose when blood glucose returns to normal, therefore preventing hypoglycaemia
		(c) Accurate recording of total insulin administered over each 24-hour period	(c) Gives initial estimation of the body's daily requirements for insulin replacement
6. Presence of infection in boil on neck	Treat infection and prevent spread	(a) Take wound swab for culture and sensitivity	(a) Identifies infecting organism and sensitivity of organism to antibiotics
		(b) Administer appropriate antibiotics intravenously initially	(b) Ensures infecting organism is rendered inactive. Intravenous route used to achieve rapid high blood levels of antibiotic
		(c) Incise abscess when pus is localised and allow free drainage. Apply clean dressing as required by aseptic technique	(c) Removes source of infection and relieves pain. Dressing prevents cross-infection
		(d) Measure and record temperature 4-hourly	(d) Estimates the effects of the infection and response to antibiotic therapy
	Minimise the systemic effects of infection	(a) Provide cool fresh bed clothes	(a), (b), (c) and (d) Promotes heat loss by convection, conduction and evaporation and so helps to reduce pyrexia
		(b) Reduce bed clothes as necessary	
		(c) Sponge patient frequently	
		(d) Give fan therapy if ordered	
7. Anxious parents	Relieve anxiety and promote positive approach to son's future	(a) Provide opportunity for parents to receive explanation of Simon's condition	(a) and (b) Helps to promote understanding of Simon's condition and prepares for provision of long-term support
		(b) Give ongoing explanation of tests and their results, and treatment	

TREATMENT TO PREPARE FOR LIFE AS A DIABETIC

Over the twenty-four hours since Simon's admission he regains full consciousness and is drinking and tolerating fluids well. His blood glucose level has returned to normal limits, urine has been containing varying amounts of glucose and traces of acetone. Simon's temperature is now normal and the wound on his neck is draining freely. The doctor now orders the treatment described below and the care plan shown in Table 6.7 is implemented.

1. Removal of intravenous infusion.
2. Soluble insulin to be given three-hourly on a sliding scale dose according to blood and urine glucose levels.
3. Fixed carbohydrate diet according to his present requirements (his age, weight and activity).
4. Antibiotics to be given orally as prescribed.
5. Patient to be taught how to regulate his diet, test his urine, give insulin injections, maintain his health.
6. A trial hypoglycaemic attack.

Table 6.7   Care plan for Simon to prepare for life as a diabetic

Problem	Objective	Plan of care	Rationale
1. Metabolic daily requirement for insulin is unknown	Estimating daily requirements of insulin	(a) Empty bladder at 3-hourly intervals. Then obtain fresh specimen of urine half an hour later and test for glucose and ketones	(a) Emptying the bladder prior to specimen being obtained for testing discards urine of the past 3 hours and ensures accurate measurement of current glucose content of urine
		(b) Record results	(b) Provides ongoing information for estimation of daily requirement
		(c) Obtain finger-prick blood samples 3-hourly and record results	(c) Provides current blood glucose level
		(d) Ensure fixed carbohydrate diet is taken	(d) This provides the basis for estimation of insulin requirements
		(e) Provide opportunity for Simon to have as near normal activity as possible	(e) This helps to estimate energy requirements for monitoring metabolic activity, normal weight and development, and to satisfy his appetite
		(f) Give soluble insulin subcutaneously 3-hourly according to prescription of sliding scale	(f) Soluble insulin has a rapid action of a short duration so needs to be given at 3-hourly intervals
		(g) Record amount given and time	(g) Provides information of daily requirement of insulin
2. Discharging abscess on his neck	Promote wound healing	(a) Continue antibiotics orally as prescribed	(a) Ensures antibiotic regime is continued after removal of intravenous line
		(b) Renew dressing by aseptic technique as required	(b) Prevents cross-infection, encourages wound healing
3. Simon is a newly diagnosed diabetic	Prepare Simon for life as a diabetic	(a) Give opportunity for explanation of the condition of diabetes	(a) and (b) To give essential information for managing at home
		(b) Provide literature that is easily understood	
		(c) Arrange for Simon and his parents to meet the dietician for explanation of his diet and carbohydrate exchanges	(c) Assists Simon to accept the need for him to keep to a fixed carbohydrate diet. (Suggested further reading: S. Davison, R. Passmore, J. F. Brock and A. S. Truswell, Human Nutrition and Dietetics, Churchill Livingstone, London, 1975)
		(d) Teach Simon and his parents how to test his urine and provide equipment for Simon to take home. Teach Simon to record result of urine test	(d) Simon will need to keep a daily record to bring to the diabetic clinic and alert him to problems of instability

Table 6.7 (cont.)

Problem	Objective	Plan of care	Rationale
		(e) (i) Teach Simon and his parents how to draw up insulin and give injections with attention to changing the sites of injection each day (ii) Teach them all how to care for glass syringes and maintain their sterility	(e) (i) Makes Simon as independent as possible. Varying sites of injection prevents the development of fat atrophy (ii) Prevents introduction of infection
		(f) Allow Simon to experience a hypoglycaemic attack under close supervision, that is by giving normal dosage of insulin and withholding his next meal. Simon is given glucose as soon as possible after experiencing symptoms of hypoglycaemia and before developing a coma	(f) Assists Simon in recognising the symptoms of a hypoglycaemic attack which are: ● sweating ● pallor ● agitation ● trembling ● nausea If untreated can result in rapid loss of consciousness

PREPARATION AND ADVICE FOR DISCHARGE

Over the next few days Simon gains confidence in giving himself injections, testing his urine and managing his diet. The doctor has changed his insulin injection to longer acting, enabling a reduction to two doses a day, morning and evening. Arrangements are made for his discharge home, including the following:

1. Informing his GP.
2. Arranging contact with his district nurse.
3. Providing ongoing dietary advice from dietician.
4. Follow-up appointment at diabetic clinic.
5. Giving the address of the British Diabetic Association.

Simon and his parents are advised to ensure that they always have an adequate supply of insulin especially to cover weekends and bank holidays. Insulin is obtainable on doctor's prescription but charges are withheld as diabetes is a long-term condition. The insulin should always be of the same kind and not altered unless by a doctor. If Simon goes abroad he should always take enough for when he is away. He needs to carry some form of identification, a card or a bracelet stating he is a diabetic, and should inform his dentist and any doctor in an emergency. He needs to carry on his person some glucose or boiled sweets in case of hypoglycaemia. If he experiences any infection or illness he needs to seek prompt medical advice and continue his insulin regime.

Simon and his parents are advised that he should resume all his usual interests and physical activities and if he feels hungry and fails to gain weight as he grows he should seek advice from his doctor or dietician. Opportunity is given to discuss the familial tendency of diabetes and the current views that diabetes has no direct genetic factor.

2 Patient history illustrating further problems related to disturbance of the metabolic function of the pancreas

This consists of a patient history, self-testing questions and guidelines for suggested answers.

An adult with diabetes mellitus of adult onset

Mrs Elsie Simmonds, aged 65 years, lives alone after the recent death of her husband. She visited her GP because of increasing lassitude, gain in weight, development of recent cramps in her legs and persistent pruritus vulvae.

Following discussion and examination the doctor discovers the following:
● Urine sample — positive to glucose, negative to ketones.
● Blood sample — raised blood glucose.

- Obesity.
- Pruritus vulvae with evidence of monilial infection.

He advises the following treatment:
1. An appointment at the local hospital outpatients' department to see a physician.
2. Starting a 1000 calories diet.
3. Recording her weight.
4. Application of antifungal ointment (nystatin) for her pruritus.

Following the outpatient visit a glucose tolerance test confirmed that Mrs Simmonds had diabetes mellitus, to be treated by controlled diabetic diet and metformin 0.5 grams twice a day.

SELF-TESTING QUESTIONS

BRIEF ANALYSIS AND GUIDELINES TO SUITABLE ANSWERS

1. Distinguish between juvenile-onset type and adult-onset type of diabetes mellitus.

Question 1
Juvenile-onset type develops within first 40 years of life in patients of normal weight. Symptoms develop acutely and patients rapidly become insulin-dependent.

Maturity-onset type appears in middle-aged or elderly patients, who are often obese and in whom hyperglycaemia can usually be controlled by dietary means alone or by oral hypoglycaemic compound.

2. Describe the action and side-effects of commonly used oral hypoglycaemic agents.

Question 2
Refer to your teacher for guidance and pharmacology textbook.

3. Describe how you would assist a patient undergoing a glucose tolerance test. Briefly explain how this investigation is helpful in the diagnosis of diabetes.

Question 3
Refer to J. Macleod (Ed.), *Davidson's Principles and Practice of Medicine*, 14th edition, Churchill Livingstone, London, 1984.

4. Discuss the possible long-term complications of this condition and describe the advice you would give to Mrs Simmonds to maintain a good approach to her health.

Question 4
Your answer should include effects on:
- The eyes.
- The blood vessels.
- The nervous system.
- The kidneys.
- The skin.

See J. Macleod (Ed.), *Davidson's Principles and Practice of Medicine*, 14th edition, Churchill Livingstone, London, 1984, or any suitable medical textbook.

For maintaining health in the elderly diabetic, refer to current literature, especially that provided by the British Diabetic Association.

(c) Disturbance of the metabolic function of the thyroid gland

1 Patient study and care plan for an adult with thyrotoxicosis

History of social, psychological and physical events leading to the present condition

The patient chosen for this section to illustrate disturbance of the metabolic function of the thyroid gland is an adult with thyrotoxicosis.

Miss Josephine Scott (Figure 6.12), aged 40 years, is a floor supervisor in a well-known department store. She owns a flat on a small development site and is involved in local community affairs, including the local ratepayers' association and photography society. Once a month she visits her parents, who live in the next county. About eighteen months ago she visited her GP complaining of:
- Loss of weight despite increased appetite.
- Sweating of face and hands.
- Intolerance of heat.
- Irritability with colleagues at work.

Following discussion and examination the doctor found:
- An anxious, talkative, active person.
- Skin moist, hair lank and greasy.
- Pulse rate rapid.
- Temperature and blood pressure normal.
- Fine tremor of hands.
- Slight exophthalmos.
- Slightly enlarged thyroid gland (goitre).

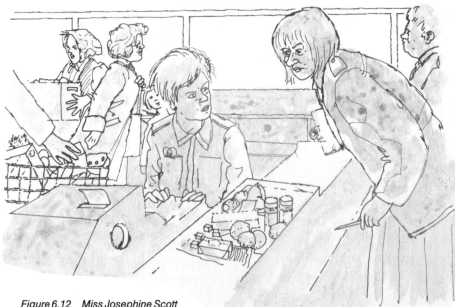

Figure 6.12   Miss Josephine Scott

He suspected an over-active thyroid gland and made arrangements for Miss Scott to attend the local medical outpatients' department for further investigations. These included blood tests such as total serum thyroxine, serum thyroid stimulating hormone levels in response to thyroid releasing hormone stimulation, and an electrocardiogram.

The results confirmed a diagnosis of thyrotoxicosis with no evidence of heart involvement and the doctor discussed the alternative treatments of antithyroid drug therapy and surgery with her. He explained that medical treatment, though prolonged, could be entirely successful but, if unsuccessful, surgery could be contemplated later.

He prescribed carbimazole 15 mg three times a day for 4 weeks, and then a reduced maintenance dose giving as little as possible to achieve a euthyroid state. He explained to her that she must report any sore throat or any other infection as it is important to stop this drug immediately and give antibiotics as carbimazole can damage the bone marrow and reduce the normal response to infection. He told her that it would take several weeks for any noticeable effect but she should start to regain weight, her appetite should return to normal and she should begin to feel less irritable and sweaty. Over the next eighteen months Miss Scott improved initially but two months ago she started to get recurrence of her original symptoms. Her doctor advised that she should be admitted to hospital for partial thyroidectomy. In the interim he increased the dosage of carbimazole and explained that this would be discontinued 10 days prior to operation when she would be given Lugol's iodine three times a day.

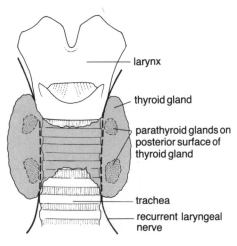

larynx

thyroid gland

parathyroid glands on posterior surface of thyroid gland

trachea

recurrent laryngeal nerve

Figure 6.13   The thyroid gland

Table 6.8

Normal physiology	Related abnormal physiology
(a) The production and release of thyroxine from the thyroid gland is dependent on:	
(i) Intake and absorption of iodine in the diet	(i) Intake and absorption of iodine is normal
(ii) Thyroid-stimulating hormone from the anterior pituitary gland	(ii) Thyroid-stimulating hormone levels are reduced but LATS (long-acting thyroid stimulators) often present
(iii) Normal functioning thyroid cells	(iii) Thyroid cells become overactive and secrete constant high levels of thyroxine
Control of serum levels of thyroxine is by feedback mechanism on the pituitary gland	Feedback mechanism control is lost
(b) (i) Thyroxine controls the rate of utilisation of oxygen by the tissue cells (metabolic rate)	(i) Excessive thyroxine increases rate of oxygen utilisation resulting in increased respirations and pulse rate; loss of weight with increased appetite
(ii) Thyroxine necessary for normal function of the nervous system	(ii) Excess causes over-excitability and nervousness. Effects on the autonomic nervous system cause tachycardia, diarrhoea, pallor and sweating. Excessive sympathetic activity can cause the eyeballs to protrude by pulling on the muscles of the upper eyelid exposing more of the eyeball than usual. In some patients exophthalmos may also be due to deposition of excess fat in the orbit behind the eye.
(iii) Thyroxine necessary for healthy skin, hair and mental activity	(iii) Excess thyroxine causes greasy skin and hair, and irritability
(iv) Thyroxine is necessary for normal red blood cell production	(iv) Unchanged in thyrotoxicosis

Explanation of abnormal physiology

It is advisable to revise the normal structure and functions of the thyroid gland, and see Table 6.8.

Care plan

PREPARATION FOR PATIENT WITH THYROTOXICOSIS

Miss Scott is admitted to the surgical ward for partial thyroidectomy. The thyroid gland (Figure 6.13) is very vascular with blood supply from the common carotid and subclavian arteries and venous drainage into the jugular veins (see pages 156–157).

Nursing history and assessment

The nurse admitting Miss Scott completes the form shown in Table 6.9.

Table 6.9   *Nursing history and assessment sheet for Miss Scott*

NURSING HISTORY AND ASSESSMENT SHEET

Record No. _____ *54541* _____

PATIENT LABEL

Mr/Mrs/Miss _____ *Josephine SCOTT* _____

Address _____ *Flat 17, Somerton Court,* ___
Langley

Male/Female   Age _____ *40 years* _____

Date of Birth _____ *2.5.46* _____

Date of admission/first visit

_____ *16.6.86* _____

Time _____

Type: ☑ Routine ☐ Emergency

Transfer from: _____

Religion _____ *C/E* _____

Practising/baptised _____ *Practising* _____

Minister _____

Telephone number _____

Next of kin (name) _____ *Mr. and Mrs R Scott* ___

Relationship to patient _____ *Parents* _____

Address _____ *The Linders, southville* _____

Telephone numbers _____ *1236* _____

Contact at night/in emergency YES/NO

Occupation (or father) _____ *Floor supervisor* ___

Marital status _____ *Single* _____

Children (or place in family) _____

Other dependants _____

Pets _____

School (children only) _____

Hobbies _____ *Local community affairs* _____

Clubs _____ *Photographic Society* _____

Favourite pastime _____

Does patient smoke? YES/<u>NO</u>

Speech difficulty/language barrier

Dysphasia   Dysarthria

Accommodation

Lives alone   <u>YES</u>/NO

Part III/EMI/Old People's Homes/Rented

Other _____ *Own flat* _____

Consultant _____ *Mr Greenland* _____

House officer _____ *Dr Smithson* _____

Presenting condition _____

History of present complaint and reason for admission

Treatment with carbimazole for
thyrotoxicosis for 18 months. Two months ago
original symptoms returned, revisited
local outpatients department.
Partial thyroidectomy

Past medical history

_____ *N/a* _____

Allergies   *None*

Current medication

Lugol's iodine 3 times a day in milk

What patient says is the reason for admission and attitude to admission

Partial thyroidectomy. Slightly
apprehensive

Patient's expectations

Any problems at home while/because patient is in hospital?

None

Relevant home conditions (e.g. stairs)

_____

_____

Visiting problems

_____

Table 6.9 (cont.)

Care at home

Community nurse _____

No. _____

Name of GP ___ *Dr Lane* ___

Address ___ *The Surgery, Somerton Rd,* ___
_____ *Langley* ___

Other services involved

Home help _____ Day hospital _____

Laundry _____ Day centre/club _____

Inco supplies _____ Health visitor _____

Aids _____ Social worker _____

Meals on wheels _____ Voluntary worker _____

Daily living

Diet

Special _____

Food or drink dislikes _____

Appetite: ☑GOOD ☐POOR

Remarks _____

Sleep

How many hours normally? ___ *6 – 7* ___

Sedation _____

What else helps? _____

Elimination

Bowels: Continent/Incontinent

How often opened? ___ *Diarrhoea occasionally* ___

Any medication? _____

Urinary: Continent/Incontinent

If incontinent; Day/Night/If not taken, how frequently? _____

Nocturia/Dysuria/Frequency/Urgency

Remarks _____

Female patients — Menstruation

Post-menopausal   Taking the pill

<u>Regular</u>   Irregular

Amenorrhoea   Dysmenorrhoea

Next period due: ___ *30·6·86* ___

Uses: <u>STs</u> Tampons

Hearing

Hearing aid: YES/<u>NO</u>

Remarks _____

Vision

Glasses/Contact lens: YES/<u>NO</u>

Remarks _____

Oral

Dentures or crowns: YES/<u>NO</u>

Any problems with mouth or teeth?

Mobility

Help needed with:

Walking/Standing/In/Out of bed/Bathing/Dressing

In/Out of chair/

Feeding/Other: _____

Remarks ___ *Normally active* ___

Prosthesis/appliance

Type of appliance _____

Help needed _____

General appearance

<u>Normal</u>   Dehydrated   Acutely ill

Obese   Thin   Emaciated

Remarks ___ *Weight fluctuating* ___

Skin

Satisfactory   Broken areas   Dehydrated

Rash   Oedematous   Jaundiced

Pallor   Other ___ *Moist and greasy* ___
                (including bruising)

Remarks ___ *Hair lank* ___

Level of consciousness

<u>Orientated</u>   Semi-conscious

Confused   Unconscious

Remarks _____

Mental assessment (if appropriate)

Mood

Elated   Irritable   <u>Agitated</u>

<u>Cheerful</u>   <u>Anxious</u>   Aggressive

Miserable   Withdrawn   Suspicious

Apathetic

Thought content

Hallucinations/Delusions/Paranoid Ideas

_____

Orientation

Time/Place/Person ___ *Yes* ___

Very confused   Slightly confused

Any particular time of day? _____

Confabulation _____

Remarks _____

Surveillance   Physical/Emotional

Information obtained from ___ *Patient* ___

Relationship to patient _____

By ___ *BDG* ___

Position/level of training _____

Date ___ *16·6·86* ___

Time _____

TREATMENT

The care plan (Table 6.10) describes the pre-operative treatment and preparation for surgery.

Table 6.10   Care plan for Miss Josephine Scott while in the surgical ward

Problem	Objective	Plan of care	Rationale
1. History of thyrotoxicosis	Maintain euthyroid state	(a) Allocate one nurse to greet and admit Miss Scott and discuss plan of care	(a), (b) and (c) Reduces stimuli and patient's anxiety and irritability
		(b) Arrange for bed in quiet area of the ward	
		(c) Encourage a calm, relaxed atmosphere in the ward	
		(d) Give night sedation and other sedatives as prescribed	(d) Promotes rest and adequate sleep
	Assess euthyroid state	(a) Measure and record sleeping pulse	(a) If sleeping pulse above 80 beats per minute surgery may be postponed
		(b) Prepare Miss Scott for electrocardiogram	(b) Assesses heart rhythm for atrial fibrillation
		(c) Measure and record temperature, pulse, respiration and blood pressure	(c) Provides baseline measurement for comparison during and after operation
		(d) Record weight	(d) For estimation of anaesthetic dosage and gives baseline for comparison
		(e) Ensure blood samples are taken for serum thyroxine	(e) Surgery will not be performed if still raised. Normal value: 244–465 nmol/l 3.1–5.9 µg/100 ml
2. Enlarged gland in neck causing pressure on nearby structures	To check for the presence of laryngeal nerve involvement and to check position of trachea	(a) Prepare Miss Scott for indirect laryngoscopy	(a) Vocal cords can be viewed with laryngeal mirror to check that both are functioning. Pressure by the enlarged thyroid gland on a recurrent laryngeal nerve can cause paralysis of a vocal cord
		(b) Prepare Miss Scott for x-ray of thoracic inlet and chest	(b) Enlarged thyroid gland may constrict trachea or push it to one side making intubation difficult
3. Treatment with carbimazole causes increased vascularity of the thyroid gland	Reduce vascularity of the thyroid gland and have blood available for replacement during or after operation	(a) Ensure carbimazole has been discontinued	(a) Carbimazole causes increased vascularity and enlargement of the thyroid gland
		(b) Give Lugol's iodine 5–10 drops in milk three times a day or other prescribed medication, e.g., potassium iodide 60 mg x 3 daily	(b) Reduces vascularity by reducing the iodine demand by the gland
		(c) Ensure blood has been grouped and cross-matched	(c) In case of haemorrhage during or after operation
4. Patient for operation under general anaesthetic	Ensure adequate preparation physically and psychologically	(a) Empty bladder, test urine for abnormalities, record result and amount	(a) Prevents involuntary emptying of bladder; checks for abnormalities of the urine
		(b) Dress patient in operation gown	(b) Reduce infection risk
		(c) Place stretcher canvas in bed	(c) Eases movement of patient
		(d) Attach identification label to patient's wrist	(d) Assists checking correct patient
		(e) Remove valuables and place in safe keeping	(e) Prevents loss or damage

Table 6.10 (cont.)

Problem	Objective	Plan of care	Rationale
		(f) Remove prostheses (including dentures) and place in labelled container	(f) Prevents swallowing/choking and prevents loss
		(g) Check consent for operation has been given by patient	(g) Legal requirement before operation
		(h) Have notes and x-rays available	(h) Required for medical staff
		(i) Give pre-medication, usually an analgesic and parasympathetic system inhibitor	(i) Reduces pain anxiety and reduces secretions
		(j) Check that fluid balance and observation charts are up to date	(j) Provides information for operating theatre staff

RETURN OF MISS SCOTT TO SURGICAL WARD

Miss Scott has a partial thyroidectomy, the surgeon's intention being to leave just sufficient gland to produce enough thyroxine for normal metabolic needs, and the parathyroid glands remain intact. She returns from the recovery unit to the ward fully conscious with an intravenous infusion in progress, having received one unit of blood during the operation. Clips are closing the neck-wound and a suction drainage tube is in position. The post-operative care plan shown in Table 6.11 is implemented for Miss Scott.

Table 6.11   Post-operative care plan for Miss Scott

Problem	Objective	Plan of care	Rationale
1. Potential shock and haemorrhage	Detect early signs of shock and haemorrhage. Prepare for emergency treatment	(a) Measure and record pulse rate and blood pressure, and observe skin colour	(a) Pulse rate rises, blood pressure falls and skin becomes pale when shock/haemorrhage occurs
		(b) Measure and record amount of wound drainage. Inspect wound for leakage of blood and/or swelling. Measure respiration rate and observe for difficulty in breathing	(b) The thyroid gland is supplied by large thyroid arteries and haemorrhage could occur due to slipped ligature when blood pressure returns to normal. Blood may drain into drainage bottle or collect under the wound causing haematoma and pressure over the trachea
		(c) Have available: (i) Means of elevating foot of bed	(c) (i) Raising foot of bed in shocked patient ensures adequate blood supply to brain
		(ii) Oxygen and suction	(ii) To clear airway and aid oxygenation of the blood
		(iii) Ensure that more blood is available for transfusion	(iii) To replace blood lost
		(iv) Provide clip removing forceps at bedside	(iv) If haematoma occurs under wound, it must be evacuated if pressure on trachea is causing respiratory difficulty, therefore skin clips must be removed
2. Potential disruption of metabolic functions of the thyroid and parathyroid glands	Detect early signs and provide for emergency treatment	(a) (i) Observe Miss Scott for signs of *thyroid crisis* by measuring and recording: ● temperature ● pulse ● respirations ● blood pressure ● mental state	(a) (i) Leakage of thyroxine into the blood stream during surgery can cause rapid uncontrolled rise in the metabolic rate: ● hyper-pyrexia ● tachycardia ● rapid respirations ● rise in blood pressure ● distress and agitation

Problem	Objective	Plan of care	Rationale
		(ii) In case of thyroid crisis occurring have available: • intravenous fluids • intravenous Lugol's iodine • propranolol • fan and prescribed sedative	(ii) Therapy to reduce metabolic rate by cooling the patient, reducing activity of remaining thyroid tissue and reducing heart activity
		(b) (i) Observe Miss Scott for signs of tetany by noting abnormal spasm and/or tingling of muscles of face, hands and feet. (Can be detected *early* in hands when blood pressure cuff is inflated and blood flow to muscles reduced—called Trousseau's sign) (ii) Have available intravenous calcium gluconate	(b) (i) Tetany is abnormal muscle spasm especially of the hands and feet (carpo-pedal spasm) and face, due to lack of parathormone normally produced by the parathyroid glands. Parathormone maintains the plasma calcium levels—calcium is necessary for normal muscle contraction (ii) To restore the plasma calcium levels. Normal 2.12–2.62 mmol/l or 8.5–10.5 mg/100 ml
3. Potential damage to recurrent laryngeal nerves	Detect early signs and provide for emergency treatment	(a) Observe for hoarseness of voice, report to doctor if it occurs	(a) Damage to one nerve causes paralysis of *one* vocal cord
		(b) (i) Observe for acute respiratory arrest (ii) Have available emergency tracheotomy set	(b) (i) Damage to both nerves causes paralysis of *both* vocal cords which approximate and completely obstruct the airway (ii) Airway has to be re-established by bypassing the obstruction
4. Pain in neck wound	Minimise pain and discomfort	(a) Sit Miss Scott upright with head well supported with pillows, avoiding over-extension of neck	(a) Relaxes the muscles of the neck and relieves tension on the wound
		(b) Give analgesia as prescribed	(b) Diminishes awareness of pain and permits mobilisation and deep breathing
		(c) Have personal belongings within easy reach	(c) Stops having to strain and stretch to reach belongings and increases independence
		(d) Support drainage tubes	(d) Prevents tension on the wound
5. Surgical incision with drainage tube	Ensure wound drainage	(a) Observe wound drainage, record amount and character	(a) Monitors fluid loss
		(b) Check and re-vacuum drainage apparatus daily or as necessary	(b) Ensures drainage tube is patent and that suction is adequate
	Ensure wound healing	(a) Redress wound aseptically as appropriate and report and record findings	(a) Monitors blood loss and reduces infection risk
		(b) Remove drainage tube when drainage is minimal and on doctor's instructions	(b) Ensures primary wound healing
		(c) Remove sutures when skin healed and/or with doctor's instructions	(c) Removes foreign body and risk of infection
	Detect early signs of infection	(a) Observe temperature and pulse 4-hourly and record	(a) The temperature and pulse rise if infection is present
		(b) Observe for changes in character of pain	(b) Local infection causes inflammation, swelling and pain
		(c) Report systemic effects, e.g., lethargy, reluctance to move	(c) Infection reduces defence mechanism of the body

Table 6.11 (cont.)

Problem	Objective	Plan of care	Rationale
6. Patient reluctant to eat and drink	Maintain nutrition and hydration	(a) Provide encouragement and support in drinking. Introduce soft diet with rapid progression to normal diet	(a) Swallowing can be uncomfortable
		(b) Remove intravenous infusion when oral intake is sufficient and risk of haemorrhage is over	(b) Patient able to maintain own hydration
7. Reluctance to move following operation	(a) To encourage mobility	(a) Help patient to sit out of bed on first day after operation	(a) and (b) Muscle pump aids venous return and prevents deep thrombosis
	(b) To reduce risk of venous stasis, pressure sores, chest infection and urinary stasis	(b) Take short walk second day and increase to full mobility by discharge	Mobility increases chest expansion and ventilation, and diffusion Mobility reduces prolonged pressure on sacrum and other pressure sites Mobility promotes good bladder emptying Mobility promotes a sense of well-being and independence

RECOVERY AND DISCHARGE

Miss Scott makes a satisfactory recovery from her operation with no complications. The drainage tube and clips are removed by the third post-operative day and she is fully mobile and taking normal diet by the fifth day when she is allowed to go home. She decides to convalesce with her parents.

She is asked to return to the outpatients' department in three weeks' time and is told that she will need regular assessment of her thyroid function to detect recurrence of thyrotoxicosis, or myxoedema if insufficient thyroxine is being secreted from the remaining thyroid tissue.

2 Patient history illustrating further problems related to disturbance of the metabolic function of the thyroid gland

This part of the chapter consists of a patient history, self-testing questions and guidelines for suggested answers.

An adult with myxoedema

Mrs Mary Henderson, aged 80 years, is a widow who lives with her 75-year-old sister in a basement flat in Pimlico. She has been an independent lady who has been involved in community visiting through her local church. Over the past two years she has had to reduce her activities due to increasing tiredness and lack of concentration. During the past month she has had to depend on her sister to do the housework and shopping and has spent most of each day dozing in a chair, wrapped in a blanket. Her sister is not over-concerned as she is aware that Mrs Henderson is getting older. However, Mrs Henderson's daughter and her family visit one Sunday and she is shocked to find such a noticeable change in her mother. She discusses her anxieties with her aunt and arranges to ring the doctor in the morning and ask him to visit.

The next day the GP visits and on examining Mrs Henderson finds:
- Skin pale and dry, hair coarse, lifeless and very sparse.
- Loss of hair on outer third of eyebrows.
- Face apparently swollen with puffy eyelids.
- Speech slow, monotonous and husky.
- Pulse rate slow.
- Temperature 36.2°C.
- Mucous membranes pale.

On questioning, Mrs Henderson admits to forgetfulness, sensitivity to cold, poor appetite but recent weight gain and severe constipation. The doctor suspects that Mrs Henderson has myxoedema.

SELF-TESTING QUESTIONS	BRIEF ANALYSIS AND GUIDELINES TO SUITABLE ANSWERS
1. Explain Mrs Henderson's symptoms by relating to the physiology of the thyroid gland.	*Question 1* Refer to normal physiology explanation, page 174, given a patient with acute thyrotoxicosis.
2. How may Mrs Henderson be treated?	*Question 2* Refer to suitable textbook for treatment regime. Your answer should also include: (a) Checking that Mrs Henderson is warm enough, maintaining her hydration and nutrition, encouraging her mobility, and attention to her personal hygiene. (b) Regular monitoring by district nurse of her response to treatment and return to euthyroid state.
3. Discuss whether you think Mrs Henderson should be treated at home or in hospital and give reasons for your choice.	*Question 3* Your answer should include attention to: (a) Mrs Henderson's wishes. (b) Risks and hazards of her remaining at home. (c) Facilities for care at home and monitoring of her progress. (d) Health of her sister. (e) Possible psychological and social effects of prolonged stay in hospital of an elderly person. (f) Financial demands of having an elderly ill person at home. (g) Whether there are means of summoning help by telephone.
4. Describe the possible outcomes if Mrs Henderson's myxoedema is untreated.	*Question 4* Refer to your teacher for guidance to a suitable medical textbook.

Chapter 7

Nursing patients with disturbances of seeing, hearing, smell or touch

The normal functions of the eye, ear, nose, tongue and skin

(a) The eye

The organ of vision is the eye (Figure 7.1), and its function is to focus light rays reflected from (or sometimes produced by) objects onto the light-sensitive *retina* at the rear of the eye, and to translate this picture into meaningful nervous signals which travel to the occipital lobes of the brain.

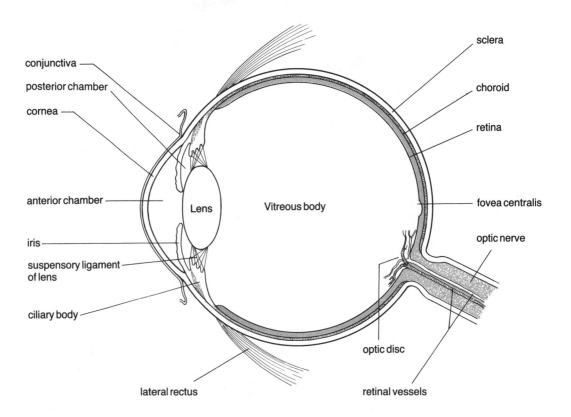

Figure 7.1   Section through an eyeball

The positioning of the two eyes (Figure 7.2) so that they face approximately the same direction enables the brain to perceive the world in three dimensions, as the two slightly different pictures detected by each eye are compared. This is the phenomenon of *binocular vision*.

1   Progress of light through the eye

The focusing of light rays depends upon the physical phenomenon of *refraction*. Light rays travelling at an angle towards a surface are bent when they pass from one medium to another of different optical density. The eye is designed so that light passes through four different surfaces where it is refracted, and these are arranged in such a way that light is focused on the retina. Greatest refraction occurs as the light leaves air and enters the transparent *cornea* which is also curved, and so receives light from a wider range of angles than if it were flat. Light is refracted again as it enters the *aqueous humour,* a fluid in the *anterior*

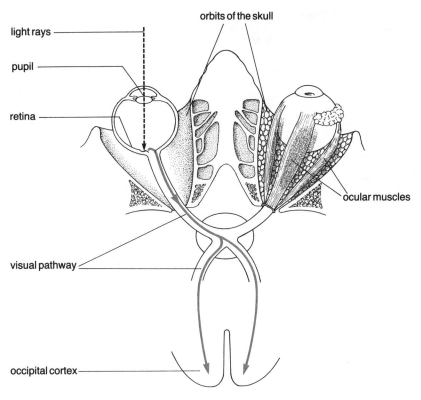

light rays

pupil

retina

orbits of the skull

ocular muscles

visual pathway

occipital cortex

Figure 7.2   Position of the eyes

chamber of the eye. Light then impinges on the *lens* which is a transparent jelly-filled structure which can change shape. Light is refracted as it enters the lens and, again, when it passes into the *vitreous humour,* a viscous fluid which fills the main chamber of the eye.

2   The retina

Light falling on the retina is detected by the light-sensitive cells, within which, as a result of the energy of light, a chemical reaction occurs. In the *rod cells, rhodopsin,* a complex protein, is split to form *retinine* (contains vitamin A) and *opsin* (a protein). This reaction stimulates the depolarisation of the rod cell membrane, and this action potential is transmitted via the optic nerve to the brain. Re-formation of rhodopsin takes a short time and requires energy. The *cone cells* of the retina detect colour, and seem to work on a similar principle. They are only stimulated by light of high intensity, and so are only in action in reasonably light conditions (e.g., daylight). They also take longer than rod cells to regenerate their visual pigment. Colour is probably perceived as a mixture of impulses from each of three different types of cone cell, each sensitive to different wavelengths of light — red, green and violet. Rod cells are much more sensitive to light than are cone cells, and so can detect low intensities of light. In conditions of high light intensity, the rods become bleached and inoperative. It takes a noticeable time for them to become adapted again on entering a dark environment.

The *fovea* is a small area of the retina directly behind the centre of the lens, and is closely packed with cones *only*. This is the optical point of greatest acuity, and has a double blood supply.

As can be seen from Figure 7.3, light passes through two layers of nerve cells before reaching the rods and cones in the retina.

3   Accommodation

A static arrangement of all the components of the eye could only bring into focus objects which are 6 metres away. To bring objects at other distances into focus, the lens is modified in shape by the action of the *ciliary muscle* which surrounds the lens, and is attached to the *suspensory ligament* which holds the lens in place. If the ciliary muscle contracts the lens is flattened and its curvature decreased. This brings *far objects* into focus. If the ciliary muscle relaxes, the lens becomes more spherical under its own elasticity, and *near*

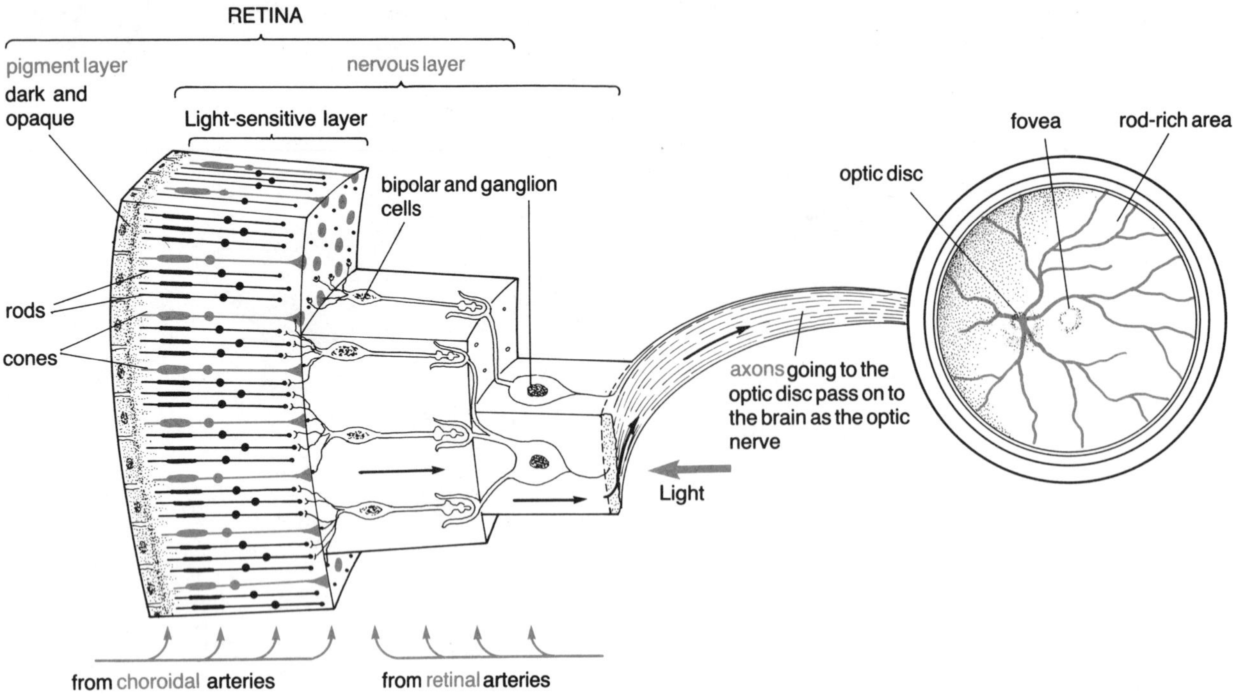

RETINA

pigment layer | nervous layer

dark and opaque

Light-sensitive layer

bipolar and ganglion cells

rods

cones

optic disc

fovea | rod-rich area

axons going to the optic disc pass on to the brain as the optic nerve

Light

from choroidal arteries | from retinal arteries

Figure 7.3   The retina

objects are focused. At the same time, the circular muscle fibres of the iris contract to reduce the size of the pupil so that light falls only on the central, most curved part of the lens.

Both ciliary and circular muscles are innervated by the parasympathetic nerves of the 3rd cranial nerve. The eyeballs are moved within the sockets by the actions of the *internal rectus muscles* around the eyeball. These are also under parasympathetic nervous control.

4   Visual acuity

This is the *clarity* of vision, which is related to the eye's ability to bring light into focus on the retina. The common defects of *myopia* and *hypermetropia* are summarised in Figure 7.4.

Astigmatism is caused by a defect in the curvature of the cornea or in the arrangement of the eye's optical parts. It results in a blurring of part of the vision, for example, one plane of vision, and can be corrected by the use of specially ground spectacles which compensate for the error.

Rays of light from a distant object are virtually parallel and, in a *normal* eye, are refracted to focus exactly on the retina. Near objects, with rays more divergent, are focused on the retina by the lens becoming more convex.

In the *myopic* (short-sighted) eye, distant rays are refracted to a point in front of the retina. This is due either to a longer or bigger eyeball than normal, or to too strong refraction. Near objects are seen clearly with little alteration of the lens. Myopia tends to get worse as the eyes (and the child) grow. After adolescence it may improve.

In the *hypermetropic* (long-sighted) eye, the focal point lies behind the retina. In the young, this can be corrected by the lens but leaves little extra refractive power for near work. Fatigue on near-vision tasks (e.g., writing, reading, sewing) or difficulty with reading presents earlier than the normal age of about 50

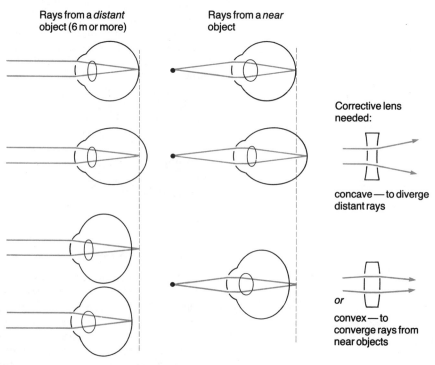

Rays from a *distant* object (6 m or more)

Rays from a *near* object

Corrective lens needed:

concave — to diverge distant rays

or

convex — to converge rays from near objects

Figure 7.4   Common refractive defects of the eye

5 Visual pathways

The pattern of the picture detected by the eye is maintained since the nerves from different parts of the retina are bundled in a strictly orderly way as they pass from the eye to the occipital cortex of the brain.

Nerves cross at the *optic chiasma* so that some information from each eye reaches each side of the brain. In the *lateral geniculate bodies* there are six layers of grey matter, and pairing of information from comparable points on each of the eyes occurs. This is thought to have a function in stereoscopic vision. The visual pathway is summarised in Figure 7.5.

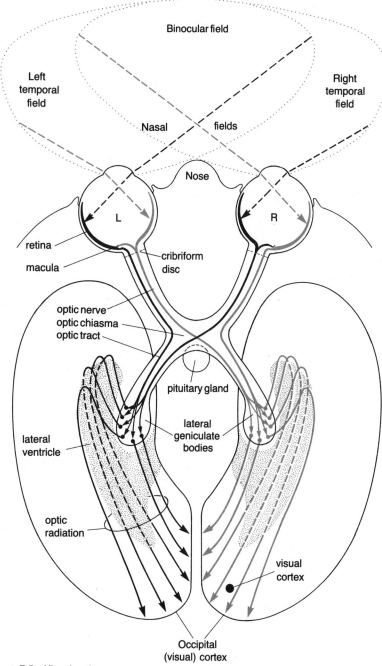

Figure 7.5   Visual pathways

Moving objects can be discerned at the periphery of vision more easily than stationary ones. You can test this for yourself: with your gaze fixed on a distant object, move a pencil down until it is just out of sight somewhere near your chest; if you then wriggle it, you'll be able to see it.

6 The psychology of vision

Recognition of the nature of objects according to the visual impression they produce (e.g., which sharp stick is a pencil) is believed to be a function of the

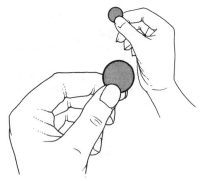

Figure 7.6 Two coins

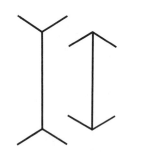

Figure 7.7 Optical illusion of two sticks of equal length appearing to be unequal

parts of the occipital cortex surrounding the visual area, and of the post-parietal region, and is called *visiopsychic function.*

The way an object is perceived varies much less than the image it produces on the retina. When looking at two coins, one held 20 cm away and the other at 40 cm, we do not perceive the further coin as half the size of the nearer one (Figure 7.6). In other words, with familiar objects, the brain eliminates the effects of perspective. (If, when holding your coin, you shut one eye and move the further hand behind the nearer, you can force your occipital cortex to admit that the images are different sizes — although it 'knows' that the objects are the same size.) Similarly with shape: a penny goes on appearing round even when its image is received 'sideways on'. These are called *constancy phenomena;* the brain is 'deceived' because of its assumptions; the two vertical lines in Figure 7.7 are the same length but the one on the left looks like the *far* corner of a room. The one on the right looks like the *near* edge of a box or building and the brain diminishes it. A similar thing happens with the coins — the nearer hand is mentally shrunk, the further one enlarged.

7 The light reflex

This is a useful test of the function of the optical nerves. If a bright light is shone into either eye of a normal person, *both* pupils constrict, as shown in Figure 7.8. If the other eye does not react this may be due to a disorder of either the *efferent* or *afferent* limb.

If a bright light is shone into *either* eye of a normal person *both* pupils constrict

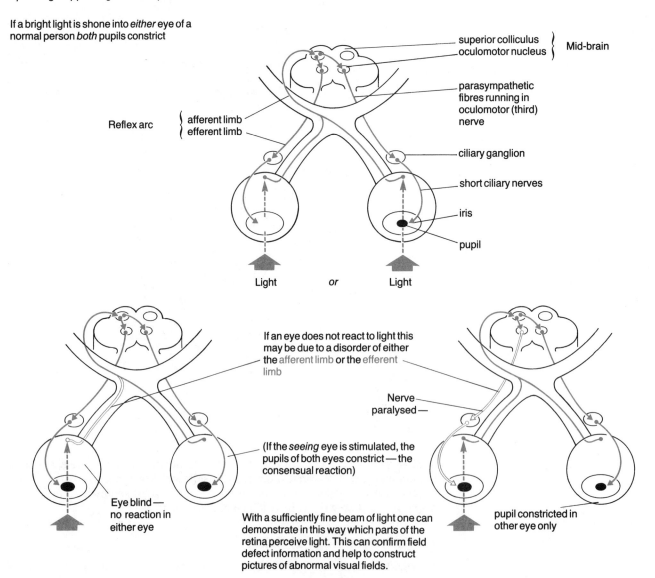

Figure 7.8 Light reflex

(b) The ear

The ear is the organ of hearing. It also plays an important role in balance. Figure 7.9 shows the general structure of the parts of the ear involved with hearing.

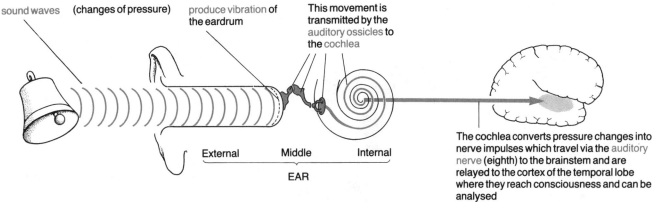

sound waves (changes of pressure)

produce vibration of the eardrum

This movement is transmitted by the auditory ossicles to the cochlea

External Middle Internal

EAR

The cochlea converts pressure changes into nerve impulses which travel via the auditory nerve (eighth) to the brainstem and are relayed to the cortex of the temporal lobe where they reach consciousness and can be analysed

Figure 7.9   The ear

1   The pinna or auricle

This is the curly, shell-like structure (Figure 7.10) which collects and focuses sound waves into the *external auditory meatus*. It consists of a leaf of fibro-cartilage which is covered by skin. The cartilage is continuous with that encircling the outer third of the auditory meatus or canal, so that pulling on the pinna moves that part of the canal. The pinna has several sensory nerves, including a branch of the *auriculo-temporal nerve* which also supplies the lower teeth, tongue and mandible. Pain can be referred to the ear from the mouth. The vagus nerve sends an auricular branch to the meatus and if this is irritated (e.g., by a foreign body or by syringing) it may produce effects relating to areas supplied by other branches of the vagus — reflex coughing or sneezing, vomiting in children, and sometimes heart failure in the elderly. The ear lobe of the pinna has few nerves, and so can be painlessly pierced.

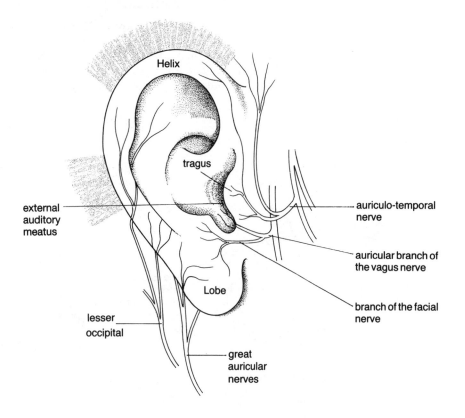

Figure 7.10   The pinna or auricle

2 External auditory (acoustic) meatus or canal

In the adult this is about 2.5 cm long, and much shorter in infants and children. Figure 7.11 illustrates the structure of the meatus.

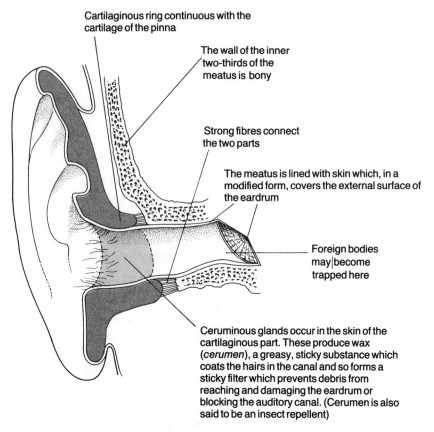

Cartilaginous ring continuous with the cartilage of the pinna

The wall of the inner two-thirds of the meatus is bony

Strong fibres connect the two parts

The meatus is lined with skin which, in a modified form, covers the external surface of the eardrum

Foreign bodies may become trapped here

Ceruminous glands occur in the skin of the cartilaginous part. These produce wax (*cerumen*), a greasy, sticky substance which coats the hairs in the canal and so forms a sticky filter which prevents debris from reaching and damaging the eardrum or blocking the auditory canal. (Cerumen is also said to be an insect repellent)

Figure 7.11   External auditory meatus

3 The eardrum (tympanic membrane)

The eardrum (Figure 7.12a, b) separates the external auditory meatus from the *middle ear.* In children, the eardrum slopes more steeply than in the adult and is more liable to damage. It is an almost oval-shaped structure attached to the *malleus,* one of the three small bones of the middle ear. It is kept tensed by the contraction of the *tensor tympani muscle* which is attached to the malleus.

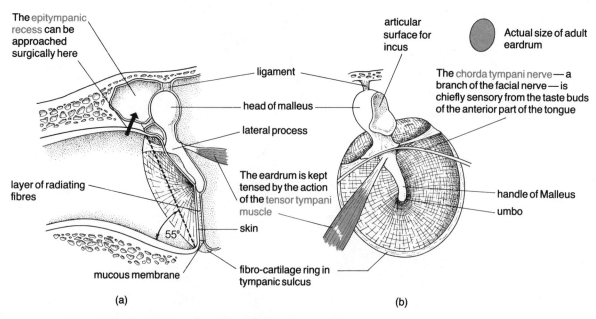

The epitympanic recess can be approached surgically here

articular surface for incus

Actual size of adult eardrum

The chorda tympani nerve — a branch of the facial nerve — is chiefly sensory from the taste buds of the anterior part of the tongue

ligament

head of malleus

lateral process

The eardrum is kept tensed by the action of the tensor tympani muscle

layer of radiating fibres

handle of Malleus

umbo

skin

55°

mucous membrane

fibro-cartilage ring in tympanic sulcus

(a)

(b)

Figure 7.12   The eardrum. (a) Transverse section of right ear and (b) eardrum viewed from the middle ear

4 The middle ear

This is an air-filled cavity in which are found the *ossicles,* the three small bones of the ear. These are the smallest bones in the body and are called the *malleus (hammer), incus (anvil)* and *stapes (stirrup)*. They articulate against each other as shown in Figure 7.13, moving when the tympanic membrane vibrates. This movement is magnified twenty-five times by the movement of the ossicles, and the sound waves are transmitted to the *oval window* of the inner ear, against which the stapes moves. The amplification of sound is necessary to set up vibrations in the *cochlea* of the inner ear, which is filled with fluid.

The 'footplate' of the stapes is attached to the rim of the oval window by the annular ligament, which is especially strong at the base, so that the stapes effectively rocks against the oval window. The *tensor tympani* and *stapedius* are tiny muscles which reflexly contract to dampen the movements of the ossicles in response to loud sounds. A further protection against loud sounds is carried out by the pivoting movement of the stapes to reduce the effect of its normal compression movements on the liquid in the cochlea.

The *auditory* or *Eustachian tube* connects the middle ear cavity with the pharynx. This equalises air pressure on either side of the eardrum and is normally closed, except during swallowing and yawning.

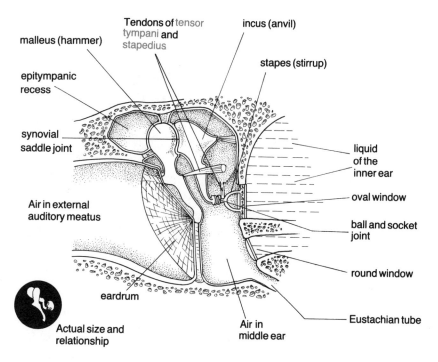

Figure 7.13   The middle ear

5 The inner ear

The inner ear (Figure 7.14 a, b) comprises the three *semi-circular canals,* the *utricle* and *saccule,* and the *cochlea*. The semi-circular canals are concerned with balance and are positioned at right angles to each other. At the end of each is a swelling called the *ampulla* which contains a receptor consisting of a group of sensory cells whose hairs are embedded in a dome-shaped gelatinous cap, the *cupula*. Because of the inertia of the fluid within the semicircular canals, it stays relatively static when the head moves and the cupula is deflected, stimulating the receptor cells. Because there is one semi-circular canal in each plane, information is available from them about movement of the head in any direction.

Utricle and saccule

The utricle and the saccule give information on the position of the head (Figure 7.15). These receptors consist of a patch of sensory cells whose free ends are embedded in a concentration of calcium carbonate called an *otolith*. The pull of gravity moves the otolith, and the effect of this on the sensory cells will vary

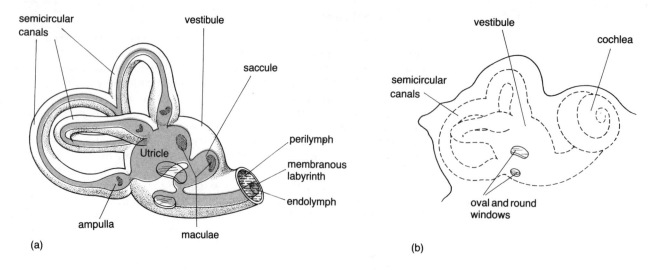

semicircular canals

vestibule

saccule

perilymph

membranous labyrinth

endolymph

ampulla

maculae

Utricle

(a)

vestibule

cochlea

semicircular canals

oval and round windows

(b)

Figure 7.14   The inner ear. (a) The vestibular apparatus and (b) the position of the vestibular apparatus and cochlea

Semicircular canals numbered 1, 2 and 3

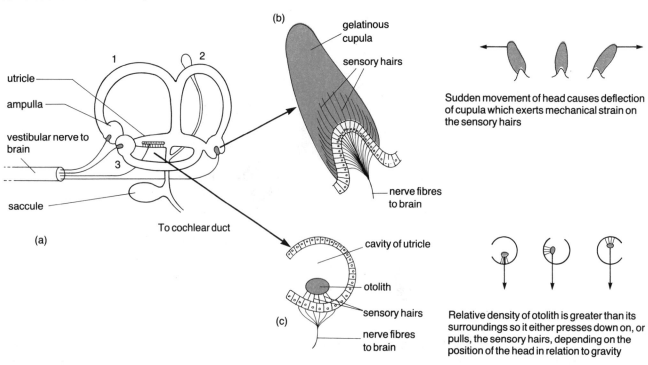

(b)

gelatinous cupula

sensory hairs

utricle

ampulla

vestibular nerve to brain

saccule

To cochlear duct

(a)

nerve fibres to brain

Sudden movement of head causes deflection of cupula which exerts mechanical strain on the sensory hairs

cavity of utricle

otolith

sensory hairs

(c)

nerve fibres to brain

Relative density of otolith is greater than its surroundings so it either presses down on, or pulls, the sensory hairs, depending on the position of the head in relation to gravity

Figure 7.15   The vestibular apparatus. (a) Positions of the ampulla organ and utricle, (b) the ampulla organ and (c) the utricle organ

with different positions of the head. This information is relayed to the brain as the sensory cells are thus stimulated.

Cochlea

The cochlea (Figure 7.16 a, b) is involved with hearing. It is a coiled bony tunnel within which is a membrane called the *cochlear duct,* filled with a viscous fluid, the *endolymph.* The cochlear duct is attached to the centre of the spiral bone, and to the outside edge. The cochlear duct stretches across the bony spiral, but does not fill it. The spaces between the bone and the duct membrane are filled with *perilymph* which is probably derived from cerebrospinal fluid.

These two cavities of perilymph are called the *scala vestibuli* and the *scala tympani* and are connected to each other at the tip or *helicotrema.* When the stapes moves against the oval window, pressure is applied to, and distributed throughout, the perilymph. This pressure is exerted on the *vestibular* and *basilar* membranes of the cochlear duct, causing them to oscillate. The alternate bulging and relaxation of the *round window* dissipates the pressure wave in the perilymph and thus adjusts the pressure in the perilymph.

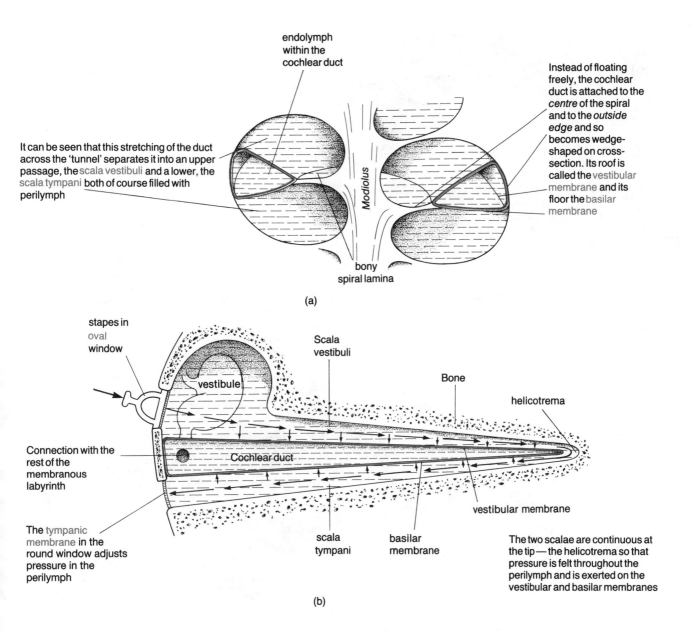

On the top figure (a):

endolymph within the cochlear duct

Instead of floating freely, the cochlear duct is attached to the *centre* of the spiral and to the *outside edge* and so becomes wedge-shaped on cross-section. Its roof is called the vestibular membrane and its floor the basilar membrane

It can be seen that this stretching of the duct across the 'tunnel' separates it into an upper passage, the scala vestibuli and a lower, the scala tympani both of course filled with perilymph

Modiolus

bony spiral lamina

(a)

On the bottom figure (b):

stapes in oval window

Scala vestibuli

Bone

helicotrema

vestibule

Connection with the rest of the membranous labyrinth

Cochlear duct

vestibular membrane

The tympanic membrane in the round window adjusts pressure in the perilymph

scala tympani

basilar membrane

The two scalae are continuous at the tip—the helicotrema so that pressure is felt throughout the perilymph and is exerted on the vestibular and basilar membranes

(b)

Figure 7.16   The cochlea. (a) Transverse section and (b) hypothetically straightened out

On the basilar membrane, within the cochlear duct, is located the *organ of Corti* (Figure 7.17). The specialised hair cells of the organ of Corti are stimulated when the basilar membrane moves in response to the pressure change in the perilymph.

Nerve fibre stimulation

Stimulation of the nerve fibres has a mechanical and electrical component.

MECHANICAL

On the basilar membrane stand the *roots of Corti,* numbering about 10 000, standing in two rigid rows along the membrane. These support the hair cells and keep them in contact with the *membrana tectoria*. These hair cells are sensitive to the shearing strains on them produced by the movements of the basilar membrane and, when moved, they stimulate nerve impulses in nerve endings at the base of the cells.

ELECTRICAL

There is a potential difference across the basilar membrane of between 50 and 100 mV, with the endolymph positive relative to the perilymph. A downward movement of the basilar membrane increases this potential difference, and an

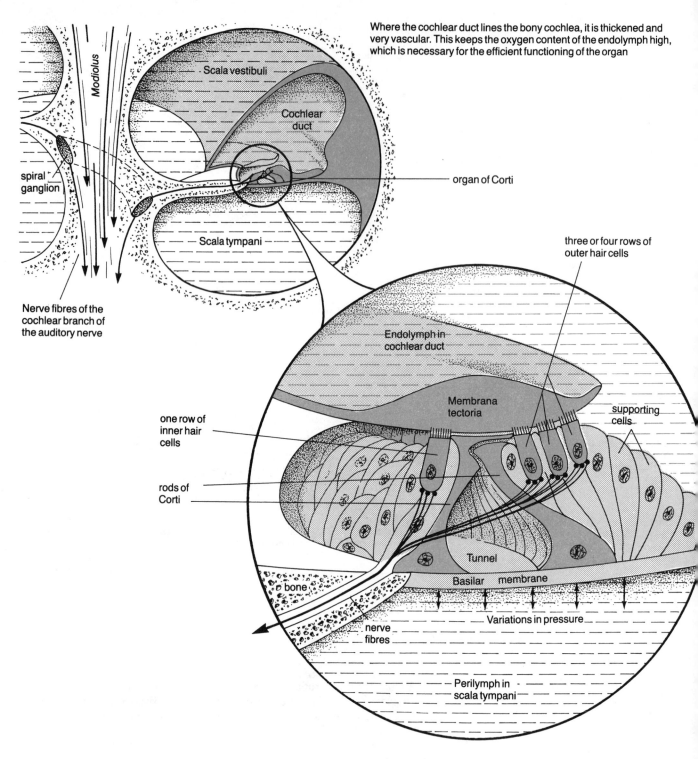

Where the cochlear duct lines the bony cochlea, it is thickened and very vascular. This keeps the oxygen content of the endolymph high, which is necessary for the efficient functioning of the organ

Figure 7.17   Section through the organ of Corti

upward movement reduces it. The *change* in potential difference stimulates nerve fibres.

6   Interpretation of sound

Different parts of the cochlea respond to different frequencies of sound: the basal turn of the spiral responds to all frequencies; the apical turn only to low ones. If the ear receives sound of a particular frequency played continuously, eventually that part of the cochlea in resonance with it degenerates and the person becomes deaf to all sounds at that frequency.

The nervous response to sounds is transmitted via the auditory nerve to the temporal lobe of the brain, where it is interpreted as sound.

Characteristics of sound

Sound has three characteristics: pitch, quality and intensity.

PITCH

This is the wavelength or frequency; the frequency range of audible sounds is from 20 to 20 000 Hz (cycles per second) in man. Dogs and bats can detect higher frequencies.

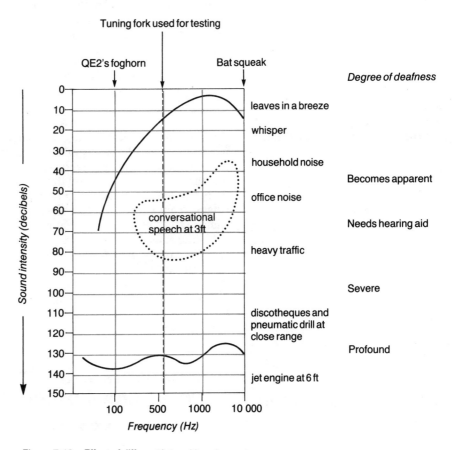

Figure 7.18   Effect of different intensities of sound

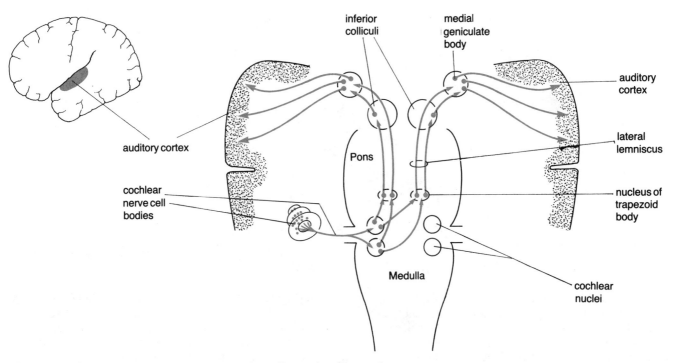

Figure 7.19   Sensory pathways from the cochlea to the auditory cortex of the cerebrum

QUALITY

This is the individual characteristic of sound which enables us to recognise an individual voice, or distinguish a violin from a piano. It comprises a mixture of sounds of slightly different frequencies and intensities.

INTENSITY

Our sensation of intensity or loudness is highly subjective because of the changes which occur in the ear to reduce the effect of loud sounds. Our perception of it also varies with the sound's frequency, as shown in Figure 7.18. The loudest tolerable sound is about 120 decibels, but this will produce deafness with prolonged exposure.

Figure 7.19 shows the pathways for the transfer of information concerning sound from the ear to the auditory cortex of the brain.

Nerve fibres from each ear travel to each side of the cerebrum.

(c) The nose, tongue and skin

The membranes lining the nasal passages contain specialised sensory cells which detect a wide variety of chemical substances inhaled as air is brought into the respiratory system. Detection of these substances is interpreted and memorised by the brain, and they can be described as odours. The substances detected have a widely differing chemical composition and range in their origins from natural sources (including the pheromones, which are chemical signals) to artificially produced flavours and perfumes.

Similar chemical-receptor cells in the surface of the tongue detect a much narrower range of chemicals which the brain interprets as either sweet, sour, bitter or salty. The reaction we normally describe as 'taste' is largely the result of chemoreception by the sensory cells of the nose.

The dermis of the skin contains a wide variety of receptors sensitive to touch, temperature, pain and pressure. These have been discussed in Chapter 5, pages 136–137.

The patients with disturbances of seeing, hearing, smell or touch

(a) Disturbance of eye function

1 Patient study and care plan for an adult with cataract

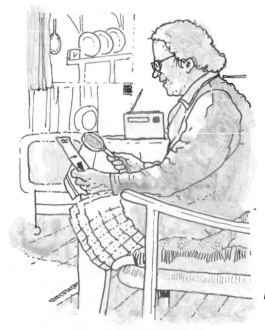

Figure 7.20   Mrs Francis Butterworth

History of social, psychological and physical events leading to the present condition

The patient chosen for this section to illustrate disturbance of the function of the eye is an adult with cataract.

Mrs Francis Butterworth (Figure 7.20), aged 70 years, lives in a flat over a shop in the high street of a busy market town. Her husband died a year ago and she has since lived alone but her son owns the shop below and he visits her regularly when on business there. Normally she does her own housework, cooking and shopping. She enjoys knitting and listening to the radio. Over the past eighteen months she has noticed that the vision of her left eye has deteriorated and her spectacles no longer seem to help. The problem with the sight of her left eye has not caused difficulty with daily activities except in reading small print in the newspaper and in knitting patterns. Her daughter-in-law noticed that the furniture was often dusty and that Mrs Butterworth, who was always houseproud, seemed unaware of this. During this period Mrs Butterworth visited her optician for sight testing and change of glasses. On examination of her eyes, the optician diagnosed a cataract in the left eye and referred her to her GP who made an appointment for her to attend the ophthalmic outpatient department. She was placed on the waiting list for admission to hospital for cataract extraction. Meanwhile, the progress of the condition was monitored.

Explanation of abnormal physiology

You are advised to revise the normal structure and function of the eye with special reference to the lens, and see Table 7.1.

Table 7.1

Normal physiology	Abnormal physiology
(a) The lens accommodates to bring visual images into focus on the retina by altering shape	Lens swells and loses elasticity and the ability to change shape. As accommodation is lost, there is increasing difficulty in focusing for near vision. Distant vision and field of vision gradually deteriorate until sight is lost
(b) The lens allows transmission of light and visual images on to the retina. It is composed of elongated epithelial cells which take up glucose from the aqueous humour for cell metabolism, having no blood supply of its own because it needs to be transparent	Lens becomes opaque due to coagulation of proteins which can be made worse in sunny climates due to excessive ultra-violet light
(c) The lens separates the two compartments of the eye containing the vitreous and aqueous humour	No change

Care plan

PREPARATION FOR PATIENT WITH CATARACT

Mrs Butterworth receives the usual preparation required for any surgical operation. It is explained to her that when she regains consciousness she will have her left eye covered with a pad and shield and she will have to remain resting in a recumbent position for the first few hours (depending on the wishes and instructions of the surgeon). Table 7.3 shows her care plan.

Nursing history and assessment
Table 7.2 shows the completed form for Mrs Butterworth.

Table 7.2 *Nursing history and assessment sheet for Mrs Butterworth*

NURSING HISTORY AND ASSESSMENT SHEET
Record No. _____ *123456* _____

PATIENT LABEL
Mr/Mrs/Miss _____ *Francis Butterworth* _____
Address _____ *2a The High Street, Dunwoody* _____
Male/Female   Age _____ *70 years* _____
Date of Birth _____ *8·12·16* _____
Date of admission/first visit
_____ *6·10·86* _____
Time _____

Type: ☑Routine ☐Emergency
   Transfer from: _____
Religion _____ *C/E* _____
Practising/baptised _____ *Practising* _____
Minister _____
Telephone number _____
Next of kin (name) _____ *Mr. B Butterworth* _____
Relationship to patient _____ *Son* _____

Table 7.2 (cont.)

Address _____ 63 Scarborough Gardens, _____ Dunwoody _____

Telephone numbers _____ 66666 _____

Contact at night/in emergency   YES/NO

Occupation (or father) _____ Housewife _____

Marital status _____ Widow _____

Children (or place in family) _____ 1 son (married) _____

Other dependants _____

Pets _____ Budgerigar _____

School (children only) _____

Hobbies _____ Knitting, listening to radio _____

Clubs _____

Favourite pastime _____

Does patient smoke?   YES/<u>NO</u>

Speech difficulty/language barrier

Dysphasia   Dysarthria

Accommodation

Lives alone   <u>YES</u>/NO

Part III/EMI/Old People's Homes/Rented

Other _____ Flat _____

Consultant _____ Mr King _____

House officer _____ Dr Jack _____

Presenting condition _____ Left cataract _____

History of present complaint and reason for admission

Deteriorating vision over past 18 months. Optician diagnosed cataract in left eye. GP referred her to Ophthalmic Outpatients.
Cataract extraction

Past medical history
None

Allergies   None

Current medication
None

What patient says is the reason for admission and attitude to admission

Patient's expectations   Improved vision after operation

Any problems at home while/because patient is in hospital?

None - son has taken budgerigar to his home

Relevant home conditions (e.g. stairs)
Flat

Visiting problems

Care at home

Community nurse _____

No. _____

Name of GP _____ Dr Brown _____

Address _____ Health Centre, High Lane, _____ Dunwoody

Other services involved

Home help _____   Day hospital _____

Laundry _____   Day centre/club _____

Inco supplies _____   Health visitor _____

Aids _____   Social worker _____

Meals on wheels _____   Voluntary worker _____

Daily living

Diet

Special _____

Food or drink dislikes _____ Dislikes fatty food _____

Appetite: ☑GOOD ☐POOR

Remarks _____

Sleep

How many hours normally? _____ 6 _____

Sedation _____

What else helps? _____

Elimination

Bowels: <u>Continent</u>/Incontinent

How often opened? _____

Any medication? _____

Urinary: <u>Continent</u>/Incontinent

If incontinent; Day/Night/If not taken, how frequently? _____

Nocturia/Dysuria/Frequency/Urgency

Remarks _____

Female patients — Menstruation

<u>Post-menopausal</u>   Taking the pill

Regular   Irregular

Amenorrhoea   Dysmenorrhoea

Next period due: _____

Uses: STs Tampons

Hearing

Hearing aid: YES/<u>NO</u>

Remarks _____

Vision

<u>Glasses</u>/Contact lens: YES/NO

Remarks _____ Difficulty in seeing people's faces unless close

Oral

Dentures or crowns: <u>YES</u>/NO

Any problems with mouth or teeth? _____

Mobility

Help needed with:

Walking/Standing/In/Out of bed/Bathing/Dressing

In/Out of chair/

Feeding/Other: _____

Remarks _____ *Normally active* _____

Prosthesis/appliance

Type of appliance _____

Help needed _____

General appearance

| Normal | Dehydrated | Acutely ill |
| Obese | Thin | Emaciated |

Skin

Satisfactory	Broken areas	Dehydrated
Rash	Oedematous	Jaundiced
Pallor	Other _____ (including bruising)	

Remarks _____

Level of consciousness

| Orientated | Semi-conscious |
| Confused | Unconscious |

Remarks _____

Mental assessment (if appropriate)

Mood

Elated	Irritable	Agitated
Cheerful	Anxious	Aggressive
Miserable	Withdrawn	Suspicious
Apathetic		

Thought content

Hallucinations/Delusions/Paranoid Ideas

_____

Orientation

Time/Place/Person   *Yes*

Very confused   Slightly confused

Any particular time of day? _____

Confabulation _____

Remarks _____

Surveillance   Physical/Emotional

Information obtained from *Mrs and Mrs B Butterworth*

Relationship to patient *Son and daughter-in-law*

By _____ *K. M. Mackay* _____

Position/level of training _____

Date _____ *6·10·86* _____

Time _____

Table 7.3   Care plan for Mrs Butterworth during her stay in hospital

Problem	Objective	Plan of care	Rationale
1. Patient with considerable sight defect being admitted to unfamiliar surroundings	To promote rapid orientation to new environment	(a) Introduce Mrs Butterworth to the different members of staff who will be involved in her care	(a) Enables her to recognise each person
		(b) Assist patient to identify furniture around her bed, and accessories such as radio, call bell and light switch. Take her to areas such as bathroom, toilet and dayroom and identify hazards on route as necessary	(b) Increases confidence and promotes independence. Minimises risks of accidental injury
2. Patient unable to focus following surgical procedure of lens extraction	Give adequate explanation of future management	Explain that she will be able to distinguish light and dark but will be unable to identify objects with the left eye until fitted with contact lens or/and glasses. Give reassurance that her right eye will be unaffected	Removal of the lens prevents focusing of images on the retina and therefore an artificial lens will be required when healing has taken place
3. Operation on the eye breeches the intact barrier to the entry of infection	Minimise risk of infection	(a) Prepare for doctor to examine the condition of the eye and eyelids	(a) Enables antibiotic therapy to be given if required
		(b) Take conjunctival swab (if required) for culture and sensitivity	(b) Identifies causative organism
		(c) Give lacrimal sac washout if required	(c) To ensure patency for adequate drainage post-surgery
		(d) Clip eyelashes (if required by surgeon)	(d) Enables easy access to the eye during operation and minimises risk of contamination

Table 7.3 (cont.)

Problem	Objective	Plan of care	Rationale
4. Risk of operation on wrong eye	Ensure correct eye is operated on	(a) Ensure surgeon indelibly marks correct eye (b) Ensure all relevant documents identify correct eye by writing *left* in full	(a) Reduces risk of wrong operation when patient unconscious (b) Draws attention of all staff involved
5. Access to the lens is via the pupil	Dilate the pupil	Instil mydriatic drops (e.g., atropine) as prescribed, prior to operation	Gives easier access to the lens during surgery

RETURN OF MRS BUTTERWORTH TO THE WARD

During the operation Mrs Butterworth's left lens is removed through an incision which is closed with five fine sutures and her eye covered with a sterile pad and cartella shield to prevent pressure being exerted on the eye. She returns to the ward and is transferred to her bed, taking care to prevent any knocking or jarring of her head or eye dressing to minimise risk of trauma to the newly operated eye. She makes an uneventful recovery from the anaesthetic and requires minimal analgesia. She is allowed up after the first renewal of dressing and inspection of the eye (see Table 7.4).

Table 7.4   Post-operative care plan for Mrs Butterworth

Problem	Objective	Plan of care	Rationale
1. Surgical intervention of the eye	Detect and prevent complications	(a) Gently remove shield and pad (b) Clean eyelids gently with sterile normal saline (c) Examine the eye with use of hand torch for: ● clear cornea ● central pupil ● normal anterior chamber (d) Instil fresh eyedrops as prescribed (e) Re-dress according to surgeon's instructions	(a) Prevents dressing pulling on the lids and/or sutures (b) Unsticks the lid margins (c) If infection or haemorrhage present the cornea could be opaque, iris prolapsed and/or discoloration present in the anterior chamber (indicating haemorrhage) (d) Prevents infection (e) May need additional protection in patients at risk

RECOVERY AND ADVICE

Mrs Butterworth is allowed to mobilise as she was able to attend to her own hygiene and daily activities, but she is advised not to bend over or shampoo her hair during convalescence. Her own spectacles are used with the left lens shielded to minimise light stimulation to the newly operated eye, pending the fitting of a contact lens. Preparation for transfer home includes the following:
1. Teaching Mrs Butterworth and her daughter-in-law how to instil eyedrops.
2. Ensuring adequate supply of eyedrops.
3. Arranging for the district nurse to visit for the first week or until Mrs Butterworth and her family are able to manage.
4. Giving advice regarding return to normal household activities, including asking neighbour to assist with heavy lifting and any tasks requiring stooping such as laying and lighting a fire.
5. Making appointment for follow-up outpatient visit and arranging hospital transport if required.
6. Sending doctor's letter to Mrs Butterworth's general practitioner giving details of treatment and future follow-up.
7. Opportunity to discuss frustrations regarding the period of waiting between operation and satisfactory provision of contact lens.

2 Patient history illustrating further problems related to disturbance of the function of the eye

Patient who is blind

Mrs Helen Smith, aged 35 years, is married with two teenage children. She has been blind since birth and is now admitted to a surgical ward for minor surgery. She is likely to be in hospital for 3 days. She has had her present guide-dog for five years and works part-time as a telephonist at a local exchange. While Mrs Smith is in hospital her husband arranges to have holiday from work to look after the children, house and dog, and allow adequate time for visiting.

SELF-TESTING QUESTIONS

1. Discuss how you would manage Mrs Smith's admission to the ward and her ongoing care during her period in hospital with reference to her blindness.

BRIEF ANALYSIS AND GUIDELINES TO SUITABLE ANSWERS

Question 1
For Mrs Smith's admission, your answer should include:
(a) Allocate one nurse to Mrs Smith.
(b) Give opportunity for her to explore her new surroundings, e.g., around her bed, ward facilities, with guidance from a nurse.
(c) Ensure all staff address Mrs Smith by name when approaching her and identifying themselves.
(d) Discover what Mrs Smith is capable of achieving, for example, daily living activities, to maintain normal independence.
For ongoing care your answer should include:
(a) Care that all staff realise the need not to move personal belongings around Mrs Smith's bedside without informing her.
(b) Be prepared to explain unfamiliar sounds and smells.
(c) Orientate to emergency exits.
(d) Allocated nurse should explain daily menu sheet to Mrs Smith.
(e) Describe each meal when given to Mrs Smith.
(f) Ensure Mrs Smith's consent for operation is witnessed.
(g) Ensure staff are particular that ward environment is safe during Mrs Smith's stay.
(h) Encourage staff to use touch as a means of communicating and avoid raising their voices and rushing to the bedside.
(i) Ensure she is included in ward activities.
(j) Allow free visiting for friends and relations.
(k) If delay in discharge occurs then consider obtaining braille or talking books.

Question 2

2. Make a summary of the facilities available (a) for those blind from birth, and (b) those who become blind.

(a) For those blind from birth:
 • Assessment for educational needs.
 • Provision of special schools and recreational activities.
 • Support for families from Royal National Institute for the Blind.
(b) For those who become blind:
 • Assessment for training for occupations (with social services and Royal National Institute for the Blind).
 • Provision of guide dogs, talking books (library and Royal National Institute for the Blind).
 • Eligibility for tax allowances and supplementary benefits.
 • Recreational facilities, e.g., special gardens and walks for the blind.

(b) Disturbance of ear function

1 Patient study and care plan for a child with otitis media

History of social, psychological and physical events leading to present condition

The patient chosen for this section to illustrate disturbance of the function of the ear is a child with a history of otitis media requiring tonsillectomy, adenoidectomy and myringotomies.

Michael Brown (Figure 7.21), aged 12 years, lives with his parents and two younger brothers on a council estate. In the past six months he has had several bouts of tonsillitis and a recurring otitis media necessitating treatment with antibiotics and keeping him away from school. His GP advises that Michael should be referred to an ear, nose and throat surgeon for further investigations and treatment. Following this visit Michael has an audiogram which revealed conductive deafness of both ears. The ear, nose and throat surgeon examined Michael's ears, nose and throat and informed his parents that Michael's difficulty in hearing was due to enlarged adenoids, which were blocking his

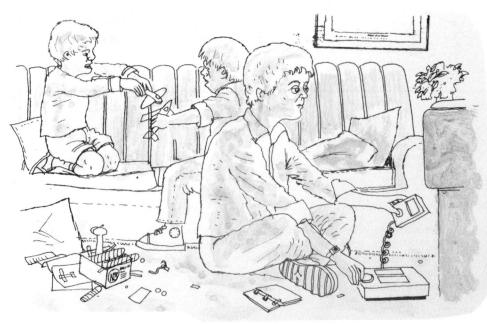

Figure 7.21   Michael Brown

Eustachian tubes. He advised that Michael's name should be placed on the waiting list for admission to hospital for removal of his tonsils and adenoids and bilateral myringotomies for restoration of his hearing and general health.

Michael and his parents arrive at the hospital as requested and are informed that Michael is to be admitted to an adult ear, nose and throat ward as he is considered too old for the children's ward at this time.

Explanation of abnormal physiology

It is advisable to revise the normal structure and function of the ear and pharynx, and see Table 7.5.

Table 7.5

Normal physiology	Abnormal physiology
(a) Sound waves are transmitted from the outside to the auditory nerve for hearing to take place by: (i) Movement of the tympanic membrane (ii) Vibration of bony ossicles in the middle ear (iii) Vibration of the oval window (iv) Disturbance of the endolymph in the inner ear which stimulates the auditory nerve (v) Nerve impulse transmitted to sensory cortex of the brain	Any interruption in the delivery of sound waves to the oval window is classified as conductive deafness. Interruption beyond the oval window is classified as sensory or nerve deafness
(b) For vibration to occur air pressure is kept the same either side of the tympanic membrane by air entering the Eustachian tube from the nasopharynx	(i) Entrance of Eustachian tube in the nasopharynx has become blocked by mass of lymphoid tissue (adenoids). Lymphoid tissue performs a protective function against infection by manufacturing lymphocytes and acts as a filter for invading organisms. Sometimes this tissue can become infected and act as a septic focus and block the Eustachian tube. Air is unable to reach the middle ear which now contains a pocket of trapped air. This air becomes absorbed into the small blood vessels lying in the walls of the middle ear with a consequent drop in the middle ear pressure. This reduced (or negative) pressure has two main effects: ● It draws the tympanic membrane inwards. ● It draws fluid into the middle ear cavity from the vessels lying in its walls. Both these factors hinder the vibration of the ossicles, producing some conductive deafness (ii) Infective organisms in the tonsils or adenoids can travel via the Eustachian tube and enter the middle ear, causing generalised inflammation and the formation of pus and eventual bulging and perforation of the tympanic membrane, producing severe earache and conductive deafness

Care plan

PREPARATION FOR MICHAEL'S TONSILLECTOMY, ADENOIDECTOMY AND MYRINGOTOMIES

Michael Brown receives all the normal preparation for surgical operation, his parents being allowed to visit and stay with him the morning of the operation (see care plan, Table 7.7). It is explained to Michael and his parents that after his operation he will have a sore throat and his hearing could return so noises might appear to be very loud at first.

Nursing history and assessment
Table 7.6 shows the nursing history and assessment sheet for Michael Brown.

Table 7.6   Nursing history and assessment sheet for Michael Brown

NURSING HISTORY AND ASSESSMENT SHEET
Record No. _____ 77777 _____

PATIENT LABEL
Mr/Mrs/Miss ____ Michael BROWN ____
Address ____ 10 St. Andrews Road ____
____ Wickton ____

Male/Female   Age ____ 12 ____
Date of Birth ____ 3·4·74 ____

Date of admission/first visit
____ 6·9·86 ____
Time _____
Type: ☑Routine ☐Emergency
    Transfer from: _____

Religion ____ R/C ____
Practising/baptised ____ Non-practising ____
Minister _____
Telephone number _____

Next of kin (name) ____ Mr and Mrs A Brown ____
Relationship to patient ____ Parents ____
Address ____ Same address ____

Telephone numbers ____ None ____
Contact at night/in emergency   YES/NO
Occupation (or father) ____ Electrician (father) ____
Marital status ____ - ____
Children (or place in family) ____ Eldest son ____
Other dependants _____
Pets _____
School (children only) _____
Hobbies ____ Cycling, football ____
Clubs _____
Favourite pastime _____
Does patient smoke?   YES/NO

Speech difficulty/language barrier

Dysphasia   Dysarthria

Accommodation
Lives alone   YES/NO
Part III/EMI/Old People's Homes/Rented
Other _____

Consultant ____ Mr Rutland ____
House officer ____ Dr Wood ____
Presenting condition ____ Conductive deafness ____

History of present complaint and reason for admission
____ Recurrent sore throats and otitis media during past 8 months. Conductive deafness (audiogram). Tonsillectomy, adenoidectomy and bilateral myringotomies ____
Past medical history
____ N/a ____

Allergies   None

Current medication
____ None (Antibiotic until 2 weeks ago) ____

What patient says is the reason for admission and attitude to admission
_____

Patient's expectations ____ Less earache and better hearing ____
Any problems at home while/because patient is in hospital?
____ None ____
Relevant home conditions (e.g. stairs)
____ N/a ____

Visiting problems
_____

201

Table 7.6 (cont.)

Care at home

Community nurse _____

No. _____

Name of GP ___ *Dr Greenfields* ___

Address ___ *The Health Centre, Wickton* ___

Other services involved

Home help _____ Day hospital _____

Laundry _____ Day centre/club _____

Inco supplies _____ Health visitor _____

Aids _____ Social worker _____

Meals on wheels _____ Voluntary worker _____

Daily living

Diet

Special _____

Food or drink dislikes _____

Appetite: ☐ GOOD ☑ POOR

Remarks ___ *Poor for past eight months* ___

Sleep

How many hours normally? ___ *10 (Poor at present – disturbed by earache)* ___

Sedation _____

What else helps? _____

Elimination

Bowels: Continent/Incontinent

How often opened? _____

Any medication? _____

Urinary: Continent/Incontinent

If incontinent; Day/Night/If not taken, how frequently? _____

Nocturia/Dysuria/Frequency/Urgency

Remarks _____

Female patients — Menstruation

Post-menopausal   Taking the pill

Regular   Irregular

Amenorrhoea   Dysmenorrhoea

Next period due: _____

Uses: STs   Tampons

Hearing

Hearing aid: YES/NO

Remarks ___ *Hearing poor. Requires people to speak v. clearly when talking to him* ___

Vision

Glasses/Contact lens: YES/NO

Remarks _____

Oral

Dentures or crowns: YES/NO

Any problems with mouth or teeth? _____

Mobility

Help needed with:

Walking/Standing/In/Out of bed/Bathing/Dressing

In/Out of chair/

Feeding/Other: _____

Remarks ___ *Normally active* ___

Prosthesis/appliance

Type of appliance _____

Help needed _____

General appearance

Normal   Dehydrated   Acutely ill

Obese   Thin   Emaciated

Remarks ___ *Slightly thin - possibly due to poor appetite* ___

Skin

Satisfactory   Broken areas   Dehydrated

Rash   Oedematous   Jaundiced

Pallor

Other _____
(including bruising)

Remarks _____

Level of consciousness

Orientated   Semi-conscious

Confused   Unconscious

Remarks _____

Mental assessment (if appropriate)

Mood

Elated   Irritable   Agitated

Cheerful   Anxious   Aggressive

Miserable   Withdrawn   Suspicious

Apathetic

Thought content

Hallucinations/Delusions/Paranoid Ideas

_____

Orientation

Time/Place/Person *Yes*

Very confused   Slightly confused

Any particular time of day? _____

Confabulation _____

Remarks _____

Surveillance   Physical/Emotional

Information obtained from ___ *Mr and Mrs Brown* ___

Relationship to patient ___ *Parents* ___

By ___ *Susan James* ___

Position/level of training _____

Date ___ *6·9·86* ___

Time _____

Table 7.7   Care plan for Michael Brown during his stay in hospital

Problem	Objective	Plan of care	Rationale
1. Anxiety of parents and Michael on being admitted to an adult ward	Minimise anxieties of Michael and his parents	(a) Encourage parents to be involved in Michael's care	(a) and (b) Assists in establishing contact with ward staff and provides suitable atmosphere for exchange of information
		(b) Give opportunity for all to express their fears and give explanation of necessary procedures	
		(c) Introduce them to other patients	(c) Encourages social interaction and settling into ward environment
		(d) Encourage parents to leave some of Michael's own books and games	(d) Prevents boredom and offers distraction
		(e) Allow parents to stay in hospital ward as much as they want to	(e) Maintains family relationships
2. Poor hearing	Minimise effects of hearing loss	(a) Attract his attention before communicating	(a) Ensures he concentrates on what is being said to him
		(b) Speak clearly and slowly	(b) Enables Michael to interpret what has been said
		(c) Ask him to repeat what you have said to him if the instructions are important	(c) Checks how much he has heard
		(d) Inform other patients and staff of Michael's difficulty in hearing	(d) Gains others' cooperation and prevents misunderstanding
3. Sleep disturbed by ear-ache	Promote sleep prior to surgery	Give analgesia and hypnotic as prescribed the night before operation	Analgesia reduces sensitivity to pain and hypnotic induces sleep

SURGERY AND RETURN TO THE WARD

Michael is taken to the operating theatre the following afternoon where his tonsils and adenoids are removed and bilateral myringotomies are performed.

Bilateral myringotomies
A myringotomy is a small incision in the tympanic membrane through which the infected fluid contents of the middle ear can be sucked out. The incision becomes closed by a blood clot within minutes and healed within one week.

On return to the ward, the post-operative care plan described in Table 7.8 is put into action.

Table 7.8   Post-operative care plan for Michael Brown

Problem	Objective	Plan of care	Rationale
1. Potential to develop reactionary haemorrhage from adenoid or tonsil bed	Detect early signs and symptoms of haemorrhage	(a) (i) Measure and record pulse rate, e.g., ½-hourly, until observations have been stable for at least four hours	(a) (i) Pulse rate rises when haemorrhage occurs
		(ii) Measure and record blood pressure, e.g., on return to ward and one hour later	(ii) Blood pressure falls when haemorrhage occurs
		(b) Observe for pallor of skin, sweating, restlessness, swallowing, pain, vomiting or spitting of blood	(b) Indicates patient is bleeding and may be swallowing the blood
		(c) Prepare for emergency treatment of haemorrhage including the following: • torch • headmirror • hydrogen peroxide • sterisponge • injection equipment	(c) Torch and headmirror give a good view of throat; hydrogen peroxide oxidises surface of mucous membrane and removes a lot of tissue debris on tonsil bed. Sterisponge acts as a fibrin mesh to promote blood clotting. Intramuscular analgesia may be given

Table 7.8 (cont.)

Problem	Objective	Plan of care	Rationale
2. Return of hearing	Prevent unnecessary distress from loud noises	(a) Explain to patient the effect of a sudden return to normal hearing (b) Speak normally but clearly	(a) and (b) Sudden return of hearing, sounds can appear to be loud and frightening
3. Surgical incision in tympanic membrane	To prevent infection	(a) Keep ears dry (b) Explain to both Michael and his parents to be careful when bathing and washing hair and avoid swimming during convalescence (c) Ensure appointment is made for check audiogram prior to out-patient visit	(a) and (b) The incision becomes closed by blood clot within minutes and healed within one week (c) Checks return of normal hearing
4. Reluctance to eat and drink following removal of tonsils	Ensure hydration and nutrition is maintained to dislodge slough from tonsil bed and aid healing. Encourage use of pharyngeal muscles	(a) Give soluble aspirin gargles before meals (b) Give normal diet and encourage completion of meals	(a) Gives an analgesic effect when swallowing (b) Assists in desloughing of tonsil bed and gives adequate nutrition and hydration
5. Potential to develop mouth sepsis	Prevent oral sepsis	(a) Check Michael cleans his teeth (b) Give him mouthwashes before and after meals (c) Encourage Michael to drink adequate fluids	(a),(b) and (c) Stimulates flow of saliva and removes debris

RECOVERY AND DISCHARGE

By the third day Michael is hearing well and has integrated well into the ward activities. His appetite has returned and temperature and pulse are normal. Mr and Mrs Brown are given the following advice prior to Michael's discharge.

1. Keep Michael indoors for a week and away from school for a further two weeks.
2. Bring him to outpatients' department in six weeks' time.
3. Contact their doctor if Michael's temperature rises and/or any bleeding occurs.
4. Keep Michael's ears dry.

2 Patient history illustrating further problems related to disturbance of the function of the ear

An adult who is deaf

Mr Reginald Kemp, aged 25 years, lives alone in a rented flat and works as an assistant to the local baker. He has been involved in a road traffic accident and sustained a fracture of his tibia. He is admitted to your ward after reduction of fracture and application of above-knee plaster of Paris. He is to stay in bed with leg elevated until his plaster dries. He is to be allowed home as soon as he is stable on crutches and able to cope with going up and down stairs safely. Mr Kemp has been profoundly deaf since birth and he attended a special school for the deaf where he had limited success in lip reading and learning to talk.

1. Discuss how you would manage Mr Kemp's admission to the ward and subsequent care during his period in hospital with reference to his deafness.

Question 1

For admission and subsequent care your answer should include:

(a) Allocating one nurse to the care of Mr Kemp.

(b) Making sure that the light is behind him when communicating with him so that he can see to lip read.

(c) Attracting Mr Kemp's attention by touch prior to speaking.

(d) Speaking slowly with normal volume.

(e) Avoiding bumping into bed and causing vibration.

(f) Maintaining pleasant, encouraging expression on face.

(g) Making sure all messages are conveyed promptly and offering to make telephone calls if required.

(h) Ensuring a friend or relative who normally communicates with him is available when vital information has to be given and/or enlist assistance from the speech therapist or Royal National Institute for the Deaf.

(i) Explain to other patients and staff Mr Kemp's difficulty and encourage them to interact with him.

2. Make a summary of the facilities for the profoundly deaf.

Question 2

Your answer should include facilities for children and adults.

For children

(a) Screening all children during the first year of life on more than one occasion.

(b) Opportunity for parents to seek assessment if worried about child's ability to hear.

(c) Provision of special schools for deaf children.

(d) Provision of teachers for the deaf in normal schools at primary and secondary level.

(e) Provision of recreational facilities.

(f) Support of parents and ongoing advice.

(g) Provision of hearing aids.

For adults

(a) Social clubs run by the Royal National Institute for the Deaf.

(b) Re-training programmes and sheltered workshops.

(c) Provision of subtitles and sign language on television.

(d) Support to deaf parents of hearing children.

(c) Disturbance of the function of the nose

History of social, psychological and physical events leading to the present condition

The patient chosen for this section to illustrate disturbance of the function of the nose is an adult with an epistaxis.

1 Patient study and care plan for an adult with an epistaxis

Mrs Phyllis Lloyd (Figure 7.22), aged 65 years, lives with her husband in a semi-detached house on the outskirts of a village. The couple live quietly because Mrs Lloyd is rather frail. In the past she has suffered from left ventricular failure due to hypertension and has received anti-hypertensive therapy and digoxin. In the last month Mrs Lloyd has felt unwell and thought her tablets were upsetting her so decided to have a rest from them. One day she developed a severe headache and two hours later started to bleed severely from her nose. Her husband became anxious and contacted their GP. The doctor examined her and advised urgent transfer to hospital for treatment, as simple measures failed to arrest the haemorrhage. Mr Lloyd travelled with his wife in the ambulance and noticed she was getting paler and was sweating.

On arrival at the accident and emergency department the following observations are made:

- Nose bleeding profusely.
- Skin pale, cold and clammy.
- Pulse rate raised, 120 beats per minute.
- Blood pressure 150/90 mmHg.
- Respirations difficult to count as she is spitting out blood.

The nurse helps Mrs Lloyd on to a couch, removes her dentures and helps her

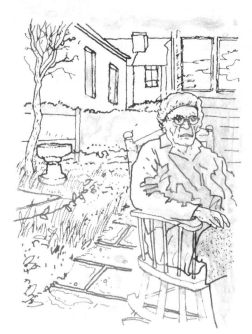

Figure 7.22　Mrs Phyllis Lloyd

to sit up, to decrease venous congestion, and lean forward so that the blood may run straight from the nose into a bowl. The doctor attempts to find the bleeding point with the help of his head mirror, a good light source and suction. He finds it impossible to discover the bleeding point so prepares to pack the nasal cavity and commences an intravenous infusion.

The nasal pack is prepared containing bismuth iodoform paraffin paste and is inserted into the bleeding nostril. He prescribes a sedative and antibiotics and arranges for her to be transferred to the ear, nose and throat ward.

Explanation of abnormal physiology

It is advisable to revise the normal structure and function of the nose, and see Table 7.9.

Table 7.9

Normal physiology	Abnormal physiology
(a) The nose provides a wide surface area for warming and moistening inspired air as it passes over the moist mucous membrane. Hairs inside the nostrils and ciliated mucous membrane filter dust particles from the inspired air	Presence of a nasal pack blocks nasal passages so preventing air to be warmed, moistened and filtered. Patient breathes through the mouth, leading to dryness of the mucous membrane and tongue
(b) Nasal mucous membrane has an abundant superficial blood supply to enable the above functions which are under the control of the autonomic nervous system	Due to hypertension superficial blood vessels can rupture but presence of arteriosclerosis prevents vasoconstriction and bleeding persists
(c) Normally, secretions of the nasal cavity pass into the nasopharynx and are swallowed	If haemorrhage occurs in the nasal cavity, the blood tends to flow into the nasopharynx and be swallowed but acts as an irritant causing the patient to vomit and feel faint
(d) Nerve endings in mucous lining convey sensation of smell via olfactory nerve to sensory cortex of the brain	Impossible for air carrying odours to reach the sensory nerve endings to deliver sensations of smells

Care plan

PREPARATION FOR PATIENT WITH AN EPISTAXIS

Mrs Lloyd is received in the ear, nose and throat ward and the care plan shown in Table 7.11 is put into action.

Nursing history and assessment
Mrs Lloyd's form is completed (Table 7.10).

Table 7.10　Nursing history and assessment sheet for Mrs Lloyd

NURSING HISTORY AND ASSESSMENT SHEET

Record No. _____ 868686 _____

PATIENT LABEL

Mr/Mrs/Miss ___ Phyllis LLOYD ___
Address ___ 36 Grange Road, Ludwick ___

Male/__Female__　Age ___ 65 ___
Date of Birth ___ 6·12·20 ___

Date of admission/first visit
_____ 5·2·86 _____

Time _____

Type: ☐ Routine　☑ Emergency
　Transfer from: _____

Religion ___ C/E ___
Practising/baptised _____
Minister _____
Telephone number _____

Next of kin (name) ___ Mr J Lloyd ___
Relationship to patient ___ Husband ___
Address ___ Same address ___
_____

Telephone numbers ___ 62784 ___
Contact at night/in emergency　YES/NO

Occupation (or father) _____ *Housewife* _____

Marital status _____ *Married* _____

Children (or place in family) _____

Other dependants _____

Pets _____

School (children only) _____

Hobbies _____

Clubs _____

Favourite pastime _____

Does patient smoke?   YES/NO

Speech difficulty/language barrier

Dysphasia   Dysarthria

Accommodation

Lives alone   YES/<u>NO</u>

Part III/EMI/Old People's Homes/Rented

Other _____ *Semi - detached house* _____

Consultant _____ *Mr Cheshire* _____

House officer _____ *Dr Martin* _____

Presenting condition _____ *Epistaxis* _____

History of present complaint and reason for admission
Unwell during past month, stopped tablets. Developed severe headache and haemorrhage.
Epistaxis, hypovolaemic shock.

Past medical history
Left ventricular failure due to hypertension. Anti-hypertensive therapy and digoxin

Allergies *None*

Current medication
None (patient discontinued it herself)

What patient says is the reason for admission and attitude to admission
N/a

Patient's expectations

Any problems at home while/because patient is in hospital?

Relevant home conditions (e.g. stairs)
Stairs

Visiting problems

Skin

Satisfactory   Broken areas   Dehydrated

Rash   Oedematous   Jaundiced

<u>Pallor</u>

Other *Cold, clammy*
(including bruising)

Remarks _____

Care at home

Community nurse _____

No. _____

Name of GP _____ *Dr Jackson* _____

Address _____ *The Surgery, Grange Lane, Ludwick*

Other services involved

Home help _____   Day hospital _____

Laundry _____   Day centre/club _____

Inco supplies _____   Health visitor _____

Aids _____   Social worker _____

Meals on wheels _____   Voluntary worker _____

Daily living

Diet

Special _____ *No added salt.* _____

Food or drink dislikes _____

Appetite: ☐ GOOD ☑ POOR

Remarks _____

Sleep

How many hours normally? *5-6 (interrupted)*

Sedation _____   What else helps? _____

Elimination

Bowels: <u>Continent</u>/Incontinent

How often opened? _____ *Daily* _____

Any medication? _____

Urinary: <u>Continent</u>/Incontinent

If incontinent; Day/Night/If not taken, how frequently? _____

Nocturia/Dysuria/Frequency/Urgency

Remarks _____

Female patients — Menstruation

<u>Post-menopausal</u>   Taking the pill

Regular   Irregular

Amenorrhoea   Dysmenorrhoea

Next period due: _____

Uses: STs Tampons

Hearing

Hearing aid: YES/<u>NO</u>

Remarks _____

Vision

<u>Glasses</u>/Contact lens: YES/NO

Remarks _____

Oral

<u>Dentures</u> or crowns: YES/NO

Any problems with mouth or teeth?

_____

Table 7.10 (cont.)

Mobility

Help needed with:

Walking/Standing/In/Out of bed/Bathing/Dressing

In/Out of chair/

Feeding/Other: _____

Remarks _Activity limited by previous heart failure_

Prosthesis/appliance

Type of appliance _____

Help needed _____

General appearance

Normal	Dehydrated	Acutely ill
Obese	Thin	Emaciated

Remarks _____

Level of consciousness

Orientated	Semi-conscious
Confused	Unconscious

Remarks _____

Thought content

Hallucinations/Delusions/Paranoid Ideas

Mental assessment (if appropriate)

Mood

Elated	Irritable	Agitated
Cheerful	Anxious	Aggressive
Miserable	Withdrawn	Suspicious
Apathetic		

Orientation

Time/Place/Person

Very confused   Slightly confused

Any particular time of day? _____

Confabulation _____

Remarks _____

Surveillance   Physical/Emotional

Information obtained from _____ Mr Lloyd _____

Relationship to patient _____ Husband _____

By _____ KPS _____

Position/level of training _____

Date _____ 5.2.86 _____

Time _____

Table 7.11   Care plan for Mrs Lloyd on admission to the ear, nose and throat ward

Problem	Objective	Plan of care	Rationale
1. Hypovolaemic shock	Restore circulation and monitor blood loss	(a) Prepare to administer packed cells as soon as available	(a) Restores red blood cell level without overloading the circulation
		(b) Reassure and explain the present treatment	(b) Reduces anxiety and promotes rest
		(c) Keep patient at rest, well supported by pillows	(c) Avoids unnecessary strain and relieves any venous congestion
		(d) Measure and record pulse rate and volume, blood pressure, fluid balance	(d) Rise in pulse, fall in blood pressure indicates further haemorrhage. Reduction in urine output indicates hypovolaemic shock and/or diminished cardiac output due to heart failure
		(e) Observe for obvious blood loss from nasal packs, from anterior nares and nasopharynx	(e) To enable prompt treatment if epistaxis persists
2. Presence of nasal pack	Minimise discomfort, prevent complications of infection and further bleeding	(a) Give antiseptic mouth washes	(a) Reduces discomfort of mouth breathing
		(b) Advise her not to blow her nose, bend her head or sneeze	(b) Minimises risk of disturbing newly formed clot
		(c) Give sedatives as prescribed	(c) Promotes rest and reduces hypertension
		(d) Give antibiotics as prescribed	(d) Nasal pack acts as foreign body and becomes a focus for infection
		(e) Advise her to avoid drinking hot fluids	(e) Hot fluids can cause vasodilation and therefore further bleeding
		(f) Encourage her to eat and drink	(f) Sensations of smell and taste are closely interlinked and if patient cannot smell, taste is diminished

Table 7.11 (cont.)

Problem	Objective	Plan of care	Rationale
3. Hypertension	Assess hypertensive state	(a) Measure and record daily blood pressure (b) Arrange for referral to a physician	(a) and (b) Provides information for assessment and reintroduction of anti-hypertensive therapy

RECOVERY AND DISCHARGE

Mrs Lloyd's condition improves and no further bleeding occurs. The nasal packs are removed after 48 hours with no further bleeding and the intravenous infusion is discontinued. Prior to her discharge the nose and postnasal space are examined to exclude any local pathology. She is seen by a physician who discusses the importance of resuming her anti-hypertensive drugs.

Mrs Lloyd goes home the next day for a period of quiet convalescence with no undue exertion, under the care of her GP.

(d) Disturbance of skin function

History of social, psychological and physical events leading to the present condition

The patient chosen for this section to illustrate disturbance of the function of the skin is an adult with psoriasis.

1 Patient study and care plan for an adult with psoriasis

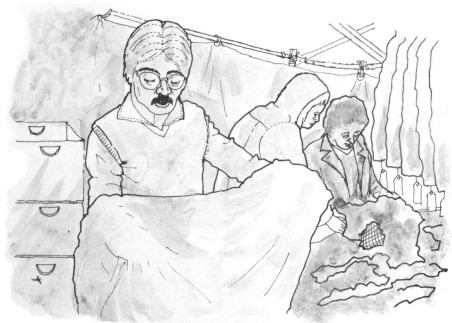

Figure 7.23   Thomas Patel

Thomas Patel (Figure 7.23), aged 21 years, lives with his mother and two sisters in a terraced house in an inner city. His parents separated ten years ago. He was born in East Africa of Indian origin and has been living in England for the past nine years. He is self-employed, working as a local market trader selling car seat covers and bedspreads. Six months ago he developed psoriasis over the whole of his body which became worse after he spent two months in India three months ago. His skin was covered with raised, red, scaly, oval lesions with clearly marginated edges. The scales were silvery-white and the skin between the lesions appeared normal. He was treated by his GP with Dermovate cream to the flexures and scalp and Betnovate N cream to the other affected areas. This treatment failed to bring about any improvement so his name was added to the waiting list for hospital admission.

On admission he appears well but has generalised psoriasis with gross involvement of his scalp and ears. Temperature, pulse, respirations and blood pressure were all within normal limits.

Explanation of abnormal physiology

It is advisable to revise the normal structure and function of the skin, and see Table 7.12.

Table 7.12

Normal physiology	Abnormal physiology
(a) Skin normally intact, barrier against infection	Skin damaged, barrier no longer intact, therefore micro-organisms can enter
(b) Skin is a barrier to loss of tissue fluid	With psoriasis, barrier is lost, and water from the tissues seeps out and evaporates as much as 3–10 times as rapidly as normal, which can result in dehydration in severe, widespread psoriasis
(c) Skin is elastic and flexible and lubricated with sebum	In the lesions, the skin loses its flexibility and develops cracks especially on the palms of the hands and soles of the feet
(d) Turnover rate of cells in the epidermis is 27–28 days as they migrate up from the dermis and are shed	Turnover rate of cells in the epidermis increases to 3–4 days and the rapid turnover causes cells of the superficial layer to retain their nuclei, giving the appearance of silvery scales which become heaped up—called hyperkeratosis
(e) Capillaries serve the dermis of skin with oxygen and nutrients	The capillaries become dilated and tortuous, causing red patches in the skin and tendency to bleed when lesions are scratched
(f) Capillaries and sweat glands in the dermis are active in the control of heat loss	In widespread psoriasis the affected skin may feel hot and patient may lose body heat. Sweat glands may become blocked, so reducing ability to sweat and keep body cool
(g) Nerve endings in the skin are sensitive to touch	Dryness and scaly skin could cause minimal irritation

Care plan

PREPARATION FOR PATIENT WITH PSORIASIS

On admission to the ward Mr Patel is settled in, in preparation for examination by the doctor.

Nursing history and assessment
Mr Patel's completed form is shown in Table 7.13.

Table 7.13   Nursing history and assessment sheet for Thomas Patel

NURSING HISTORY AND ASSESSMENT SHEET
Record No. _____ 61616 _____

PATIENT LABEL
Mr/Mrs/Miss ___ Thomas PATEL ___
Address ___ 68 Forecourt Road, Lonchester ___

Male/Female   Age ___ 21 ___
Date of Birth ___ 10·2·65 ___

Date of admission/first visit
___ 25·5·86 ___

Time _____
Type: ☑ Routine ☐ Emergency
  Transfer from: _____

Religion ___ Hindu ___
Practising/baptised ___ Practising ___
Minister _____
Telephone number _____

Next of kin (name) ___ Mrs P Patel ___
Relationship to patient ___ Mother ___
Address ___ Same address ___
Telephone numbers _____
Contact at night/in emergency   YES/NO

Occupation (or father) ___ Market trader (self-employed) ___
Marital status ___ Single ___
Children (or place in family) _____
Other dependants ___ Mother and 2 sisters ___
Pets _____
School (children only) _____
Hobbies _____
Clubs _____
Favourite pastime _____
Does patient smoke?   YES/NO

Speech difficulty/language barrier

No difficulty but mother speaks

Dysphasia   Dysarthria *limited English*

Accommodation

Lives alone   YES/<u>NO</u>

Part III/EMI/Old People's Homes/Rented

Other _____ *Terraced House* _____

Consultant _____ *Mr Mackie* _____

House officer _____ *Dr Stone* _____

Presenting condition _____ *Generalised psoriasis* _____

History of present complaint and reason for admission

Developed psoriasis over whole body 6 months ago, became worse 3 months ago after visit to India. Dermovate and Betnovate failing to improve. Intensive treatment for psoriasis

Past medical history

N/a

Allergies *None*

Current medication

Dermovate and Betnovate N creams to body and scalp

What patient says is the reason for admission and attitude to admission

Scaly skin

Patient's expectations *Anxious to recover fully a.s.a.p.*

Any problems at home while/because patient is in hospital?

Concerned about financial situation as self-employed. Mother (separated from husband) and two sisters at home.

Relevant home conditions (e.g. stairs)

Visiting problems _____

Care at home

Community nurse _____ No. _____

Name of GP _____ *Dr Gupta* _____

Address _____ *50 Forecourt Terrace, Lonchester* _____

Other services involved

Home help _____   Day hospital _____

Laundry _____   Day centre/club _____

Inco supplies _____   Health visitor _____

Aids _____   Social worker _____

Meals on wheels _____   Voluntary worker _____

Daily living

Diet

Special _____ *Vegetarian* _____

Food or drink dislikes _____

Appetite: ☑GOOD   ☐POOR

Remarks _____

Sleep

How many hours normally? _____ *8* _____

Sedation _____

What else helps? _____

Elimination

Bowels: <u>Continent</u>/Incontinent

How often opened? _____ *Daily* _____

Any medication? _____

Urinary: <u>Continent</u>/Incontinent

If incontinent; Day/Night/If not taken, how frequently? _____

Nocturia/Dysuria/Frequency/Urgency

Remarks _____

Female patients — Menstruation

Post-menopausal   Taking the pill

Regular   Irregular

Amenorrhoea   Dysmenorrhoea

Next period due: _____

Uses: STs   Tampons

Hearing

Hearing aid: YES/<u>NO</u>

Remarks _____

Vision

Glasses/Contact lens: YES/<u>NO</u>

Remarks _____

Oral

Dentures or crowns: YES/<u>NO</u>

Any problems with mouth or teeth?

Mobility

Help needed with:

Walking/Standing/In/Out of bed/Bathing/Dressing

In/Out of chair/

Feeding/Other: _____

Remarks _____ *Normally active* _____

Prosthesis/appliance

Type of appliance _____

Help needed _____

General appearance

Normal   Dehydrated   Acutely ill

Obese   Thin   Emaciated

Remarks _____ *See skin condition* _____

Table 7.13   (cont.)

Skin

Satisfactory	Broken areas	Dehydrated
Rash	Oedematous	Jaundiced
Pallor		

Other _Widespread psoriasis_
(including bruising)

Remarks _Body, scalp and ears affected_

Level of consciousness

Orientated	Semi-conscious
Confused	Unconscious

Remarks _____

Mental assessment (if appropriate)

Mood

Elated	Irritable	Agitated
Cheerful	Anxious	Aggressive
Miserable	Withdrawn	Suspicious
Apathetic		

Thought content

Hallucinations/Delusions/Paranoid Ideas
Fear of spreading psoriasis to rest of family

Orientation

Time/Place/Person _Yes_

Very confused   Slightly confused

Any particular time of day? _____

Confabulation _____

Remarks _____

Surveillance   Physical/Emotional

Information obtained from _Patient_

Relationship to patient _____

By _C. Robinson_

Position/level of training _____

Date _25·5·86_

Time _____

TREATMENT

Mr Patel is examined by the doctor who prescribes the following topical and systemic treatment to be carried out as part of the care plan (see Table 7.14).

Table 7.14   Care plan for Mr Patel while a patient in the dermatology ward

Problem	Objective	Plan of care	Rationale
1. Patient is to embark on an intensive treatment regime	Plan treatment to allow time for rest and recreation	(a) Explain the need for the treatment regime	(a) To gain his cooperation and to start teaching him to give his own treatment
		(b) Arrange treatment in following way: (i) Bath and shampoo after breakfast (ii) Arrange for physiotherapist to give ultraviolet light treatment (iii) Apply ointments as prescribed taking care to limit application to lesions following (i) and (ii) each morning and evening	(b) (i) To remove previous day's ointment and prepare skin for ultraviolet light and application of fresh ointment (ii) Possibly increases sensitivity of lesions to ointments and has a therapeutic effect (iii) Dithranol can burn healthy skin and heal psoriatic lesions. Hydrocortisone cream can be absorbed and cause striae and other systemic side-effects
	Prevent ointment damaging own clothing	Provide hospital gowns and stockinette socks as needed	Dithranol stains clothing and this can lower morale
2. Patient has fears and anxieties about his condition	Relieve anxiety and offer reassurance and explanation	(a) Give opportunity to express fears and receive explanation, i.e., psoriasis is not infectious	(a) He will feel happier living with his family and mixing with friends
		(b) Disease does not lead to permanent scarring	(b), (c) and (d) Patient informed of the nature of his condition
		(c) Treatment will be in an intensive form for the next three weeks	
		(d) Psoriasis tends to recur but with prompt treatment effects can be minimised	
		(e) Introduce him to other patients with psoriasis	(e) and (f) Minimises feeling of isolation
		(f) Inform him of the Psoriasis Association	

Problem	Objective	Plan of care	Rationale
3. Difficulty in selecting vegetarian diet from hospital menu	To provide adequate diet	(a) Allow him to choose his own meals from menu	(a) Maintains independence
		(b) Refer to dietician if there is an inadequate choice	(b) and (c) Increases the range of choice available
		(c) Make provision for him to keep his own food in the refrigerator	
4. Boredom	Provide stimulation	(a) Introduce him to other patients	(a),(b) and (c) Provides opportunity for him to interact and maintain outside interests
		(b) Show him where games, cards and television are in the ward for his use	
		(c) Arrange for him to go out on visits	
5. Patient concerned about his financial situation, being self-employed	Relieve concern, provide advice	Arrange for him to see the social worker for advice	Patient may be eligible for receipt of financial aid and/or help with rent

Topical treatment
1. Hydrocortisone 2.5% ointment to face, flexures and ear pinnae twice a day.
2. Polytar bath daily.
3. Ultraviolet light daily.
4. Polytar plus shampoo, pomade to scalp after shampoo.
5. Coal tar 3% in arachis oil to inside ears twice a day.
6. Dithranol 0.25% in Lassar's paste to all lesions on body and legs twice a day.

Systemic treatment
1. Brompheniramine LA 24 mg as required 12-hourly.
2. Paracetamol 1 g as required 8-hourly.

RECOVERY AND DISCHARGE

After three weeks of this treatment regime the lesions on Mr Patel's face have cleared and his scalp, ears and body are very much improved. It is decided that he can manage at home but this needs to be reviewed in a week's time.

2 Patient history illustrating further problems related to disturbance of the function of the skin

An adult with dermatitis

Miss Susan Foster, aged 31 years, lives with her married sister and family in a council flat. She is unemployed and has a brother currently in prison. She has a history of persistent obesity and in the past has had her jaws wired in an attempt to control her weight. The weight problem has contributed to periods of depression. One month ago she fell and fractured her left humerus and this is being treated by supporting her arm in a sling. Five years ago she developed irritating rashes on her arms and legs and during the past two months the skin rash has started to 'weep' and become more widespread, affecting the scalp, hands and feet. She has allergies to penicillin, Elastoplast and cleaning fluids. Over the past five years she has had intermittent systemic and local medication for the rash. She is to be admitted to the dermatology ward for treatment.

On admission to the dermatology ward the doctor prescribes the following treatment for her dermatitis:
1. Daily bath with Oilatum emollient (contains liquid paraffin and aims to soothe rash and reduce risk of secondary infection).
2. Twice daily application of topical hydrocortisone ointment 1% to ears and flexures, especially the axillae, under breasts, groins and behind the knees.

3. Betnovate 25% in yellow soft paraffin to be applied to all other lesions.
4. Potassium permanganate soaks to 'weeping' lesions on legs for 10 minutes.
5. Coal tar pomade to lesions on scalp.

SELF-TESTING QUESTIONS

1. Devise a daily care plan for Miss Foster.

2. What further care and support may be needed for Miss Foster on her return home?

3. Discuss other factors which can cause dermatitis.

BRIEF ANALYSIS AND GUIDELINES TO SUITABLE ANSWERS

Question 1
Your answer should include attention to:
(a) Intensive treatment regime to allow adequate rest and recreation.
(b) Management of an obese patient having a daily bath with an injured arm.
(c) Patient's depression due to skin condition, obesity and social problems.
(d) Patient's psychological needs of privacy.
(e) Opportunity to talk about herself.
(f) Encouragement in choosing appropriate reducing diet.
(g) Assessing the need for night sedation, analgesia and anti-pruritic medications.

Question 2
Your answer should include:
(a) Continuation of prescribed medications.
(b) Assistance from the district nurse to continue baths.
(c) Follow-up appointment at orthopaedic clinic for her arm.
(d) Follow-up by dietician and GP for her obesity.
(e) Follow-up appointment at dermatology clinic.
(f) Referral for assessment by a psychiatric social worker for joining a group therapy class.

Question 3
Refer to your teacher for guidance to a suitable dermatology textbook.
They can be divided into two groups of causes:
(a) Extrinsic, due to contact with irritant or sensitising agents such as soaps, oils, metals, dyes, cement and cosmetics.
(b) Intrinsic, as associated with asthma or hay fever.

Further reading

L. Fry, *Dermatology–An Illustrated Guide*, Update Books, London, 1978.
R. Marks, *Psoriasis–A Guide to One of the Commonest Skin Diseases*, Martin Dunitz, London, 1981.

Chapter 8

Nursing patients with a communicable condition

Defence systems of the body

The body is continuously being invaded by micro-organisms, primarily bacteria and viruses, which enter via the body's orifices, including the mouth and nose. They will also enter wounds. These pathogens either feed on the tissues or release toxic chemicals into the blood stream and bring about disease.

The body is equipped with various defence mechanisms designed to prevent the entry of micro-organisms, and to destroy them if they do enter.

(a) Preventing entry

Figure 8.1   Leucocytes

The skin acts as an effective barrier to bacteria and viruses, with its hard keratinised outer layer. Other parasitic organisms, including pathogenic amoebae and intermediate stages in the life cycle of flukes and tapeworms, can, however, penetrate the skin.

The alimentary canal and respiratory tract are more vulnerable, but the respiratory tract is defended by the *cilia* (moving hair cells) which line it, and the *mucus* secreted onto the cilia, which traps particles. Coughing, sneezing and vomiting all expel micro-organisms from the body, and the acid environment of the stomach also destroys some bacteria and viruses.

When wounds occur, entry of micro-organisms is cut down by the clotting of blood, which is discussed in Chapter 3, pages 86–87.

Pathogens do, however, succeed in entering the body and there are two important mechanisms for dealing with them. Both mechanisms are carried out mainly by the five types of *leucocyte* (white blood cell), as shown in Figure 8.1.

1. *Phagocytosis*   This is mainly performed by the *neutrophils* which are amoeboid cells, and engulf bacteria. Once engulfed, the bacteria are digested by *lysozyme* enzymes. Neutrophils are not confined to the blood system but can squeeze out into the extracellular environment.
2. *Action by macrophages*   In addition to phagocytic white blood cells, many tissues possess *macrophages* which are also phagocytic in function and are part of the body's *reticulo-endothelial* system. They are most frequently found in the liver and lymph but move actively to the site of infection.

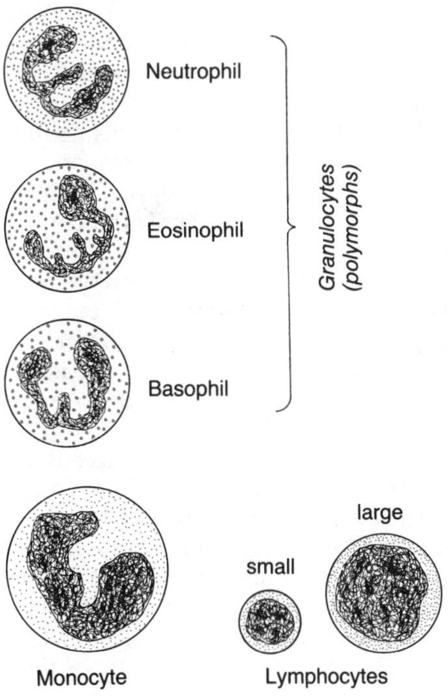

(b) The immune system

All organisms have chemical substances which are characteristic of them and unique to them. These may act as *antigens* if the organism enters the body. The presence of these antigens stimulates the production of a corresponding and antagonistic protein called an *antibody* which is formed by cells derived from lymphocytes. The antibody combines with, and in some way neutralises, the antigen, destroying the micro-organism in the process. Generally, the invading micro-organisms then clump together and are ingested by phagocytes.

Production of antibodies in response to an antigen is the *immune response*: once an antibody has been produced against a particular bacterium, *immunity* is established for some time. These antibodies can pass across the placenta from the mother to foetus, conferring *passive immunity* on the baby for a short period after birth.

Artificial immunity can be generated if the body is injected with small quantities of an antigen or a modified antigen. This process is called *immunisation*. This stimulates the relevent lymphocytes to produce the necessary antibody so that the pathogen will be fought vigorously if it enters the body. Short-lived and artificial 'passive' immunity can be conferred by injecting the body with antibodies already prepared against certain antigens, including tetanus. The protection is short-lived because the antibodies are broken down by the body, and in this case are not being replaced. (See Sheila Collins and Edith Parker's book in this series entitled *An Introduction to Nursing*, pages 44–49.)

Interferon is a protein produced by the body, which prevents the multiplication of *viruses*. Unlike antibodies, it is non-specific, and thus effective against a wide variety of viruses.

As well as the antibody reaction to foreign organisms, there is another response, the *cell-mediated immune response*, in which small lymphocytes attack the foreign body organism or material directly. This is the reaction involved in *hypersensitivity (allergies)* and also in the rejection of transplanted tissue.

Material from another body is identified as 'foreign' because some proteins in the cell membranes are identified as unfamiliar, and stimulate the immune response. By using tissue from close relatives, or by 'tissue-typing', tissue transplants can be more successful as closely similar tissue may not stimulate the immune response. The efficiency of the immune response can be lowered using cytotoxic drugs, steroids or x-rays; this, of course, renders the body less able to cope with infections, but may be necessary in treating certain conditions.

1 Blood groups

A particular example of the different identity of tissue from different people is the phenomenon of *blood groups*. The entire human population can be divided into four groups: A, B, AB and O, on the basis of the reaction between the blood of different individuals when mixed. They correspond to different antigens present in the red blood cells. Corresponding antibodies carried in the plasma are represented by: a, b, ab and o. Group O blood contains neither antigen, but both antibodies. Group AB contains both antigens but no antibodies, and Group A contains A antigens and b antibodies; Group B contains B antigens and a antibodies. If transfusion is required, the correct blood type must be chosen, as shown in Figure 8.2.

In addition to the ABO system there are several other blood group systems. One is the *Rhesus system*. The majority of people have blood which contains the Rhesus antigen, and which is described as *Rhesus positive*. Others lack this antigen and are *Rhesus negative,* and will produce an antibody to it if Rhesus positive blood is transfused into them, causing agglutination of the donor's red cells.

This can be a problem during pregnancy, causing *haemolytic disease of the newborn* if a Rhesus negative mother carries a Rhesus positive child. In the later months of pregnancy, fragments of the foetal red blood cells may pass across the placenta into the mother's blood stream. Her blood responds by producing antibodies which pass across the placenta into the foetus's blood, destroying the red blood cells both before and after birth. This is usually not a problem in the first child, as the antibodies are not formed sufficiently quickly, but second and subsequent children are at risk, if they are also Rhesus positive. It may be fatal unless the child's blood is replaced by transfusion, which can be carried out while the foetus is still in the womb. It can also be prevented by treating the mother with an anti-Rhesus globulin which coats foetal cells and blocks the Rhesus antigen.

universal donor   universal recipient

	Recipient			
	O ab	A b	B a	AB o
O ab	—	—	—	—
A b	+	—	+	—
B a	+	+	—	—
AB o	+	+	+	—

Donor (left axis label)

Figure 8.2 Summary of the reactions that occur when bloods of different groups are mixed

The patients with communicable conditions

(a) Sexually transmitted diseases

1 Patient history, self-testing questions and guidelines to suitable answers

A young adult with gonorrhoea

Simon Parker, aged 19 years, is completing his first year at University. Over the last few days he has experienced pain on passing urine with increased frequency. Today he noticed a yellowish discharge from his urethra, and as he has been sexually active he suspected an infection and seeks medical advice from the department of genito-urinary medicine at the local hospital.

The following examination is made:
(a) Skin of the trunk and thighs inspected for spots, rashes or scratch marks.

(b) Pubic hair for pubic lice.
(c) Inguinal fold for adenitis.
(d) Testes palpated for swelling and tenderness.
(e) Skin of scrotum and penis for warts, rashes, ulcers or scratch marks.
(f) Specimen of discharge for screening of gonorrhoea by Gram stain and culture.

Specimen of urine for the following tests:
- Clarity or haze due to pyuria.
- Microscopy for presence of leucocytes, red blood cells, organisms.
- Culture and sensitivity.
- Presence of protein and sugar.

The doctor discusses his findings with Simon and informs him of the diagnosis of gonorrhoea and of its contagious nature. He advises him to avoid sexual intercourse for at least 2–4 weeks until clear of infection, and prescribes and gives procaine penicillin.

Arrangements are made for contacting and treating of sexual partners.

SELF-TESTING QUESTIONS

BRIEF ANALYSIS AND GUIDELINES TO SUITABLE ANSWERS

1. List alternative treatment regimes the doctor could have prescribed Simon.

Question 1
For other treatment regimes refer to your teacher for guidance to suitable textbook or journal.

2. Describe the effects on Simon if left untreated.

Question 2
Your answer should include:
(a) Chronic infection leading to urethral strictures, chronic prostatitis and sterility.
(b) Spread to sexual partners.

3. Describe the possible clinical features of this condition in women.

Question 3
(a) Gonorrhoea is often asymptomatic but women can develop dysuria, frequency of micturition, and whitish-yellow vaginal discharge and, if untreated, cervicitis, salpingitis and sterility.
(b) An infected pregnant woman can transmit infection to the conjunctiva of the newborn during delivery (ophthalmia neonatorum, now rare in Britain).

4. List other common sexually transmitted diseases and their causative organisms.

Question 4
Other commonly sexually transmitted diseases:
- Trichomoniasis — *Trichomonas vaginalis* (a protozoan).
- Genital herpes — *Herpes simplex* virus type II.
- Genital candidiasis — *Candida albicans* (a fungus).

5. Describe the clinical features and give an outline of the treatment required for common sexually transmitted diseases (as listed in answer to question 4).

Question 5
Trichomoniasis
(a) Clinical features:
- Can be asymptomatic in men and women.
- Slight urethral or vaginal discharge — if present green, frothy and offensive.
- Vulva and perineum can become inflamed.
- Pain during intercourse (dyspareunia).
- Occasionally dysuria and frequency.
- Discomfort in sitting and walking in severe cases.

NB This condition is not always sexually transmitted and can occur in young children and the elderly.
(b) Treatment:
- Treat with an anti-protozoan agent such as metronidazole (Flagyl).
- Treat sexual partners.

Genital herpes
(a) Clinical features:
- Patch of erythema on skin of labia or glans penis upon which appears a group of small, moist vesicles.
- Erosions tender until healing occurs in about 10 days.
(b) Treatment:
- Chronic and recurring infection with no known cure at present.
- Abstain from sexual contact while lesions are present.

Genital candidiasis

(a) Clinical features:
- In women, vulval irritation and copious white, cheesy or purulent vaginal discharge; or watery, scanty discharge.
- Commoner during pregnancy or while taking contraceptive pill or prolonged antibiotic therapy.

(b) Treatment:
- Fungicidal preparations such as nystatin pessaries.
- Treat sexual partners.

6. Identify the causative organisms of syphilis and describe the possible clinical manifestations and treatment of this condition.

Question 6
Refer to suitable textbook, e.g. J. Macleod (Ed.), *Davidson's Principles and Practice of Medicine*, 14th edition, Churchill Livingstone, London, 1984.

7. Discuss the changes in sexual attitudes and their effects on the incidence of sexually transmitted diseases.

Question 7
Refer to any recent publications, including Anne Roberts, The pox and the people, *Nursing Times*, July 14th, 1982, page 1177.

8. How would you explain to a first year student nurse how to allay public anxiety concerning Auto Immune Deficiency Syndrome (AIDS)?

Question 8
Refer to recently published literature, local policies and DHSS guidelines.

(b) Airborne transmitted diseases

1 Patient histories, self-testing questions and guidelines to suitable answers

An adult with pulmonary tuberculosis

Mr Percy Roberts, aged 58 years, lives with his daughter, son-in-law and family in a council flat in a city centre. He works for the local bus company as a driver in a one-man-operated bus. Previously, Mr Roberts has enjoyed good health but last winter he suffered from influenza-like symptoms (which never cleared up completely). Since this time he has had a dry cough, which more recently has become productive of mucoid sputum. His daughter notices that her father appears to be losing weight and has a tendency to tire easily, and advises him to visit his doctor. Mr Roberts is reluctant to do this but became frightened when he started to wake each morning feeling weak and ill and with his clothing soaked with sweat.

One morning he agrees with his daughter to visit the doctor for advice. The doctor obtains a history, and examines Mr Roberts, and asks him to have a chest x-ray at the local hospital and to produce three early morning sputum specimens for identification of acid-fast tubercle bacilli.

The results of the investigations confirm a diagnosis of active pulmonary tuberculosis. The doctor explains this diagnosis to Mr Roberts and his daughter and advises that he should be admitted to hospital for treatment.

SELF-TESTING QUESTIONS

BRIEF ANALYSIS AND GUIDELINES TO SUITABLE ANSWERS

1. State the likely medical treatment for Mr Roberts.

Question 1
Using anti-tuberculosis drugs in combination to prevent resistance and for a sufficient period of time to ensure a cure and prevent a relapse:
- Isoniazid 300 mg daily
- Rifampicin 600 mg daily   } for 2 months
- Ethambutol 15 mg/kg daily

After this time ethambutol omitted and the other two continued for a further 7 months. Sometimes streptomycin 1 g daily intramuscularly replaces the ethambutol.

2. Mr Roberts has been admitted to your ward; devise a care plan for his stay in hospital.

Question 2
Your answer should include identification and management of the following problems:
(a) Anxious gentleman, e.g., nearing retirement.
(b) Has infectious disease which is airborne spread by droplets.

(c) Has productive cough containing *Mycobacterium tuberculosis*.
(d) Potential for haemoptysis.
(e) Recent weight loss, anorexia and tiredness.
(f) Recurrent night sweats.
(g) Receiving medication with potential unwanted as well as wanted effects.
(h) Rehabilitation physically, psychologically and socially.

3. Describe what further action the doctor will undertake following arrangements for Mr Robert's admission.

Question 3
As pulmonary tuberculosis is a notifiable disease, the GP notifies the Medical Officer of Health or Community Physician, who arranges for tracing of all contacts of family and work colleagues. Immediate family including the children have chest x-rays and Heaf Tests, e.g., Mantoux (if negative, BCG is given).

4. How long is Mr Roberts likely to spend in hospital?

Question 4
Mr Roberts will remain only while sputum specimens are positive for the causative organism. (See Fact Sheet 3, page 220, for characteristics of sputum.)

A child with whooping cough

Jimmy Saunders, aged 3 years, attends a local playgroup. He developed a mild fever with catarrh and a cough which lasted for about a week. The fever subsided but Jimmy was left with the cough which became more severe at night. His mother suspected whooping cough when during a bout of coughing Jimmy ejected sticky mucus through his nose and mouth and his face became congested and his eyes streamed. At the end of the coughing bout he 'whooped' as he took a breath in. He had several more paroxysms after which he vomited and appeared exhausted.

Jimmy's mother arranges for the doctor to call and he confirms the diagnosis of whooping cough by nasal swab. On questioning, Mrs Saunders reminds the doctor that she declined the opportunity of vaccination against whooping cough for Jimmy due to her fears of complications.

The doctor notifies the Community Physician, as whooping cough is a notifiable disease. He also arranged for the health visitor to call and advise Mrs Saunders how to care for Jimmy.

SELF-TESTING QUESTIONS

1. Describe the advice which Mrs Saunders would be given to help her care for Jimmy during the course of his illness. This could last an average of 4-6 weeks, but could be considerably longer.

BRIEF ANALYSIS AND GUIDELINES TO SUITABLE ANSWERS

Question 1
Your answer should include attention to the following:
(a) Care and comfort of a sick child.
(b) Calm approach during paroxysms.
(c) Careful disposal of infective sputum and material.
(d) Isolation from other children initially.
(e) Ensure feeding is done immediately following a paroxysmal bout of coughing.
(f) Hydration and micturition.
(g) Return to normal activities as symptoms subside.

2. Discuss the possible complications of whooping cough.

Question 2
Your answer should include the detection of early signs and symptoms of the following:
- Pulmonary atelectasis
- Bronchopneumonia (usually due to secondary bacterial infection)
- Convulsions
- Prolapse of the rectum
- Subconjunctival or periorbital haemorrhage

3. Discuss whether vaccination against whooping cough should be compulsory.

Question 3
Your answer should include:
(a) Consideration of the rights of the individual, both the adult person and the child.
(b) The place of health education.
(c) The role of the well-baby clinics.
(d) The feasibility of legislation in health matters.

A child with measles

Mandy Phillips, aged 6 years, comes home from school irritable and lethargic. She refuses her tea and vomits soon afterwards. Her mother puts her to bed earlier than usual when she finds Mandy feverish with runny eyes and nose. The next morning, after a restless night, Mandy is obviously still unwell and her mother calls the doctor. After taking a history the doctor examines Mandy and finds the diagnostic Koplik's spots on the buccal mucosa and tells Mrs Phillips to expect the rash of measles to appear within the next couple of days. He describes the appearance as a reddened raised rash starting on the neck and spreading to the face, trunk and finally limbs.

The doctor calls again the next day and finds Mandy with quite severe conjunctivitis and slight photophobia. He suggests that Mandy may be more comfortable if kept in a shaded room. He notifies the disease to the Community Physician and arranges to see Mandy a week later, if there is no further cause for concern.

SELF-TESTING QUESTIONS

1. Discuss measures to minimise spread of this disease.

2. Identify the major problems that may be encountered during Mandy's illness at home.

3. Discuss the complications which may occur during the illness and indicate how you would detect these.

BRIEF ANALYSIS AND GUIDELINES TO SUITABLE ANSWERS

Question 1
Your answer should include attention to the following:
(a) Restriction of visitors.
(b) Keeping Mandy at home from school until she is clinically well.
(c) Care of infected fomites, bed linen and secretions.
(d) Discussion of immunisation programmes.

Question 2
Your answer should include:
(a) Difficulty in maintaining hydration and nutrition.
(b) Photophobia.
(c) Febrile state.
(d) Irritable/bored child in bed.
(e) Isolation from friends and family.

Question 3
Your answer should include attention to the following:
(a) Acute obstructive laryngitis (croup) causing inflammation and oedema of the larynx, vocal cords and epiglottis, plus audible laryngeal stridor with a hoarse squeaky voice.
(b) Secondary bacterial infection such as bronchitis, pneumonia, otitis media (see Chapter 7).

Fact Sheet 3 Characteristics of sputum

MUCOID SPUTUM

This is like raw white of egg and occurs in *chronic bronchitis* between acute exacerbations.

A very sticky tenacious mucoid sputum occurs in *asthma*. This may block small bronchi during an attack and be coughed up afterwards.

MUCOPURULENT SPUTUM

Thick, sticky or slimy, and green or yellow, this occurs during acute exacerbations of chronic bronchitis and in other respiratory tract infections.

PURULENT SPUTUM

This is pus from infective lung conditions. It is thick and yellow or green but not sticky or slimy. It may occur in any lung infection such as bronchopneumonia, but very large amounts are produced in bronchiectasis or lung abscess.

FROTHY SPUTUM

Often this is coughed up in pulmonary oedema. It may be white, or if tinged with blood, pinkish.

This comes from larynx, trachea, bronchi or lungs, is bright red and frothy, and the patient is likely to go on coughing up blood for a few days after the original episode. The following are possible causes:

1. Carcinoma of bronchus. This is the cause of death in one in 12 of all males who die in England and Wales. More than half of all cases of carcinoma of the bronchus have haemoptysis which occurs usually as regular daily staining rather than as a massive haemoptysis or with the production of clots.
2. Tuberculosis. This is one of the most commonly occurring notifiable infections but 1 in 5 cases are only diagnosed after death, probably because the disease is wrongly believed to be rare nowadays. This is especially unfortunate because it is curable, may be fatal, and is infectious if untreated. Recurrent haemoptyses of small volumes of blood is the most common type in tuberculosis.
3. Pulmonary embolism.
4. Bronchiectasis (with large volumes of purulent sputum).
5. Mitral stenosis.
6. Pneumonia — when the sputum is classically said to be 'rusty'.

(c) Intestinal transmitted diseases

1 Patient history, self-testing questions and guidelines to suitable answers

An adult with salmonella

Susan Wilkins, aged 20 years, has been out with friends for an evening meal. The following morning, about eight hours later, Susan wakes up with abdominal discomfort and colic. She has a headache and feels feverish, and vomits. Later in the morning she starts to experience watery diarrhoea and feels unwell. She stays at home and contacts her work place and visits her GP that evening. In the meantime she hears that two friends who were with her the previous evening have been admitted to hospital with severe food poisoning.

Her doctor obtains a history and examines Susan, and advises her to go home to bed and drink plenty of fluids. He obtains a rectal swab for identification of the causative organism which is later confirmed as *Salmonella typhimurium*.

Salmonella is spread by the intestinal route and is transmitted by infected humans, domestic animals and birds such as cattle, pigs, poultry, domestic pets and eggs. Sources include frozen poultry and exposed foods contaminated by vermin.

SELF-TESTING QUESTIONS

1. Describe the action taken to identify the source of Susan's infection.

BRIEF ANALYSIS AND GUIDELINES TO SUITABLE ANSWERS

Question 1
(a) Notification to the Environmental Health Department who will investigate the restaurant where Susan and her friends had a meal. Samples of foods, if still available, are taken for examination; standard of hygiene of equipment and premises is checked; staff are screened for presence of infecting organism (carriers).
(b) Any personnel with symptoms of diarrhoea are excluded from work until tests are negative.

Question 2
2. How can Susan minimise risk of spread to her family and others?
(a) Susan should pay meticulous attention to handwashing after going to the toilet.
(b) The rest of the family should do likewise.
(c) If Susan's work entails handling food, she will have to stay away until three consecutive rectal swabs are clear of the infecting organism.

Question 3
3. List the possible complications of *Salmonella* poisoning.
Your answer should include:
(a) Dehydration due to severe vomiting leading to electrolyte imbalance and possible renal failure (see Chapters 1 and 2).
(b) Septicaemia: in severe cases the organisms can enter the bloodstream.
(c) Colitis: with bloody diarrhoea and/or toxic dilation of the colon.

1 Patient history, self-testing questions and guidelines to suitable answers

An adult with scabies

Mr Harry Stokes, aged 80 years, has lived in a warden-controlled flat for the past two years. The warden notices that he has been neglecting himself lately and that he appears to have scratch marks on his hands. On closer inspection she finds greyish pencil lines on the sides and backs of his fingers and across the front of his wrists. There is some scaling and occasional small vesicles. She contacts the local GP who examines Mr Stokes and diagnoses infestation with scabies. As Mr Stokes shares communal activities with other residents the doctor prescribes treatment for Mr Stokes, all residents and the warden. He arranges for the district nurse to call and carry out the treatment.

SELF-TESTING QUESTIONS

1. Describe the current treatment used for scabies.

2. (a) Why is it necessary to treat all the residents and staff?
   (b) How can this be done without causing embarrassment and loss of self-esteem to Mr Stokes?

3. Describe the life cycle of *Sarcoptes scabiei (Acarus scabiei)*.

BRIEF ANALYSIS AND GUIDELINES TO SUITABLE ANSWERS

Question 1
Application of one of the following:
- 10% sulphur ointment.
- 1% gammabenzene hexachloride cream or lotion.
- 25% benzyl benzoate emulsion.

Instructions for treatment must be carried out to the letter; failure to do so will result in failure to cure.

Question 2
(a) It is necessary to treat all residents and staff because this infection is spread by direct skin contact. Therefore, it is essential that all persons in close contact with the infected person are treated promptly to prevent recurrence.
(b) To minimise psychological effects on Mr Stokes attention must be given to reassurance, explanation and privacy for all residents.

Question 3
Refer to your teacher for guidance to suitable dermatology or communicable diseases textbook.

Chapter 9 Nursing patients with immobilisation from disease or prescribed treatment

Normal physiology of the skeletal and muscular systems

(a) The skeletal system

The skeleton provides the body with a supporting framework, and provides protection, e.g., for the brain and spinal cord. It provides a firm base for muscle movement, which may also use parts of the skeleton as levers.

The skeletal system is made up of hard *bones* which resist both tension and compression. These are numerous and very varied in size and shape, and are related to each other by several different types of *joint*.

1 Bones

Bone tissue consists of an organic matrix (Figure 9.1 a, b) packed with calcium salts, primarily calcium phosphate, which is secreted by star-shaped cells called *osteoblasts* (Figure 9.1 c). These arrange themselves in concentric rings around nerves and blood vessels. Ninety-nine per cent of the total calcium content of the body (about 1 kg) is contained in the bones; 500 mg of calcium are exchanged between bone and blood each day, 8400 mg are filtered by the kidneys, and most is retained, under the control of *parathyroid hormone* produced by the parathyroid glands.

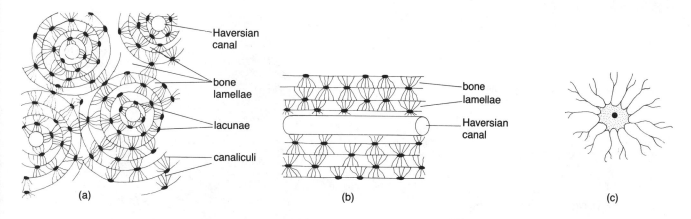

Figure 9.1   Structure of compact bone. (a) In transverse section and (b) in longitudinal section. (c) Single bone-secreting osteoblast

Bone is living tissue and has a constant, dynamic metabolism comparable to any other part of the body. Bone material is constantly being broken down (by osteoclast cells) and regenerated (by osteoblasts), and bone tissue has several important metabolic functions, including the production of red blood cells.

The growth and development of bone is stimulated by the *growth hormone* produced by the pituitary glands. Uptake of calcium and phosphate from the blood and extracellular fluid by the bones is stimulated by the thyroid hormone *calcitonin*, and requires the presence of vitamin D. The development of bone begins with cartilage, and this progressively becomes ossified as shown in Figure 9.2.

The bone is surrounded by a fine membrane, the *periosteum*, in which runs a fine network of blood vessels (supplying compact bone) and nerves (Figure 9.3). Arteries also supply the interior of the bone, in which lies the *marrow*. The marrow cavity is maintained in shape by the action of osteoclasts.

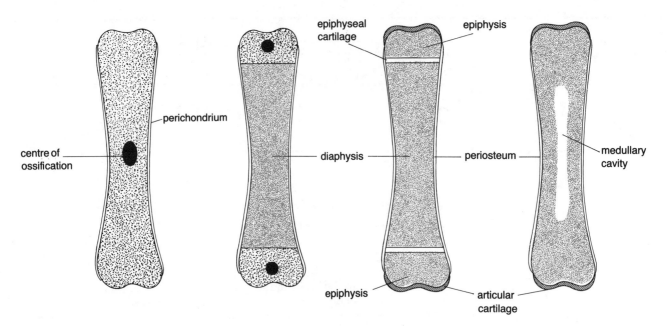

Figure 9.2   Development of bone

2   Joints

Joints occur at any place in the body where two or more bones touch. Some are fixed and ossified, such as the joints (sutures) between the bones of the adult skull. Others may be slightly movable, such as the *cartilaginous* joints between the bodies of the vertebrae, or at the pubic symphysis of the pelvis.

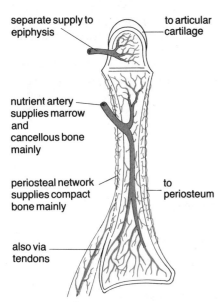

Figure 9.3   Blood and nerve supply to bone

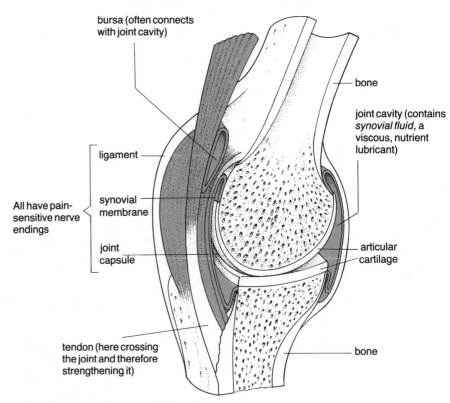

Figure 9.4   A synovial joint

The third type of joint is of importance in locomotion, and is free moving (Figure 9.4). The articulating surfaces must be smooth, and match each other in shape. The surfaces are made even more smooth by a covering of tough and resilient cartilage, which also acts as a shock absorber. The bones are held together by tough bands of fibres called *ligaments,* and the whole joint is encased in an envelope of fibrous tissue called the *joint capsule* which is strengthened by *capsular ligaments.*

Freely moving joints are lubricated by *synovial fluid* which is a clear and viscous liquid, secreted by the *synovial membrane* which lines the joint cavity. Figure 9.5 illustrates some of the movements possible at freely movable joints.

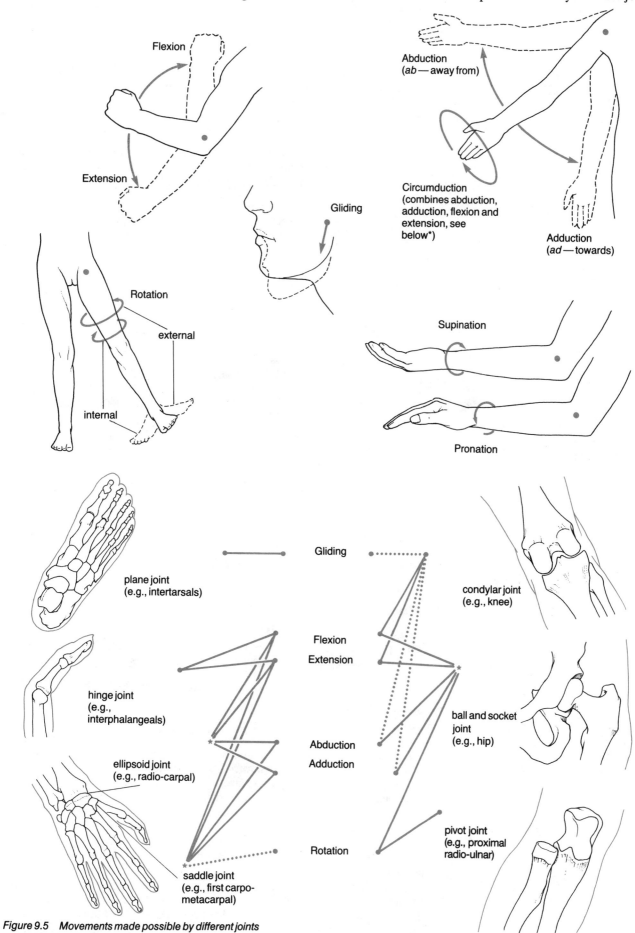

Figure 9.5 Movements made possible by different joints

(b) Muscular system

1 Types of muscle

Muscle is contractile tissue designed to effect movement of and within the body. There are three types: voluntary, involuntary and cardiac muscle.

Voluntary or skeletal muscle

This is attached to the skeleton, and is concerned with movement and locomotion. It is innervated by the voluntary part of the nervous system. It has a striped appearance under the microscope, and so is also called *striated muscle*. It contracts and fatigues rapidly.

Involuntary or visceral muscle

This is found throughout the body (see Figure 9.6) and is innervated by the autonomic (involuntary) part of the nervous system. Its unstriated fibres are arranged in sheets or bundles, and it contracts and fatigues slowly.

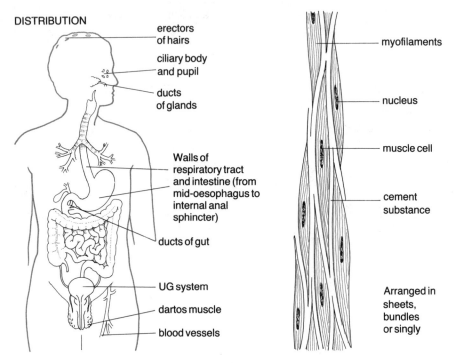

DISTRIBUTION

erectors of hairs

ciliary body and pupil

ducts of glands

Walls of respiratory tract and intestine (from mid-oesophagus to internal anal sphincter)

ducts of gut

UG system

dartos muscle

blood vessels

myofilaments

nucleus

muscle cell

cement substance

Arranged in sheets, bundles or singly

Figure 9.6   Structure and location of involuntary muscle

Cardiac muscle

This is found only in the heart and at the cardiac ends of the great vessels. Its special properties have been discussed in Chapter 3 (see page 90). Of major importance is its innate rhythmical activity. It contracts without fatigue.

2 Structure and functioning of skeletal muscle

A whole muscle is made up of numerous *muscle fibres* of varying lengths. The fibre is filled with a specialised cytoplasm called *sarcoplasm* and contains numerous nuclei which are spaced out evenly just below the outer membrane or *sarcolemma*. If stained, the muscle fibre appears to have lateral stripes, when viewed under the light microscope (see Figure 9.7).

Within each muscle fibre there are very fine threads or *myofibrils* running along the length of the fibre. The fine structure of the myofibrils is visible by use of the electron microscope and consists of repeating sets of interlinking thick and thin filaments as shown in Figure 9.8.

The thick filaments are composed of the protein *myosin,* and the thin filaments consist of a second protein, actin. Using high-magnification electron microscopy, fine *bridges* can be observed between the actin and myosin filaments where they overlap. Actin and myosin can combine to form a third protein, actomyosin, and it is thought that actomyosin is formed at the contact point between the myosin bridges and the actin filaments. If these bridges then contract simultaneously, the actin filaments will be pulled along and overlap

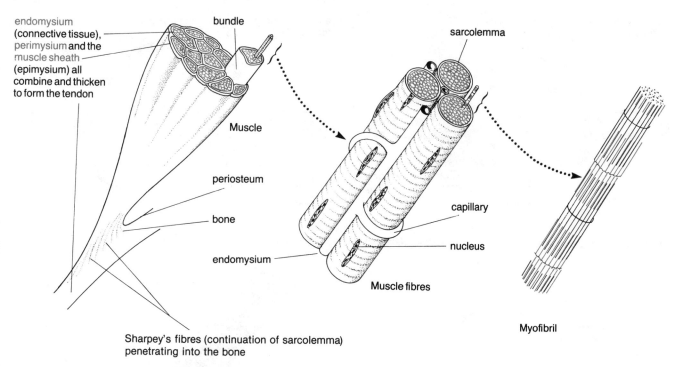

endomysium
(connective tissue),
perimysium and the
muscle sheath
(epimysium) all
combine and thicken
to form the tendon

bundle

Muscle

periosteum

bone

endomysium

Sharpey's fibres (continuation of sarcolemma)
penetrating into the bone

sarcolemma

capillary

nucleus

Muscle fibres

Myofibril

Figure 9.7   Detailed structure of voluntary muscle

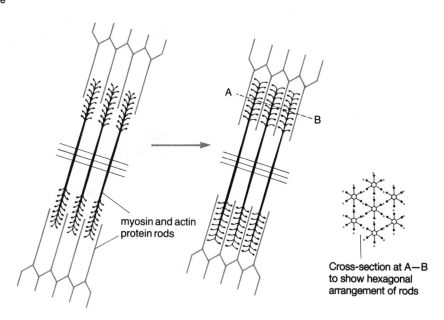

myosin and actin
protein rods

A

B

Cross-section at A—B
to show hexagonal
arrangement of rods

Figure 9.8   Fine structure of voluntary muscle as elucidated by use of the electron microscope

the myosin further. The bridges then detach and re-attach at a new point on the actin filament, and contract again; then the actin filaments will be moved further, and the overall effect will be to *contract* the myofibril.

The effect described above is thought to be the basis of muscle contraction. This muscle contraction is stimulated by electrical activity at the sarcolemma. At rest, the sarcolemma has a potential difference across it, which depolarises if stimulated, in a manner similar to that of nerve cells. This *action potential* is transmitted along and around the sarcolemma, and may be carried into the fibres, via fine transverse tubules which run from the sarcolemma.

Contraction of muscle requires energy, and this is derived from glucose, or its storage product, *glycogen*. These are converted to *pyruvic acid* in the muscle fibres, and then to either *lactic acid* (if oxygen is in short supply) or carbon dioxide and water via the *citric acid cycle* if oxygen is available. Heat is produced in both cases. Pain and fatigue in muscles are due to lack of oxygen and the accumulation of waste products of metabolism including lactic acid.

When muscle is relaxed, the blood supply to it flows through the capillary network within the bundle of fibres (Figure 9.9a). But on contraction this blood

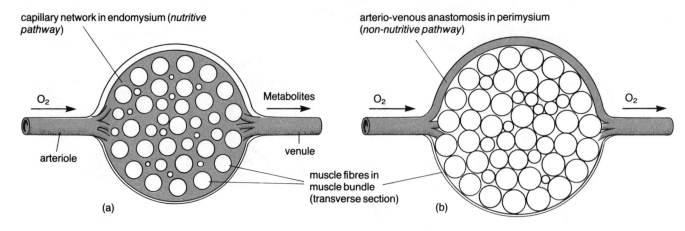

Figure 9.9 *Blood supply to voluntary muscle. (a) Muscle relaxed and (b) muscle contracted*

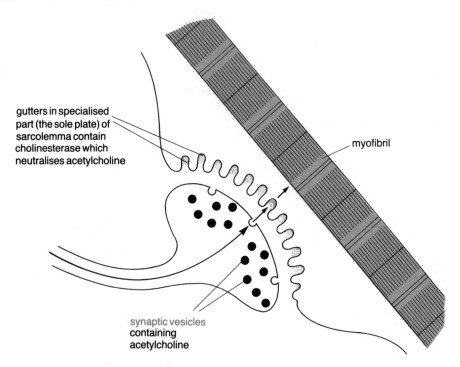

Figure 9.10 *Neuromuscular junction*

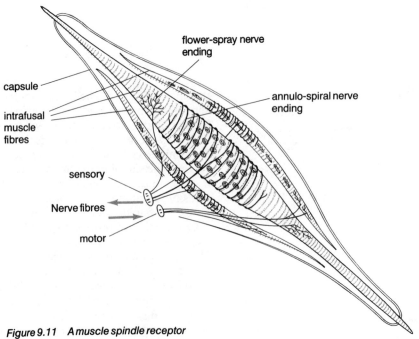

Figure 9.11 *A muscle spindle receptor*

is forced to by-pass that system, and travels along vessels in the *perimysium,* the membrane system surrounding the muscle block (Figure 9.9b). Thus blood supply to the individual fibres is limited.

Muscles are richly innervated. Motor neurons bring stimulation from the central nervous system which results in muscle contraction. The impulse is transferred to the muscle at the *neuromuscular junction* (Figure 9.10) or *motor end plate,* at which the neuron releases acetylcholine, and this causes depolarisation of the sarcolemma.

Within the muscle there are numerous *muscle spindles* (Figure 9.11) which are receptors sensitive to muscle length and speed of contraction. These, and the tendon organs, send important information to the central nervous system, so that *muscle tone* is maintained (see page 116).

Voluntary muscles perform numerous functions throughout the body, including the maintenance of posture, sphincter function, speech, facial expressions and locomotion. Muscles cannot relax in isolation, but must, instead, be pulled in the direction opposite to that of their contraction. This is effected by a set of antagonistic muscles, which work in the opposite direction, as shown in Figure 9.12.

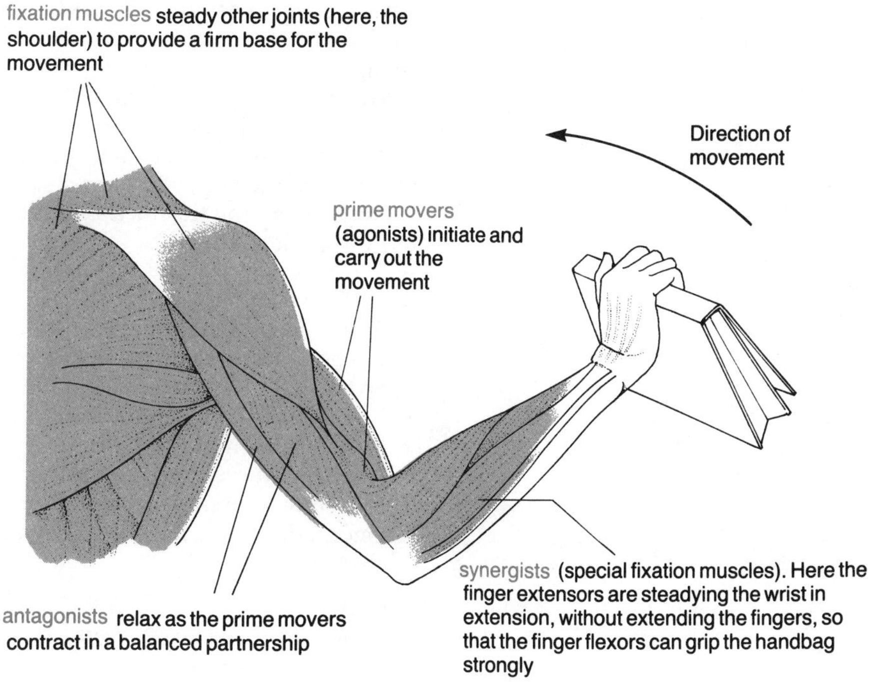

fixation muscles steady other joints (here, the shoulder) to provide a firm base for the movement

Direction of movement

prime movers (agonists) initiate and carry out the movement

synergists (special fixation muscles). Here the finger extensors are steadying the wrist in extension, without extending the fingers, so that the finger flexors can grip the handbag strongly

antagonists relax as the prime movers contract in a balanced partnership

Figure 9.12   Antagonistic muscle systems in the arm

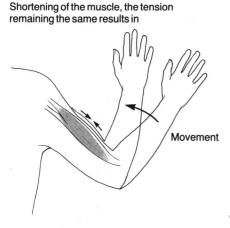

Shortening of the muscle, the tension remaining the same results in

Movement

Figure 9.13   Isotonic contraction

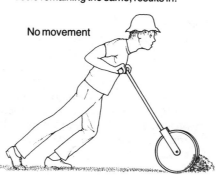

Increasing the tension, the length of the muscle remaining the same, results in:

No movement

Figure 9.14   Isometric contraction

Muscle contraction, when it results in movement, is called *isotonic* contraction (Figure 9.13); if it does not result in movement, but instead increases the tension within the muscle, it is termed *isometric* contraction (Figure 9.14).

The patients with immobilisation from disease or prescribed treatment

(a) Immobilisation from disease

1 Patient histories, self-testing questions and guidelines to suitable answers

An adult with rheumatoid arthritis

Mrs Sylvia Cooper, aged 55 years, lives with her husband, who is a local machine operator. They live in a small maisonette in a suburb of a city near to where their two married children live with their families. From the age of 30 years, she started to suffer from early symptoms of pain and stiffness of the small joints of her hands and feet which progressed with intermittent remission to the present day. Steroid therapy was commenced at this time and has been continued in varying doses in an attempt to reduce the inflammatory response in the joints. Over this period Mrs Cooper's activities have gradually become less, and her dependence on others has increased.

The disease has affected her hands so that she cannot grip items such as cutlery, saucepan handles, hairbrush, or do up buttons and zips. The effect on her spine and knees and feet has caused difficulties with getting in and out of the bath, and moving up and down stairs. Her husband has been able to help her to get up and dress in the morning when her stiffness is worse and at the weekends assist her with getting in and out of the bath.

One day her joints became suddenly painful, swollen and stiff to the extent that she contacts her doctor, suspecting that she is experiencing an exacerbation of her condition.

On examination the doctor finds the following:
- Low grade pyrexia.
- Tachycardia.
- Stiff, swollen, painful joints.
- Pale mucous membranes.
- Cushingoid appearance — moonshaped face.
- Sparse hair, large trunk with thin arms and legs, purple striae on abdomen.
- Features of slight hypertension.
- Features of slight glycosuria.
- History of increasing tiredness.

The doctor obtains a blood sample for haemoglobin, estimation of sedimentation rate, full blood count, blood glucose. Following discussion he advises:

1. Bed rest.
2. Support for painful joints.
3. Nourishing diet.
4. Recommencement of aspirin tablets, 4–6 grams daily.
5. Mefenamic acid tablets 600 grams daily.

He contacts the district nurse to assess and care for Mrs Cooper and arranges to give Mrs Cooper intramuscular iron injections.

SELF-TESTING QUESTIONS

1. Briefly explain the pathology and abnormal physiology of rheumatoid arthritis.

BRIEF ANALYSIS AND GUIDELINES TO SUITABLE ANSWERS

Question 1
You are advised to revise the normal structure and function of a synovial joint, including the normal range of movements. Your answers should include:
(a) Brief description of the condition, i.e., a systemic disease characterised by polyarthritis affecting mainly the small joints. It runs a chronic course with exacerbations and remissions leading to eventual destruction of the joints.
(b) The local effects on joints include: inflammation of the synovial membrane; production of excessive synovial fluid causing pain and swelling of the joint; and overgrowth of synovial membrane on to the articular cartilage (pannus) which it destroys, producing pain and stiffness, disruption and occasionally dislocation of the joint. The characteristic deformity in the hands is anterior subluxation of the metacarpophalangeal joints and ulnar deviation of the fingers.

2. Devise a care plan for Mrs Cooper's care during the acute exacerbation of her illness.

Question 2

Management of Mrs Cooper during the *acute phase* of the illness should include:
(a) Resting the patient.
(b) Resting and immobilising the affected joints.
(c) Relieving pain and inflammation.
(d) Attention to personal hygiene.
(e) Attention to nutrition and hydration.
(f) Prevention of complications of bed rest in a person who is already disabled and has limited mobility.

Particular emphasis should be given to the use of aids to relieve pressure and possible deformity of feet and toes, e.g., flexion deformity of toes and/or drop foot can be prevented by use of splints, pillows and bedcradles. A firm base to the bed is preferable with a suitable backrest to support the spine. Splints can be used at night on wrists and hands to prevent wrist drop.

Active movements of the affected joints should be minimised during the acute phase but passive exercises may be advised to prevent adhesions within the joint, and to minimise muscle wasting and atrophy. Mrs Cooper should be helped to lie prone twice a day to prevent flexure deformities of hips and knees.

Monitoring of the effects of medication both wanted and unwanted is important. Refer to a pharmacology textbook for effects of aspirin, mefenamic acid and iron.

3. Describe what could be necessary in rehabilitating Mrs Cooper after recovering from the acute phase of her illness.

Question 3

Your answer should include:
(a) Reassessment of her capabilities, home aids and environment.
(b) Discussion with Mrs Cooper and her husband on the necessity for return to as full and active a life as possible, perhaps with help from the occupational therapy and physiotherapy departments of the local hospital.
(c) Attention to the psychological and social needs of Mrs Cooper, including Mr Cooper and their family.
(d) Physical assessment kept under review in case reconstructive surgery on selected joints becomes necessary.

4. Describe the abnormal physiological effects to a patient who is taking therapeutic doses of corticosteroids.

Question 4

Refer to Fact Sheet 4.

Fact Sheet 4 Steroid therapy

Normally the adrenal glands produce:
(a) Cortisol – affects:
- Utilisation of carbohydrates.
- Conversion of amino acids to glucose.
- Deposition of body fat.
- Inflammatory response.
- Mental state.
(b) Aldosterone – affects:
- Balance of sodium/potassium.
- Maintenance of blood pressure.
(c) Androgens/oestrogens – affect:
- Secondary sexual characteristics.

Therapeutic doses of cortisone can cause:	Due to:
Short-term effects: Raised blood sugar levels	Abnormally rapid conversion of amino acids to glucose
Thin arms and legs, purple striae in skin	Loss of body protein, therefore loss of muscle and dermis
Moonface, large trunk with 'buffalo hump'	Abnormal distribution of body fat
Osteoporosis	Loss of protein and calcium from bone
Reduced inflammatory response to infection or injury	Excessive anti-inflammatory action (the reason for giving a therapeutic dose)
Euphoria	Excessive stimulation of mental function
Long-term effects: Long-term administration of cortisone can cause interference with aldsosterone and androgen/oestrogen production causing:	
Hypertension and oedema	Excessive retention of sodium and water
Growth of facial hair and deepening of voice	In females due to increase of androgens over oestrogens
Loss of beard and body hair and occasionally enlargement of the breasts	In males due to increase of oestrogens over androgens

An adult with osteoarthritis of the hip

Mr Arthur Small, aged 60 years, is a long-distance lorry driver who lives with his wife in a council house on the outskirts of a county town. His main leisure interest is in his garden where he grows sufficient vegetables for family use and has a small but colourful flower garden and lawn. He has always been active but in recent years has started to put on weight which he attributes to spending long hours in the driving seat and irregular cafe meals. When he was young he was a keen rugby player and during several season's play he suffered injuries including a dislocated right hip.

Over the past year he has complained of pain and stiffness in his right hip which is getting worse so that he is finding considerable difficulty in getting up into the cab of the lorry. By the end of the day the hip is painful and he is starting to limp. Movement in the joint is becoming very limited: he can no longer bend to tie his shoe laces and has had to give up digging his garden.

Mr Small feels that his disability is increasing and affecting his normal activities to such an extent that he visits his doctor for advice. The doctor examines Mr Small and finds a stiff, painful hip joint with severe reduction in range of movement. He orders an x-ray which reveals osteoarthritic changes and advises Mr Small that he should be examined by an orthopaedic surgeon with a view to hip replacement.

SELF-TESTING QUESTIONS

1. What do you understand by the term osteoarthritis?

2. What measures will be taken to reduce Mr Small's symptoms while he is waiting for hip replacement.

3. Discuss the specific problems associated with mobility in the post-operative period following hip replacement.

BRIEF ANALYSIS AND GUIDELINES TO SUITABLE ANSWERS

Question 1
Osteoarthritis is a degenerative condition affecting mainly the weight-bearing joints of the lower limbs and spine. It is characterised by destruction of the articular cartilages exposing the underlying bone, causing pain, stiffness, swelling and loss of function.

Question 2
Your answer should include:
(a) Pain relief in the form of analgesics, anti-inflammatory medication, e.g., indomethacin.
(b) Dietary advice: calorie controlled diet to reduce weight.
(c) Physiotherapy to prevent muscle atrophy, poor posture and encourage movement (aids may be necessary such as stick, walking frame).
(d) Involvement of the medical social worker concerning his long-term disability, while awaiting surgery.
(e) Discussion with disablement resettlement officer may be required.

Question 3
Your answer should include attention to the following:
(a) Positioning in bed.
(b) Management of hygiene, toilet needs, pressure areas, nutrition and hydration in relation to movement in bed.
(c) Specific measures necessary to prevent disclocation of the prosthesis which may include:
- Use of abduction pillow.
- Prevention of rotation or flexion of the hip.
(d) Introduction of mobility as patient is rehabilitated and prepared for discharge.
(e) Involvement with physiotherapist and occupational therapist.

An adult with prolapsed intervertebral disc

Mrs Elizabeth Clarke, aged 26 years, is married with two small children. They live in a country cottage in a small community. She has had a history of recurrent back pain since her first pregnancy. In the past this has been treated with a period of bed rest, analgesics and, on one occasion, with a plaster jacket. She has attended the physiotherapy department in the local hospital where she has been taught exercises to improve her posture, strengthen her muscles supporting her spine, and the correct method of lifting. She experienced very severe pain six months ago when attempting to carry her 3-year-old child upstairs. The pain radiated down the right side of her buttock and down the back of her right thigh (sciatica). Her doctor became concerned when over the next few months the sciatica persisted and sensory and motor changes in the lower limb became obvious.

X-ray of spine reveals reduced disc space between lumbar vertebrae 1 and 2, consistent with prolapsed intervertebral disc. Her doctor advises referral to an orthopaedic surgeon, who advises laminectomy.

Mrs Clarke makes arrangement for the care of her children and is admitted for laminectomy and removal of the protruding nucleus pulposus which is causing pressure on a nerve root. The post-operative management after laminectomy includes:

(a) Lying flat on a firm mattress for the first 24 hours.
(b) Careful repositioning of Mrs Clarke to relieve pressure but taking care to turn her body in one piece and avoid twisting at the hips.
(c) Observation of bladder and bowel function.
(d) Observation of feet and legs for normal sensation and movement.
(e) Observation of blood pressure; this may be labile if there has been any interference of the sympathetic nervous system activity.
(f) Early ambulation with Mrs Clarke permitted to walk but not to sit to prevent complications such as retention, distension, deep vein thrombosis and hypostatic pneumonia.
(g) Back extension exercises are taught by the physiotherapist.

SELF-TESTING QUESTIONS

1. Explain the abnormal physiology resulting from a prolapsed intervertebral disc.

2. What do you understand by the following terms:
   • Lordosis
   • Scoliosis
   • Myelogram
   • Laminectomy?

3. What arrangements need to be made prior to Mrs Clarke's return home?

4. Find out and discuss the current information on back injuries in relation to number of working days lost, occupational status, age, sex and body build.

5. Discuss the place of health education in the prevention of back injuries in nurses.

BRIEF ANALYSIS AND GUIDELINES TO SUGGESTED ANSWERS

Question 1
Refer to your teacher for guidance.

Question 2
Refer to dictionary or orthopaedic textbook.

Question 3
Your answer should include attention to the following:
(a) Continuation of back strengthening exercises.
(b) Education of Mrs Clarke to avoid lifting until she is seen at a follow-up appointment in the outpatients' department.
(c) Obtaining a firm-based bed.
(d) Ensuring she keeps her weight within normal limits.
(e) Period of convalescence or help in looking after the children until she is fit.

Question 4
Refer to the Department of Health and Social Security statistics.

Question 5
Your answer should include attention to the following:
(a) Correct lifting techniques.
(b) Maximum loads for height and build.
(c) Health and Safety at Work legislation.

An adult with multiple sclerosis

Margaret and Graham Patterson, a couple in their thirties, live in a bungalow on the outskirts of a city. Margaret has severe multiple sclerosis and is confined to a wheelchair. Graham is a teacher at the local secondary school and is able to come home at lunchtimes. Margaret's disabilities include:
• Some clumsiness and lack of coordination in her hands and arms with intention tremor.
• Complete paralysis of lower limbs with foot drop and spontaneous jerks of legs.
• Incontinence of urine and faeces.
• Double vision.

● Some dysphasia.

Graham is distressed to find that she is getting progressively worse but Margaret is slightly euphoric and appears unaware of the seriousness of her condition. It is getting increasingly difficult for Graham to manage while still having to work and he seeks advice from his doctor. The doctor agrees that he has to have some help and arranges for the district nurse and medical social worker to visit.

Refer to pages 113–114.

SELF-TESTING QUESTIONS

1. What do you understand by the term multiple sclerosis?

2. Explain the normal physiology of nerve impulse.

3. Devise a care plan for Margaret so that her problems can be dealt with by the district nurse and her husband.

BRIEF ANALYSIS AND GUIDELINES TO SUGGESTED ANSWERS

Question 1
Multiple sclerosis is due to demyelination of nerve fibres and can occur at random throughout the central nervous system, including the brain and spinal cord. This causes interruption of the electrical impulses and results in loss of function, i.e., reduced sensation, loss of motor power, coordination of movement.

Question 2
Refer to pages 113–114.

Question 3
Your answer should include:
(a) Discussion with both partners of Margaret's special needs and difficulties.
(b) Establishment of a daily routine for attention to hygiene, nutrition, hydration, toilet needs, relief of pressure, occupation, maintenance of morale, involvement of those available to help (home care assistant, bath attendants).
(c) Use of aids/facilities, laundry service, cradles, maintenance of wheelchair, adaptation of the home, talking books, special adaptation of the telephone to summon aid in emergency.
(d) Medication to alleviate spontaneous jerky movements of limbs.
(e) Care of limbs to prevent contractures and deformity.
(f) Marriage guidance counselling.

An adult with Parkinson's disease

Mr George Harris, aged 70 years, lives alone and has been advised to be admitted to hospital for reassessment of his present condition, which has gradually deteriorated since he was diagnosed as having Parkinson's disease five years ago.

On admission, the nurse's assessment reveals an elderly gentleman with a blank, inexpressive face and unblinking stare. He has rhythmical tremor of both hands and a shuffling rapid gait with some unsteadiness. Mr Harris's voice appears rapid and monotonous. She observes that the muscles of his trunk are rigid, with slight flexion of trunk and limbs, and that he has restricted rotary movement of the spine.

SELF-TESTING QUESTIONS

1. Parkinson's disease is a disease of the basal ganglia causing impairment of movement (hypokinesis), muscle rigidity and tremor. State where and what are the basal ganglia?

2. Parkinson's disease is thought to be due to lack of production of dopamine, a chemical transmitter for the basal ganglia. State the current treatment for this condition.

BRIEF ANALYSIS AND GUIDELINES TO SUGGESTED ANSWERS

Question 1
Refer to pages 116–117, and to J.H. Green, *Basic Clinical Physiology*, 3rd edition, Oxford University Press, London, 1979.

Question 2
Dopamine orally cannot cross the blood/brain barrier but its precursor L-dopa does. Therefore patients can be given Levodopa (L-dopa) by mouth in doses ranging from 2 to 8 grams daily. It is particularly beneficial for the hypokinesis.

3. Devise a care plan for the period of Mr Harris's stay in hospital during his reassessment.

Question 3

Your answer should include:

(a) Giving him sufficient time to carry out activities.
(b) Care of joints and muscles to prevent further rigidity and contractures.
(c) Psychological support and care in understanding that Mr Harris is mentally able, although he appears slow and unresponsive.
(d) Explanation of investigations and trials of medication, and observations and monitoring of effects.
(e) Attention to assistance with eating and drinking with emphasis on maintaining dignity.
(f) Discussion and agreement as to whether any member of Mr Harris's family should be informed of his admission.
(g) Arrangements for return home.

(b) Immobilisation from prescribed treatment

1 Patient histories, self-testing questions and guidelines for suitable answers

A young adult with a fractured tibia

Simon Matthews, aged 18 years, has Down's Syndrome. He lives at home with his parents but works a few hours each day in a sheltered workshop. His mother meets him from work each day but today, because she was a few minutes late, he attempted to cross the road and was knocked down by a cyclist. He damaged his leg and was unable to walk, an ambulance was called and he was admitted to the Accident and Emergency Department where an x-ray revealed a fractured tibia involving the ankle joint.

The nurse admitted Simon in the Accident and Emergency Department made the following assessment:

- Young adult with Down's Syndrome accompanied by his mother who explained that Simon was quite severely retarded.
- Tearful and disturbed but easily distracted and reassured.
- Short for his age and rather obese.
- Movements appeared clumsy and poorly coordinated.

Following examination by the doctor he advised Mrs Matthews that Simon would need a general anaesthetic and reduction of his fracture. She agreed to give consent for this to be done and stayed with Simon while he was prepared for operation. In the operating theatre Simon's fracture was reduced under x-ray control and an incomplete (possible backslab) plaster of Paris splint was applied. He was transferred to the ward and his leg was elevated to minimise swelling and the circulation to the toes was monitored. He is to stay in bed until the plaster of Paris splint is completed, planned for the next day, and until it is completely dry.

SELF-TESTING QUESTIONS

1. Identify the problems likely to be encountered in caring for Simon after the application of the plaster of Paris.

BRIEF ANALYSIS AND GUIDELINES TO SUITABLE ANSWERS

Question 1

Your answer should include identification of the following:

(a) A young Down's Syndrome adult in strange new surroundings, separated from his family and usual routine.
(b) Simon's limited intelligence makes it difficult for him to understand instructions regarding care of his plaster, having to stay in bed, use of crutches.
(c) Plaster of Paris on a lower limb requiring to dry, and careful handling while it dries.
(d) Observations need to be attentive to detail with careful assessment of alteration of pain, colour, sensation of toes.
(e) Clumsiness and uncoordinated movements will increase the difficulty of regaining balance and of using crutches on the non-weight-bearing affected leg.
(f) Difficulty in being socially accepted in the ward area by others.

2. How could Simon's behaviour alter following admission and how could this be minimised?

Question 2

(a) Simon's behaviour could change to him being bad-tempered, irritable and uncooperative, and he could regress to being unable to achieve things he could previously accomplish, e.g., feeding himself.

(b) This behaviour could be prevented or minimised by keeping as near as possible to his normal routine, for example:
  • Reduction of the number of persons caring for Simon as much as possible.
  • Encouragement of mother's participation in his care and in being near at hand.
  • Encouragement of diversional therapy.
  • Careful, patient and repeated explanation before undertaking any procedures.

Question 3

3. How would you prevent Simon developing possible complications due to the enforced immobility of his leg?

Possible complications are:

(a) Reluctance to straighten and eventual difficulty in straightening the knee.

(b) Likelihood of development of deep vein thrombosis due to reluctance to exercise toes and keep leg elevated when sitting.

In order to avoid these complications, supervised physiotherapy in a manner that gains Simon's cooperation is needed from all staff concerned.

An adult with fractured neck of femur

Mrs Grace Anderson, aged 76 years, is admitted to the ward with a fractured neck of left femur after falling at home. She is very frail and has been under the care of her own GP for mild heart failure and anaemia. She is to have Hamilton Russell skin traction (Figure 9.15) applied to her left leg to relieve the muscle spasm and immobilise the fracture until she is physically fit to undergo surgery to internally fix the fracture.

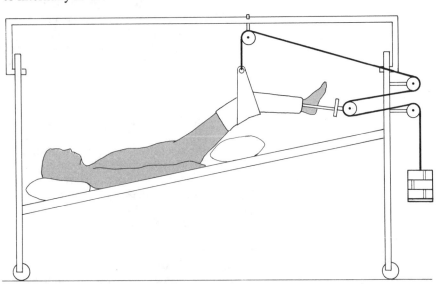

Figure 9.15   Hamilton Russell traction

SELF-TESTING QUESTIONS

BRIEF ANALYSIS AND GUIDELINES TO SUGGESTED ANSWERS

1. Devise a care plan for Mrs Anderson while she is immobilised in traction.

Question 1

Your answer should include attention to the following:

(a) Positioning.

(b) Management of pressure areas including those affected by the traction apparatus and the elbow and heel of unaffected side.

(c) Management of eating and drinking with foot of bed elevated.

(d) Management of bladder and bowels and maintenance of continence.

(e) Maintenance of orientation to time and place.

(f) Monitoring of cardiac function with observation of fluid balance.

(g) Management of traction apparatus.

(h) Physiotherapy to chest and all joints and muscles.

(i) Correction of anaemia.
(j) Assessment of home circumstances.
(k) Preparations for surgery.

Question 2

2. (a) Discuss the problems of wound and bone healing in the elderly patient.

(a) The problems of wound and bone healing include:
- Poor nutrition.
- Anaemia.
- Poor heart function resulting in poor perfusion of tissue.
- Problems with mobility.

(b) What factors are necessary for healing to occur?

(b) Factors necessary for healing include:
- Prevention of infection.
- Good blood supply to the area including oxygen carrying capacity.
- Skin edges and bone ends in apposition.
- Good nutritional state including extra vitamin C, calcium and protein for the bones.
- Fracture site immobilised until healing takes place (in this instance internal fixation allows mobilisation of the patient while ensuring immobilisation of the fracture).

Further reading

Books

Bell, G. H., Leslie-Smith, D. and Paterson, C. R., *Textbook of Physiology and Biochemistry*, 10th edition, Churchill Livingstone, London, 1980.

Capra, L. G., *The Care of the Cancer Patient*, 2nd edition, Macmillan Education, London, 1986.

Davidson, S. *et al.*, *Human Nutrition and Dietetics*, 7th revised edition, Churchill Livingstone, London, 1979.

Fry, L., *Dermatology — An Illustrated Guide*, 2nd edition, Medical Update Books, London, 1978.

Green, J. H., *Basic Clinical Physiology*, 3rd revised edition, Oxford University Press, London, 1979.

Henderson, V., *Basic Principles of Nursing Care*, revised edition, International Council of Nurses, Switzerland, 1969.

Houston, J. C. *et al.*, *Short Textbook of Medicine*, 7th revised edition, Hodder and Stoughton, London, 1982.

Macleod, J. (Ed.), *Davidson's Principles and Practice of Medicine*, 14th edition, Churchill Livingstone, London, 1984.

Ministry of Agriculture, Fisheries and Food. *Manual of Nutrition*, 9th edition, HMSO, London, 1985.

Marks, R., *Psoriasis — a Guide to One of the Commonest Skin Diseases*, Martin Dunitz, London, 1981.

Tiffany, R., *Oncology for Nurses and Health Care Professionals*, volume 2, *Care and Support*, George Allen and Unwin, London, 1978.

Thal, A. P., *Shock. A Physiological Basis for Treatment*, Year Book Medical Publishers, Chicago, 1971.

Thomson, W. A. R., (Ed.), *Black's Medical Dictionary*, 34th edition. A and C Black, London, 1984.

Journal

Roberts, A., 'The pox and the people', in *Nursing Times*, July 14th, 1982, pages 1177–1185, Macmillan Journals, London.

Index